Atlas of Dermatology in Internal Medicine

Néstor P. Sánchez
Editor

Atlas of Dermatology in Internal Medicine

Springer

Editor
Néstor P. Sánchez
Professor of Dermatology and
Dermatopathology and Chairman
Department of Dermatology
University of Puerto Rico School of Medicine
Medical Sciences Campus
San Juan, Puerto Rico
nestor.sanchez@upr.edu

Associate Editors
Adisbeth Morales-Burgos, MD
Assistant Professor, Department of Dermatology
University of Puerto Rico School of Medicine
Medical Sciences Campus
San Juan, Puerto Rico

Mark Pittelkow, MD
Professor of Dermatology
Mayo Graduate School of Medicine
Mayo Clinic, Rochester, Minnesota

Martin Charles Mihm, MD
Professor of Pathology
and Dermatology
Department of Dermatology
and Department of Pathology
Massachusetts General Hospital
Harvard Medical School
Boston, Massachusetts

Lilliam S. Chiqués Colón, MD
Assistant Professor
Department of Medicine
University of Puerto Rico
School of Medicine
Medical Sciences Campus
San Juan, Puerto Rico

ISBN 978-1-4614-0687-7 e-ISBN 978-1-4614-0688-4
DOI 10.1007/978-1-4614-0688-4
Springer New York Dordrecht Heidelberg London

Library of Congress Control Number: 2011938858

Printed on acid-free paper

Springer is part of Springer Science+Business Media (www.springer.com)

This book is dedicated to my loving family, especially to my wife, Nelly, my children, Dara, Fitz and Vannesa, and to my grandchildren, Diego, Hugo, Néstor, Gustavo, Natalia, and Marco. Furthermore, to the families of all the contributing authors and associate editors who illuminated this book with knowledge and wisdom.

Preface

Dermatology is a fascinating field based in the skills of clinical observation and clinicopathologic correlation to diagnose diseases. We wish to bring the art and science of dermatology into a practical resource. In this spirit, we created *Atlas of Dermatology in Internal Medicine*.

Skin reflects the health of the body and its diseases are often a manifestation of systemic conditions. To know skin disorders is of paramount importance for other specialties. We are committed to creating an excellent tool to assist in the diagnosis and management of common cutaneous manifestations of systemic diseases.

Atlas of Dermatology in Internal Medicine is organized to reflect current knowledge in dermatology relevant to Internal Medicine. It provides a comprehensive review and updated information on the diagnosis and treatment of common cutaneous manifestations of systemic diseases. To facilitate the diagnosis of frequently encountered skin diseases, a gallery of illustrations combined with disease descriptions and their current therapeutic information are included. This book welcomes internists and other specialists in medicine interested in learning more about clinical dermatology.

We are proud to present our work. We hope this text will provide a timely addition to the field of Internal Medicine.

We would like to thank the authors who contributed in this book.

Néstor P. Sánchez
Adisbeth Morales

Acknowledgments

I was extremely fortunate to have extraordinary teachers who enlightened the path of my training in Dermatology and Dermatopathology.

Dr. Rodolph L. Baer – Master of Dermatology, Professor Emeritus of NYU Skin and Cancer. My late Professor and mentor during my Residency in NYU.

Dr. A. B. Ackerman – Master of Dermatology and Dermatopathology. My early inspiration in the jungle of Dermatology. A spectacular human being.

Dr. Alfred Kopf – Master of Dermatology and role model.

Dr. Thomas B. Fitzpatrick – Master of Dermatology and innovator. My late mentor while at Harvard. Source of knowledge, inspiration and leadership.

Dr. Martin Charles Mihm – Master of Dermatology and Dermatopathology. My dear teacher, friend and role model. Physician by excellence and humanitarian.

Dr. Harold Perry – Master of Dermatology. Great inspiration for me while at Mayo Clinic.

Dr. Richard Winkelmann – Master of Dermatology and Dermatopathology. My mentor and innovator. Great physician and thinker.

Dr. Arnold Schroeter – Master of Dermatology and Dermatopathology, who trusted me during my early years in dermatology. A great mentor.

Dr. Mark Pittelkow – Master of Dermatology. Friend, extraordinary thinker and exceptional human being.

Dr. Jorge L. Sánchez – Master of Dermatology and Dermatopathology. Role model, who first inspired me.

Contents

Cutaneous Manifestations of Connective Tissue Diseases 1
Lesliane E. Castro-Santana, José González Chávez, Jennifer Rullán, and Rachelle E. Seijo-Montes

Cutaneous Manifestations of Pulmonary Disease 17
Jennifer Rullán, Rachelle E. Seijo-Montes, Annie Vaillant, and Néstor P. Sánchez

Cutaneous Manifestations of Renal Disease 31
Lilliam S. Chiqués Colón and Rosbel González Rivera

Cutaneous Manifestations of Gastrointestinal Diseases 41
María I. Vázquez-Roque and Wilfredo E. De Jesús-Monge

Cutaneous Manifestations of Common Endocrine Disease 53
Inés M. Hernández and Yanira Marrero

Cutaneous Manifestations of Internal Malignancy and Paraneoplastic Syndromes 59
Zelma C. Chiesa-Fuxench, Liliana Ramírez, and Néstor P. Sánchez

Cutaneous Manifestations of Infectious Diseases 77
Elena Montalván Miró and Néstor P. Sánchez

Cutaneous Manifestations of HIV Disease 121
Humberto M. Guiot, Carlos G. Sánchez Sergenton, Carlos J. Sánchez Rivera, and Rosbel González Rivera

Cutaneous Disorders in the Intensive Care Unit 129
Tania M. González Santiago and Jacobo M. Orenstein Cardona

Index 143

Contributors

Jacobo M. Orenstein Cardona, MD, PhD Candidate Center for Translational Science Activities, Mayo Clinic Rochester, MN
jorenstein@yahoo.com

Lesliane E. Castro-Santana, MD Department of Rheumatology, University of Puerto Rico School of Medicine, Medical Sciences Campus, San Juan, Puerto Rico
c_lesliane_e_@hotmail.com

José González Chávez, MD Department of Dermatology, University of Puerto Rico School of Medicine, Medical Sciences Campus, San Juan, Puerto Rico
pepepiel@aol.com

Lilliam S. Chiqués Colón, MD Department of Medicine, University of Puerto Rico School of Medicine, Medical Sciences Campus, San Juan, Puerto Rico
lchiques@gmail.com

Zelma C. Chiesa-Fuxench, MD Department of Dermatology, University of Puerto Rico School of Medicine, Medical Sciences Campus, San Juan, Puerto Rico
chifu14@hotmail.com

Humberto M. Guiot, MD Department of Medicine, University of Puerto Rico School of Medicine, Medical Sciences Campus, San Juan, Puerto Rico
humberto@guiot.com

Inés M. Hernández, MD Department of Medicine, University of Puerto Rico School of Medicine, Medical Sciences Campus, San Juan, Puerto Rico
ineshndez@hotmail.com

Wilfredo E. De Jesús-Monge, MD, MSc Department of Medicine, University of Puerto Rico School of Medicine, Medical Sciences Campus, San Juan, Puerto Rico
wilmedresearch@yahoo.com

Yanira Marrero, MD Department of Endocrinology, University of Puerto Rico School of Medicine, Medical Sciences Campus, San Juan, Puerto Rico
yani109@hotmail.com

Martin Charles Mihm, MD Professor of Pathology and Dermatology, Department of Dermatology and Department of Pathology, Massachusetts General Hospital, Harvard Medical School, Boston, Massachusetts

Elena Montalván Miró, MD Department of Dermatology, University of Puerto Rico School of Medicine, Medical Sciences Campus, San Juan, Puerto Rico
elena.montalvan@upr.edu

Adisbeth Morales-Burgos, MD Department of Dermatology, University of Puerto Rico School of Medicine, Medical Sciences Campus, San Juan, Puerto Rico
adismorales@yahoo.com

Mark Pittelkow, MD Professor of Dermatology, Mayo Graduate School of Medicine, Mayo Clinic, Rochester, Minnesota

Liliana Ramírez, MD Department of Medicine, University of Puerto Rico School of Medicine, Medical Sciences Campus, San Juan, Puerto Rico
lmramirez@onelinkpr.net

Carlos J. Sánchez Rivera, MD Department of Medicine, University of Puerto Rico School of Medicine, Medical Sciences Campus, San Juan, Puerto Rico
cjsanchez99@prtc.net

Rosbel González Rivera, MD Department of Dermatology, University of Puerto Rico School of Medicine, Medical Sciences Campus, San Juan, Puerto Rico
rg94@cornell.edu

Jennifer Rullán, MD Department of Dermatology, University of Puerto Rico School of Medicine, Medical Sciences Campus, San Juan, Puerto Rico
rullanmed@yahoo.com

Néstor P. Sánchez, MD Professor of Dermatology and Dermatopathology and Chairman, Department of Dermatology, University of Puerto Rico School of Medicine, Medical Sciences Campus, San Juan, Puerto Rico
nestor.sanchez@upr.edu

Tania M. González Santiago, MD Mayo Clinic Department of Dermatology Residency, Rochester, MN
tania2009@gmail.com

Rogelio Mercado Seda, MD Department of Dermatology, University of Puerto Rico School of Medicine, Medical Sciences Campus, San Juan, Puerto Rico
rogelio.mercado@upr.edu

Carlos G. Sánchez Sergenton, MD Department of Medicine, University of Puerto Rico School of Medicine, Medical Sciences Campus, San Juan, Puerto Rico
csanchez@coqui.net

Rachelle E. Seijo-Montes, MD Department of Dermatology, University of Puerto Rico School of Medicine, Medical Sciences Campus, San Juan, Puerto Rico
rachelleseijo@hotmail.com

Annie Vaillant, MD Department of Obstetrics and Gynecology, San Juan City Hospital, Medical Sciences Campus, San Juan, Puerto Rico
availlant0628@gmail.com

María I. Vázquez-Roque, MD, MSc Department of Medicine, University of Puerto Rico School of Medicine, Medical Sciences Campus, San Juan, Puerto Rico
vazquezroque.maria@mayo.edu

Cutaneous Manifestations of Connective Tissue Diseases

Lesliane E. Castro-Santana, José González Chávez, Jennifer Rullán, and Rachelle E. Seijo-Montes

Most connective tissue diseases are characterized by a diversity of systemic and cutaneous manifestations. In this chapter, we focus on the unique cutaneous manifestations that characterize systemic lupus erythematosus, dermatomyositis, and scleroderma. Observation and histopathologic evaluation of the skin can assist the clinician in initiating therapy in a timely manner, even before the onset of systemic disease. A detailed discussion of these cutaneous and histopathological manifestations is presented.

Introduction

Lupus erythematosus, dermatomyositis, scleroderma, and rheumatoid arthritis are connective tissue diseases characterized by a diversity of systemic and cutaneous manifestations. In some cases, the skin changes may precede the development of overt disease and may, in fact, be the only indicator of the patients' disease [1, 2]. It is important to recognize these signs early to institute adequate and timely therapy.

Systemic Lupus Erythematosus

Systemic lupus erythematosus (SLE) is an autoimmune inflammatory disease, which can affect multiple organ systems, including the skin [3, 4]. There is a wide variation in the natural history of SLE among different ethnic and geographic groups [5]. The cutaneous manifestations of SLE can be classified as specific or nonspecific [3, 4]. The specific skin manifestations can be further subdivided into acute, subacute, and chronic cutaneous lupus erythematosus (CCLE) [4]. Bullous lupus erythematosus is categorized as a nonspecific blistering skin manifestation of SLE [4]. These will each be discussed in detail in the remainder of the chapter.

Acute Cutaneous Lupus Erythematosus

Malar erythema is commonly the first manifestation of SLE, and the most common manifestation of acute cutaneous lupus erythematosus (ACLE). It can precede other systemic manifestations of SLE by weeks or months, and frequently coincides with disease exacerbations. The rash is characterized by erythema, edema, and occasionally fine scales in a malar distribution, along the bridge of the nose, with characteristic sparing of the nasolabial folds (Fig. 1). It is often called a "butterfly" rash because of the appearance. This generally resolves without any residual scarring or hyperpigmentation. Histopathologic findings show atrophy of the epidermis and marked liquefactive degeneration of the basal layer [3]. A maculopapular lupus rash is an uncommon manifestation and frequently occurs after sun exposure. The lesions are pruritic and may be located anywhere on the body, although they have a predilection for occurring above the waistline. The colors of the lesions are usually red, dull red, or livid [3].

Subacute Cutaneous Lupus Erythematosus

Subacute cutaneous lupus erythematosus (SCLE) is a distinctive subset of lupus erythematosus. Patients can develop cutaneous lesions with two different morphologies: papulosquamous and annular, polycyclic lesions. There is no induration or telangiectasias. The distribution of the lesions is generally on sun-exposed areas, particularly the dorsal surface of upper extremities, upper back, and chest [3, 4].

L.E. Castro-Santana (✉)
Department of Rheumatology, University of Puerto Rico School of Medicine, Medical Sciences Campus, San Juan, Puerto Rico
e-mail: c_lesliane_e_@hotmail.com

J.G. Chávez • J. Rullán • R.E. Seijo-Montes
Department of Dermatology, University of Puerto Rico School of Medicine, Medical Sciences Campus, San Juan, Puerto Rico

N.P. Sánchez (ed.), *Atlas of Dermatology in Internal Medicine*,
DOI 10.1007/978-1-4614-0688-4_1,

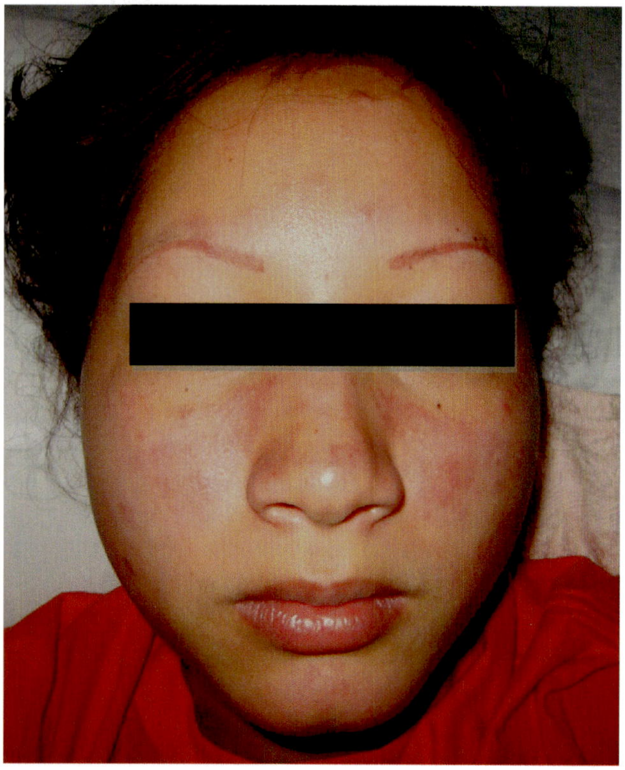

Fig. 1 Acute cutaneous lupus erythematosus associated with systemic lupus erythematosus

Histopathologically, the lesions are very similar to those of discoid lupus erythematosus (DLE); however, SCLE lesions have minimal hyperkeratosis and follicular plugging. Instead, they are characterized by more prominent epidermal atrophy and liquefaction degeneration of the basal cell layer. The inflammatory infiltrate in contradistinction to DLE tends to be scattered throughout the reticular dermis, but similar to DLE, is composed of activated T-cells [3, 4].

Chronic Cutaneous Lupus Erythematosus

The wide spectrum of CCLE includes the classical discoid lesions that can be localized or generalized, chilblain, hypertrophic, verrucous, lichenoid, lupus panniculitis (profundus), mucosal discoid, palmoplantar erosive, or lupus erythematosus tumidus lesions [4]. We will discuss the most commonly seen.

The lesions of DLE are characterized by well-defined, disk-shaped, erythematous plaques with epidermal atrophy, telangiectasias, and scaling (Fig. 2). The scale adheres to the skin and causes plugging of hair follicles. Removing the scale is very painful due to hyperalgesia of the skin. Healing of the lesions leaves atrophy, scaling, and changes in skin pigmentation (can be hypo- or hyper-pigmented) [3, 4]. The distribution of DLE presents most frequently on areas exposed to sunlight, and affect women more often than men [4]. DLE occurs with a frequency of 44% on the ears, 60% on the scalp, and 85% on the face. The atrophy and scarring can result in a significant amount of alopecia and disfiguration. Histopathological examination of active lesions reveals marked hyperkeratosis, orthokeratosis, epidermal atrophy, vacuolar degeneration of basal keratinocytes, and perivascular as well as perifollicular mononuclear cell infiltrate, scattered throughout the papillary and/or reticular dermis [3, 4].

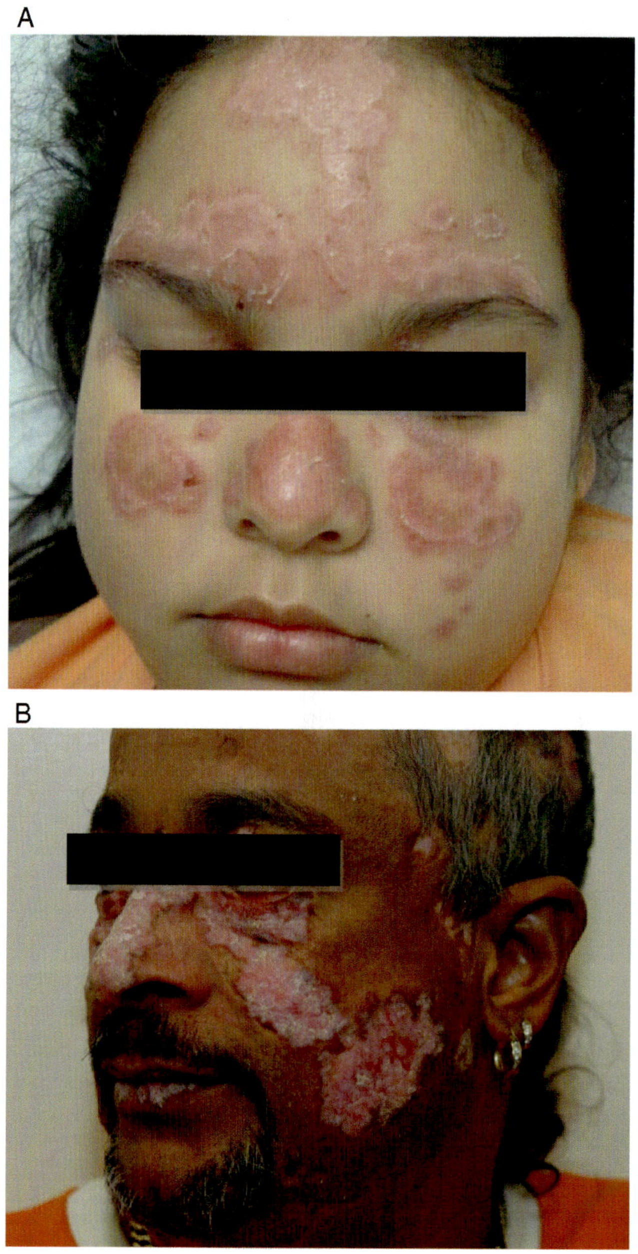

Fig. 2 (**a**, **b**) Discoid lesions of lupus erythematosus (chronic cutaneous lupus erythematosus)

Hypertrophic DLE is a distinct form of DLE, which is characterized by hyperkeratotic plaques that typically are

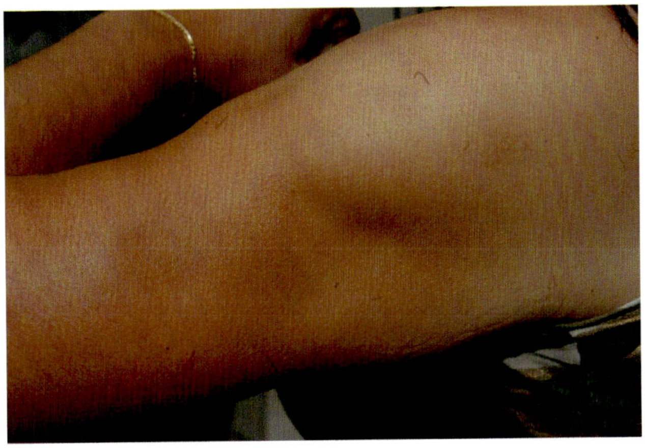

Fig. 3 Lupus panniculitis (lupus profundus): Well-demarcated depressed plaques with atrophy located on the upper extremity of a patient with lupus panniculitis

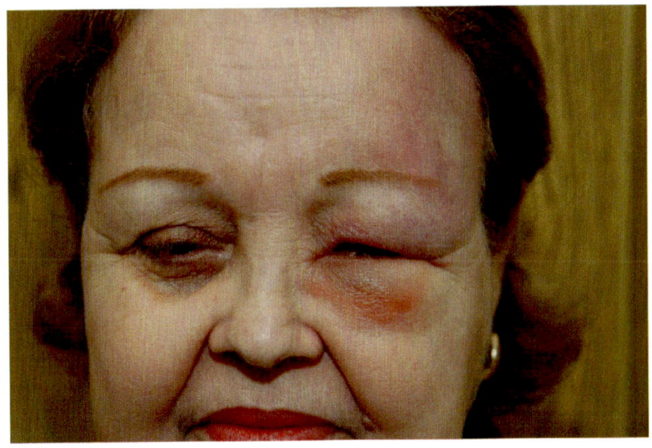

Fig. 4 Lupus erythematosus tumidus. Succulent, erythematous plaque involving left upper forehead

observed over the face, extensor surfaces of the arms, legs, and upper trunk [6]. Hypertrophic DLE lesions are dull, red, indurated, and covered by several layers of keratin (white or yellow scales). These lesions typically occur concurrently with the lesions of DLE. Histopathologic findings include marked acanthosis, hyperkeratosis and hypergranulosis, and a mononuclear cell infiltrate [3].

Lupus panniculitis (also known as lupus profundus) is a condition characterized by multiple firm, well-demarcated subcutaneous nodules or plaques that are persistent and painless (Fig. 3). The sites most frequently involved are the arms, face, and buttocks. Resolution of the lesions leaves atrophic scars and rarely, ulceration [3]. Skin biopsy reveals lymphocytic infiltrate around blood vessels and in the subcutaneous tissue. Calcification, hyalinized vessels, and fat necrosis may be present [3, 4].

Chilblain lupus is a rare manifestation of CCLE consisting of lesions induced by cold in acral areas. They are pruritic or painful and can have erythematous papules that ulcerate or become hyperkeratotic [3]. The most common histological findings are an atrophic epidermis, a vacuolated dermal–epidermal junction, and a dermal mononuclear cell infiltrate around blood vessels and pilosebaceous appendages [3].

Lupus erythematosus tumidus is characterized by marked photosensitivity and a tendency to occur in the male sex (Fig. 4). The lesions have a swollen, succulent appearance with the absence of clinically visible follicular plugging. The lesions develop mainly on the face and upper extremities as single or multiple raised erythematosus plaques with a bright red or violaceous smooth surface. The borders are sharply demarcated, and often there is swelling in the periphery and flattening in the center [3]. Histologic features are characterized by minimal follicular hyperkeratosis with basal layer vacuolization, dermal lymphocytic infiltrate, and interstitial mucin deposition [3].

The differential diagnosis of cutaneous lupus erythematosus includes sunburn, rosacea, seborrheic dermatitis, allergic contact dermatitis, phototoxic drug eruption, polymorphous light eruption, tinea faciei, granuloma faciale, sarcoidosis, alopecia mucinosa, and benign lymphocytic infiltrate of Jessner [2].

Bullous Systemic Lupus Erythematosus

The bullous lesions of lupus erythematosus are predominantly located on the face, neck, and upper trunk. They tend to be tense and may rupture leaving erosions, crusts, and changes in pigmentation (Fig. 5). A number of primary blistering diseases have been reported in association with SLE and should be differentiated from bullous lupus erythematosus. These include dermatitis herpetiformis, bullous pemphigoid, pemphigus vulgaris, pemphigus foliaceous, epidermolysis bullosa acquisita, and linear IgA disease. The most important histopathologic feature is the finding of a subepidermal blister with predominance of neutrophil inflammation in the papillary dermis [3, 4]. A linear deposition of immunoglobulins (IgG, IgA, and/or IgM) or complement is detected at the basement membrane zone on direct immunofluorescence testing [3, 4].

Classification and Treatment

The American College of Rheumatology has developed criteria for the classification of SLE (Table 1). A patient that meets four or more of these criteria is considered to have SLE [7]. Initial patient evaluation for a patient who presents with skin lesions should be aimed at the identification of these criteria and includes a thorough history and physical

A

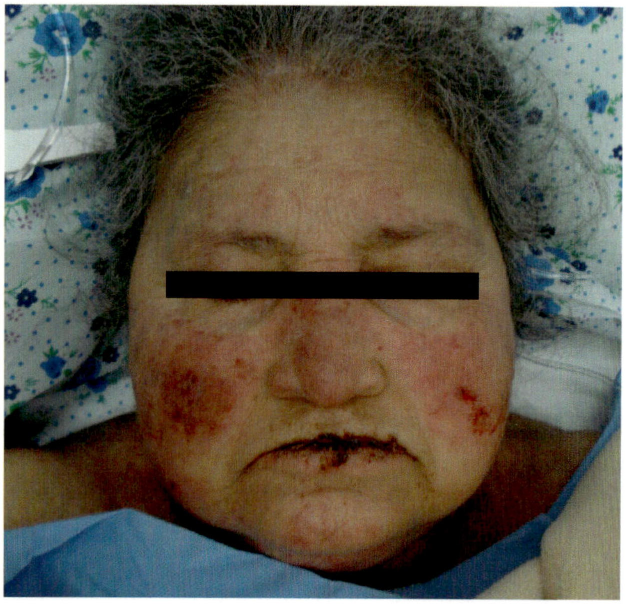

B

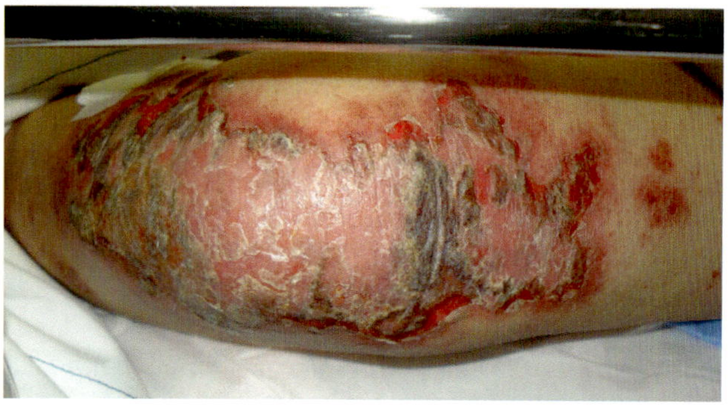

Fig. 5 (**a**, **b**) Exacerbation of systemic lupus erythematosus presenting clinically with bullaes and erosions in skin and mucous membranes. Blistering usually indicate a more severe systemic disease

Table 1 ACR criteria for the classification of systemic lupus erythematosus

1.	Malar rash
2.	Discoid rash
3.	Photosensitivity (by patient history or physician observation)
4.	Oral ulcers (painless, observed by physician)
5.	Arthritis (non-erosive, two or more peripheral joints)
6.	Serositis (pleuritis or pericarditis)
7.	Renal disorder (proteinuria >500 mg/day or 3+; or cellular casts)
8.	Neurologic disorder (seizure or psychosis)
9.	Hematologic disorder (hemolytic anemia, leucopenia, or thrombocytopenia)
10.	Immunologic disorder (+ LE cell preparation, anti-DNA antibodies, anti-Smith antibodies or False-positive serologic test for syphilis)
11.	Antinuclear antibody

The patients must meet at least four of these criteria to be diagnosed SLE

Adapted from Tan EM, Cohen AS, et al. The 1982 revised criteria for the classification of systemic lupus erythematosus. Arthritis Rheum. 1982;25:1271–7

examination, biopsy of lesions for evaluation, complete blood count with differential, antinuclear antibodies, VDRL, erythrocyte sedimentation rate, urinalysis, creatinine clearance, and complement levels [2].

It has been confirmed that the different subtypes of cutaneous LE can be triggered and exacerbated by ultraviolet (UV) irradiation [8]. Therefore, every patient should be advised to avoid sun exposure, use protective clothing, and apply sunscreen daily. Therapeutic options for patients with cutaneous lupus erythematosus can be topical or systemic, depending upon the severity of symptoms. Topical options include low potency corticosteroids creams or lotions or intralesional corticosteroid injections [2]. First-line systemic therapy includes antimalarials such as chloroquine (250–500 mg/day), hydroxychloroquine (200–400 mg/day), mepacrine (100–200 mg/day), and dapsone (100–200 mg/day). Second line agents include gold compounds such as oral auranofin (6–9 mg/day) or parenteral aurothiomalate or aurathioglucose; oral prednisone (0.5–1.5 mg/kg/day); retinoid derivatives such as isotretinoin (1 mg/kg/day) and etretinate (0.5–1 mg/kg/day); and thalidomide (100–200 mg/day). Third line therapeutic agents include intravenous corticosteroids (1 g/day for 3 days) and cytotoxic immuno-suppressive agents such as azathioprine (1–2 mg/kg/day), methotrexate (7.5–25 mg/week), cyclophosphamide (1–2 mg/kg/day), and cyclosporine (2.5–5 mg/kg/day) [3].

Dermatomyositis

Dermatomyositis (DM) is an inflammatory myopathy with characteristic skin manifestations [1, 9, 10]. The average age at diagnosis is 40, and it occurs more commonly in women [1, 10]. The cutaneous manifestations of DM are generally categorized into the following groups: pathognomonic, characteristic, compatible, less common and rare [10]. We will discuss the pathognomonic, characteristic and compatible lesions.

Pathognomonic manifestations of DM include Gottron's papules and Gottron's sign [10]. Gottron's papules are violaceous papules or small plaques overlying the dorsal or dorsolateral aspects of the interphalangeal or metacarpophalangeal areas [9, 10] (Fig. 6). When fully formed, they become slightly depressed at the center and can assume a whitish appearance. There is usually an associated scale, pigmentation changes, or telangiectasias [9]. Gottron's sign is when there are erythematosus or violaceous macules (with or without scale, changes in pigmentation or telangiectasias) involving the extensor aspects of the knuckles, elbows, knees, or medial malleoli [9, 10] (Fig. 7).

Characteristic findings in DM include the heliotrope rash, shawl sign, V-sign, and periungual telangiectasias [10]. The heliotrope rash is characterized by a macular and violaceous erythema of the eyelids that can be associated

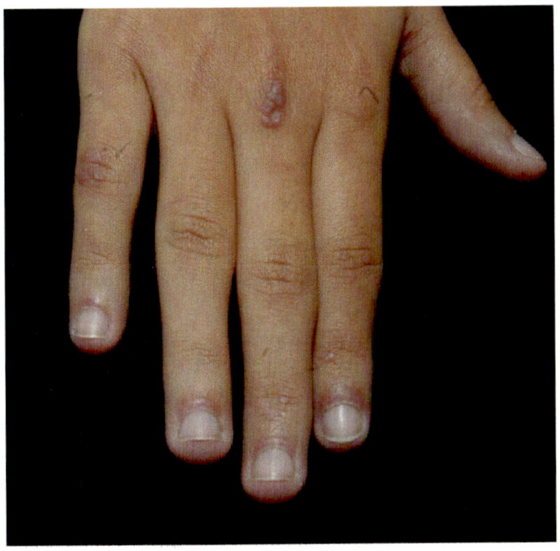

Fig. 6 Gottron's papules on the dorsal aspect of the hand involving the metacarpals and the proximal and distal interphalangeal joints

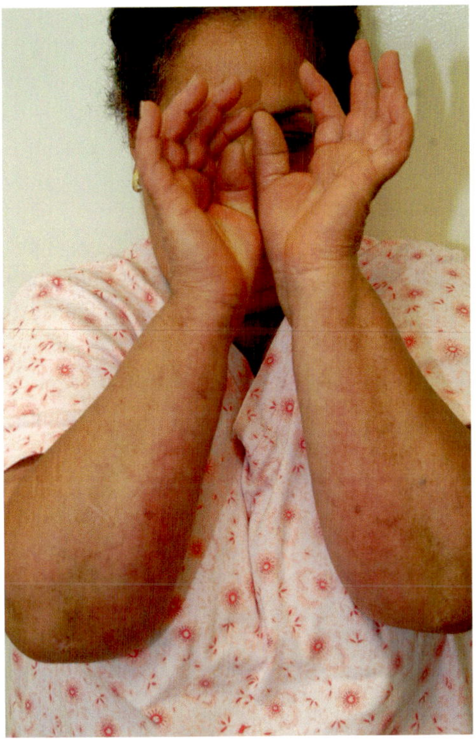

Fig. 7 Gottron's sign: Violaceous, poorly demarcated patches involving the extensor surface of the arms and elbows in a patient with dermatomyositis

with periorbital edema, scales, pigmentary changes, or telangiectasias. The characteristic lesions of the shawl sign and the V-sign appear as erythematous, poikilodermatous (variegated hyperpigmentation and telangiectasias followed by atrophy) macules distributed in a shawl pattern over the shoulders, arms, and upper back and a V-shaped distribution over the anterior neck and chest, respectively [9, 10] (Fig. 8). Periungual telangiectasias may also be seen.

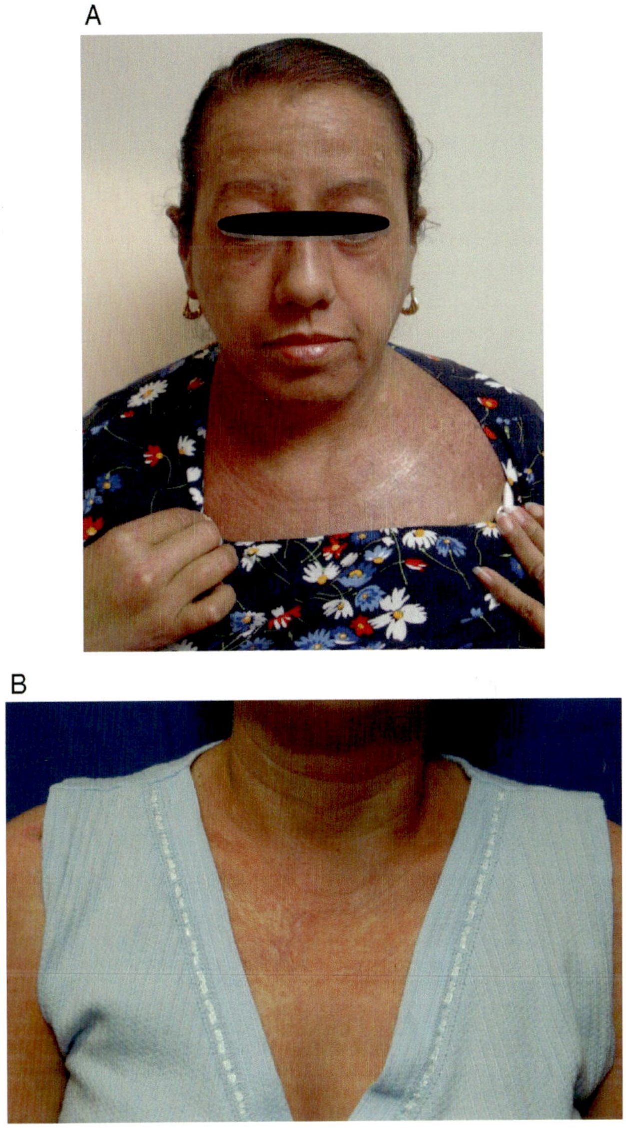

Fig. 8 (**a**, **b**) Dermatomyositis. Poikilodermatous macules on the anterior chest and face with accompanying periocular erythema

The manifestations recognized to be compatible with DM are poikiloderma atrophicans vasculare and calcinosis cutis [10]. Poikiloderma atrophicans vasculare is a circumscribed violaceous erythema with associated telangiectasias, hypopigmentation, and superficial atrophy, most commonly found over the posterior shoulders, back, buttocks, and in a V-shaped area of the anterior neck and chest. Poikiloderma atrophicans vasculare is usually a late finding in the disease. Calcinosis cutis (calcium deposition) occurs in 10% of adult cases. It most commonly presents on the buttocks, elbows, knees, or traumatized areas, and is associated with increased disease activity and duration [9, 10]. The deposits of calcium are firm, irregular, and generally nontender, ranging in diameter from one millimeter to several centimeters. They can become inflamed, infected, or ulcerated and may discharge a chalky, white material [9, 10].

Table 2 Classification criteria for polymyositis and dermatomyositis

1.	Skin lesions (heliotrope rash, Gottron's sign, erythema on the extensor surface of extremity joints)
2.	Proximal muscle weakness
3.	Elevated serum creatine kinase or aldolase levels
4.	Muscle pain on grasping or spontaneous pain
5.	Myogenic changes in electromyography
6.	Positive anti-Jo antibody
7.	Nondestructive arthritis or arthralgias
8.	Systemic inflammatory sings (fever, elevated ESR, or CRP)
9.	Pathologic findings compatible with inflammatory myositis.

ESR erythrocyte sedimentation rate, *CRP* C-reactive protein
Patients presenting with the first plus four of the findings from two to nine are said to have dermatomyositis. If skin changes are absent, then the patient has polymyositis
Adapted from Koler RA, Montemarano A. Dermatomyositis. Am Fam Physician. 2001;64:1565–72

Classification and Treatment

When DM is suspected, the diagnosis can be made on clinical grounds alone if there are typical skin manifestations or classical patterns of muscle involvement [9]. The classification criteria for dermatomyositis are depicted in Table 2.

The definitive diagnosis of an inflammatory myopathy, however, requires a muscle biopsy [9, 11]. In 80% of cases, the biopsy shows chronic inflammatory cells in the perivascular and interstitial areas surrounding myofibrils. The pathognomonic finding of polymyositis is lymphocytic invasion of non-necrotic fibers. More common than inflammatory infiltrates is the degeneration and regeneration of myofibrils with phagocytosis of necrotic fibers [11]. The serum creatinine kinase is usually elevated. Electromyography allows confirmation of myopathy by the presence of early recruiting motor unit potentials of low amplitude and short duration in the limbs and paraspinal muscles. Electromyography also shows prominent spontaneous muscle fiber potentials in patients with active myositis [9]. A skin biopsy should be taken from the lesions of the skin to show vacuolar degeneration of the basal cell layer and a mild mononuclear cell infiltrate in the upper dermis and dermal–epidermal junction. There may be basement membrane thickening, edema, and increased mucin in the dermis, which can be better appreciated if the specimen is stained with periodic acid schiff (PAS) stain [9].

The use of sunscreen is recommended for all patients with DM. They should also be referred for physical therapy to prevent atrophy and contractures. For the control of severe pruritus, antihistamines and doxepin are recommended [10]. The core therapeutic approach remains daily high-dose oral corticosteroid therapy, along with adjunctive steroid-sparing immunosuppressive therapies, which are used to treat disease activity, prevent mortality, and attempt to reduce long-term disability [12]. Oral or intravenous corticosteroids are used in a single daily dose of 0.5–1.5 mg/kg/day, until the serum creatinine kinase levels is normalized and then slowly tapered down over the following 12 months [1, 10]. If no improvement occurs after 3 months of therapy, another immunosuppressive agent should be considered, for which, methotrexate is the first-line adjuvant therapy. Such immunosuppressive medications often allow corticosteroid dosages to be reduced, but monitoring is required for their own side effects [13]. Oral therapy should be initiated at a dose of 7.5–10 mg/week and increased by 2.5 mg until the goal of 25 mg/week is reached. Intravenous immunoglobulin is used in refractory cases [10].

There is an increase risk of malignancy in adults with DM, and it should always be excluded as the cause of these manifestations. The risk appears to be higher in patients diagnosed with DM after 45 years. The most common malignancies associated with this disease are ovarian cancer, gastric cancer, and lymphoma. Other reported malignancies include lung cancer, carcinoma of the male genital organ, nonmelanoma skin cancer, malignant melanoma, Kaposi's sarcoma, and mycosis fungoides [10]. Thus, the diagnosis of this condition warrants a work up for malignancy initially aimed at the most commonly associated forms of cancer and should at least include a complete history and physical examination, chest radiograph, AST, ALT, CBC with differential, routine serum chemistry, stool guaiac, and urinalysis (including myoglobulin) [10]. Poor prognostic factors include recalcitrant disease, delayed diagnosis, older age, malignancy, fever, asthenia, anorexia, pulmonary interstitial fibrosis, dysphagia, and leukocytosis. Malignancy, cardiac dysfunction, pulmonary dysfunction, and infection are the most common causes of death. With early treatment, however, survival rates are as high 80% at 5 years [10].

Scleroderma

Scleroderma is a multisystem disorder of unknown etiology, which presents major challenges for clinical management [14]. The sclerodermoid disorders comprise a heterogeneous group of conditions linked by the presence of thickened, sclerotic skin lesions [15]. These disorders can be divided into localized and systemic forms.

Systemic Sclerosis

Systemic sclerosis (SSc) is a systemic disease with the potential for multiple organ system involvement, including the gastrointestinal, cardiac, renal, and pulmonary systems [16]. There are three phases of skin thickening in systemic sclerosis: the edematous phase, the indurative phase, and the atrophic phase [15]. Raynaud's phenomenon is observed in 90–98% of scleroderma patients [17].

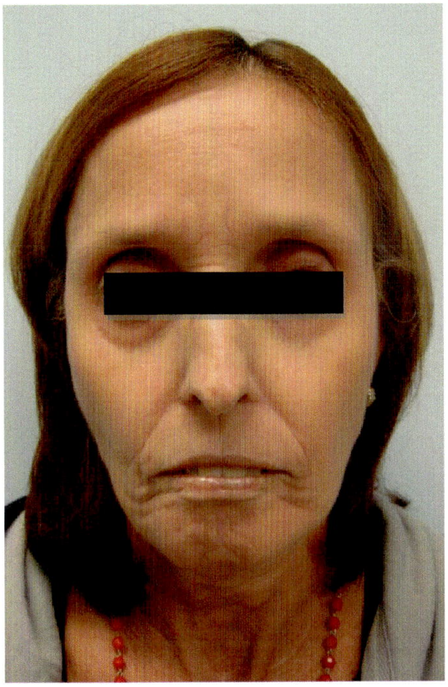

Fig. 9 Patient with systemic scleroderma: tightly pursed lips with perioral furrowing

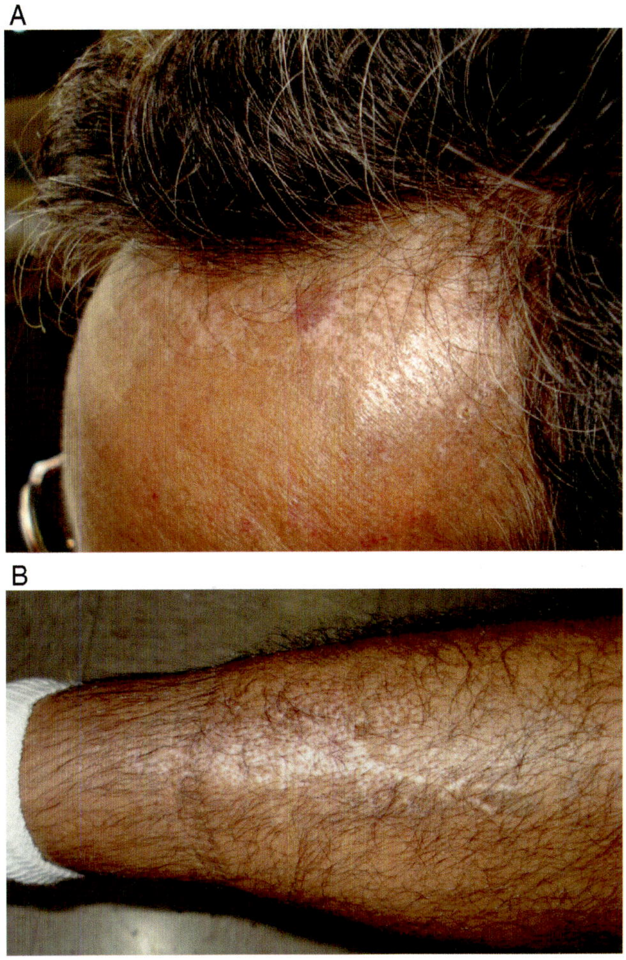

Fig. 10 (**a**, **b**) Patient with systemic scleroderma presenting with the characteristic salt and pepper pattern of pigmentation (leukoderma)

In the edematous phase, there is edema (both pitting and non-pitting) of the fingers, dorsum hands, forearms, legs, feet, and face. This swelling is usually painless and may be associated with pruritus and hyper- or hypo-pigmentation. The patients complain of puffy fingers, especially in the morning [15].

The indurative phase is characterized by tightened thick skin. The affected skin becomes increasingly shiny, taut, and tightly adherent to the subcutis. Transverse creases on the dorsum of the fingers disappear, and skinfolds over joints become widened. There is thinning of the epidermis leading to hair loss and decreased sweating. Facial changes include tightly pursed lips that lose their fullness, perioral subcutaneous fibrosis, and temporomandibular joint involvement that contribute to reduced oral aperture and radial furrowing around the mouth [18] (Fig. 9). Another characteristic finding is leukoderma with perifollicular pigment retention (Fig. 10).

After several years, patients undergo an atrophic phase in which the thickened dermis softens and reverts to a normal thickness. At this stage, the dermis becomes firmly bound to the subcutaneous fat. The skin of the fingers may look normal, but on palpation, the skin is very taut [18].

Systemic sclerosis can be further classified into limited and diffuse disease based on the extent of skin involvement. Limited SSc is so named because skin involvement is limited to the hands and face, while a wider extent of skin involvement is observed in diffuse SSc [19]. CREST syndrome is included in the limited scleroderma spectrum and is composed of the combination of calcinosis, Raynaud's phenomenon, esophageal dysmotility, sclerodactyly, and telangiectasias, with skin involvement mainly limited to the face or fingers (Figs. 11 and 12). Diffuse cutaneous scleroderma involves larger areas of skin and progress more rapidly from the edematous phase to the indurative phase [18]. Rapidly progressive diffuse scleroderma carries a poor prognosis and involves facial, truncal, extremity, and acral skin involvement along with extensive visceral organ involvement. Survival is approximately 50% at 10 years [18].

The skin affected by scleroderma is prone to ulceration and necrosis most commonly at the fingertips, secondary to ischemia from the obliterative vasculopathy and vasospasm associated with Raynaud's phenomenon. Raynaud's phenomenon is distinguished by cold-induced changes, typically a blanching that is followed by cyanosis and then a reactive hyperemia (Fig. 13). Patients with CREST syndrome or late stage diffuse systemic sclerosis frequently have subcutaneous

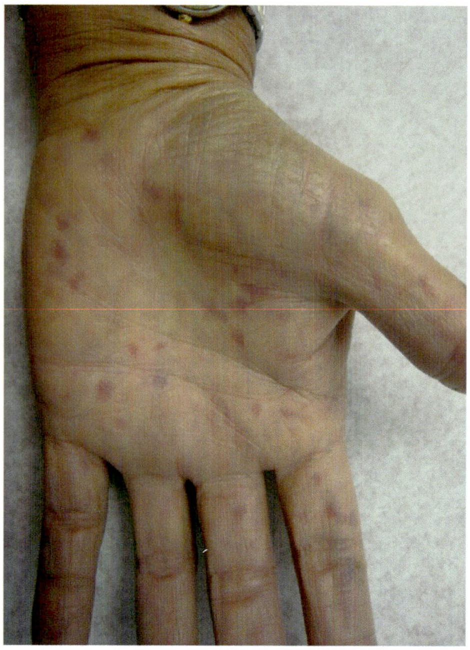

Fig. 11 Patient with systemic scleroderma presenting with telangiectasias of the hands

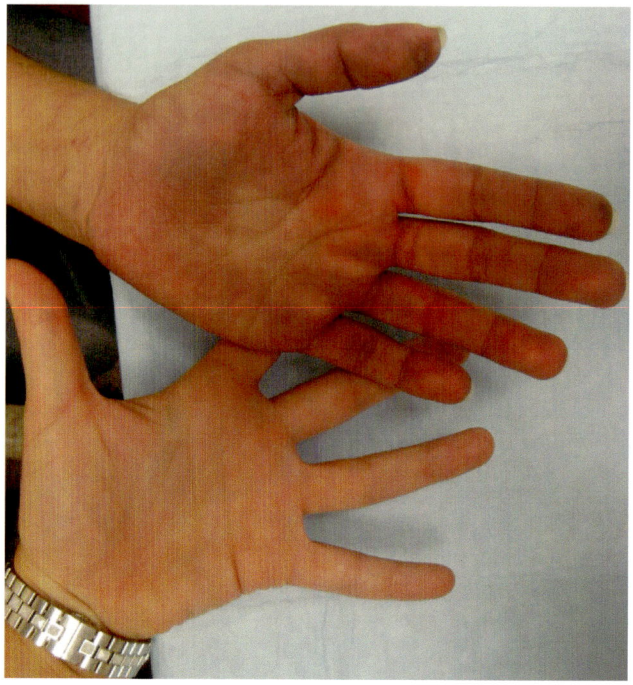

Fig. 13 Raynaud's phenomenon. Affected patient presents with a persistent bluish discoloration of the digits (*above*) compared with an unaffected person (*below*)

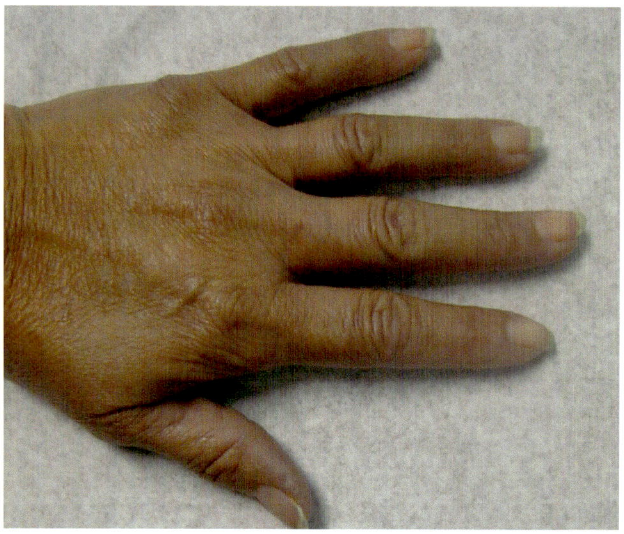

Fig. 12 Sclerodactyly

or infracutaneous calcinosis. These deposits occur mainly in the digital pads, but can also be found on other sites of repetitive trauma [18]. The antinuclear antibody (ANA) is present in 90–95% of patients with systemic sclerosis. In diffuse systemic sclerosis, anti-topoisomerase I (Scl-70) is more common than limited systemic sclerosis (20–30% versus 10–15%), whereas anti-centromere antibody is more common in limited systemic sclerosis (50–90% versus 5%) [18].

Morphea or Localized Scleroderma

Morphea has multiple distinctive clinical presentations and different subsets, of which we will discuss the most common. There are many scleroderma-like diseases that can make the diagnosis difficult: eosinophilic fasciitis, connective tissue overlap syndromes, phenylketonuria, amyloidosis, scleromyxedema, carcinoid syndrome, insulin-dependent diabetic cheiroarthropathy, lichen sclerosis et atrophicus, and infiltrating carcinomas [15].

The different types of morphea include plaque and linear. Plaque morphea is the most common presentation and is characterized by one or a few oval, rounded areas of induration. They are usually located on the trunk or proximal extremities. Mild-to-moderate hyperpigmentation may be present in the early indurated phase. The plaques begin with erythema, and then develop a nonpitting edema and central loss of pigment, and finally dermal and fat fibrosis ensues, but the tissue remains freely movable. Limited plaque morphea is defined as involving only one or two anatomic sites, whereas generalized morphea involves more than two anatomic sites or plaques that start to become confluent in some areas. The acral areas are almost never involved [18] (Fig. 14).

Linear morphea occurs on the extremities or scalp as single, linear, and unilateral bands. "En coup de sabre" is a form of linear morphea that referring to the involvement of the frontoparietal skin and is characterized by furrowing

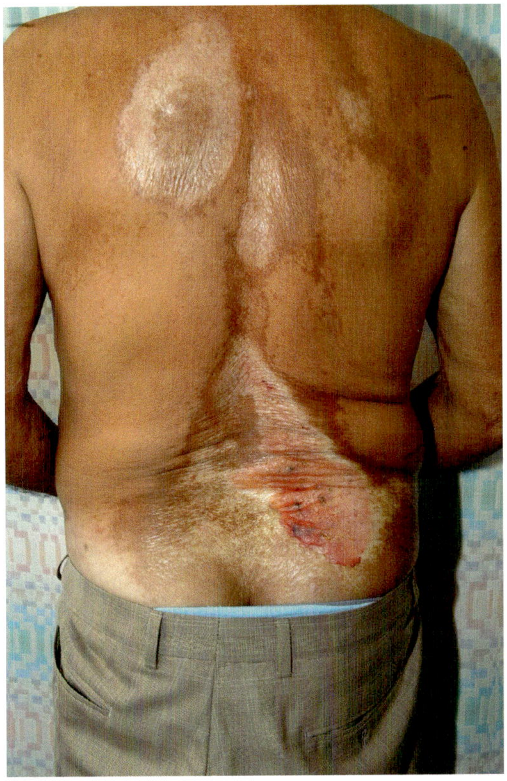

Fig. 14 Generalized morphea. The atrophic plaques are widely distributed so as to become confluent in some areas

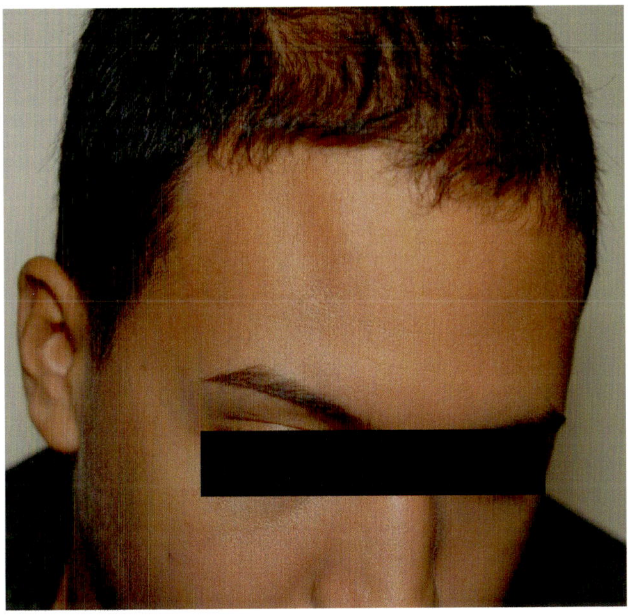

Fig. 15 Linear morphea ("en coup de sabre")

of the skin of the scalp and forehead, usually in a vertical fashion [18] (Fig. 15).

The histopathologic features of localized scleroderma/morphea show variations depending on the stage of the disease and the biopsy site. The peripheral violaceous border may show numerous inflammatory cells, comprised chiefly of lymphocytes and histiocytes scattered throughout the collagen bundles. Initial changes in collagen are seen in the lower part of the dermis and subcutaneous tissues, but later affect the entire dermis; these changes include eosinophilia of the collagen, broadening of the collagen bundles, and diminished interbundle spaces. The progression of the disease is heralded by the disappearance of inflammatory changes followed by hyalinization of the connective tissue. Sebaceous glands and hair structures become completely absent. Atrophic sweat glands (eccrine glands) become reduced in number and trapped between sclerotic collagen bundles in the dermis as the subcutaneous fat is replaced by collagen. Dermal blood vessels display thickened walls and narrowed lumens. Excessive sclerosis and hyalinization of connective tissue extends to the underlying fascia [20] (Fig. 16).

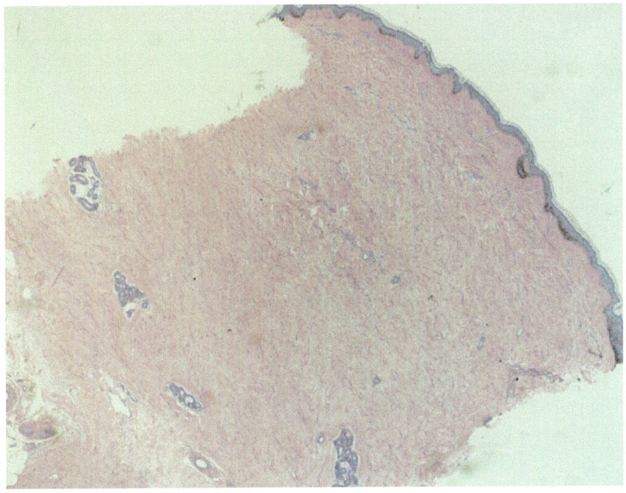

Fig. 16 Biopsy of a lesion of morphea shows that the biopsy maintains a "square" shape. There are superficial and deep perivascular infiltrates of lymphocytes and plasma cells (not visible at this magnification). The inflammation can extend to the septa of the fat and the fascia. The collagen bundles in the reticular dermis are thickened and arranged in a parallel fashion to the skin surface

Classification and Treatment

The American College of Rheumatology has developed a classification criterion that is 97% sensitive and 98% specific for the diagnosis of systemic sclerosis. These criteria are summarized in Table 3.

General measures, such as regular massages, warm compresses, protection from trauma and cold, avoidance of smoking, and reassurance are very important. For the treatment of localized sclerotic skin, the use of ultraviolet A (UVA) appears to reduce the induration of these lesions.

Table 3 ACR classification criteria for systemic sclerosis

Major criterion
1. Proximal diffuse (truncal) sclerosis (skin tightness, thickening, non-pitting induration)
Minor criteria
1. Sclerodactyly (only fingers and or toes)
2. Digital pitting scars or loss of substance of the finger pads (pulp loss)
3. Bilateral basilar pulmonary fibrosis

The patient should fulfill the major criterion or two of the three minor criteria
Adapted from Masi AT, Rodnan GP, et al. Preliminary criteria for the classification of systemic sclerosis (scleroderma). Arthritis Rheum. 1980;23:581–90

Other treatment options include psoralen plus UVA irradiation, topical photodynamic therapy, systemic corticosteroids, and oral calcitriol. D-Penicillamine, low-dose methotrexate, sulfasalazine, topical calcipotriene, diphenylhydantoin (phenytoin), clonidine hydrochloride, and antimalarials are also effective [20].

There is no proven curative therapy for systemic sclerosis to date. Therapy is aimed at treating organ-specific complications of the disease. The most common include gastroesophageal reflux disease, for which proton pump inhibitors are recommended to aid in the prevention of strictures; scleroderma renal crisis, which should be suspected when patients develop hypertension, and is treated with angiotensin receptor blockers; Raynaud's phenomenon, which responds to calcium channel blockers, and pulmonary hypertension, for which bosentan is most commonly employed [18]. The survival rate of localized scleroderma/morphea is comparable to that of the general population [20].

Rheumatoid Arthritis

Introduction

Rheumatoid arthritis (RA) is a systemic disease that affects the joints originally, with a gradual development of extra-articular manifestations involving other organs, particularly, the skin [21]. It is a chronic autoimmune inflammatory arthritis, in which the extra-articular manifestations are generally related to a poor prognosis and more severe disease. RA affects 1% of the US adult population. It is a multifactorial disease where environment and genetics plays an essential role [22–24]. Extra-articular features of RA, such as pericarditis, pleuritis, neuropathy, glomerulonephritis, interstitial lung disease, anemia, thrombocytosis, etc. need to be recognized early and managed promptly. The cutaneous manifestations of different inflammatory origins include vasculitis, neutrophilic processes, and granulomatous dermatoses. Most of the cutaneous manifestations correlate with disease activity, while others are nonspecific and unpredictable in nature. Occasionally, RA may overlap with other collagen diseases, most commonly with SLE and Sjogren's syndrome [25, 26].

The most important specific cutaneous lesions associated with rheumatoid arthritis are the classic rheumatoid nodules (CRN), rheumatoid nodulosis, accelerated rheumatoid nodulosis (ARN), and vasculitis. Other less common lesions include pyoderma gangrenosum, interstitial granulomatous dermatitis with arthritis (IGDA), palisaded neutrophilic and granulomatous dermatitis, and neutrophilic dermatitis associated with RA [26]. Nonspecific changes of the skin in RA include atrophy, fragility, easy bruisability, and the nails show longitudinal ridging (onychorrhexis), clubbing, telangiectasia, periungual erythema, onycholysis, or inversion of the pterygium [26–28].

Most of the cutaneous lesions associated with RA have characteristic features that distinguish them and facilitates prompt clinical diagnosis which can be correlated with the histopathological changes. It is in this setting that the dermatologist can provide early assessment and contribute together with other specialties towards an expedient work-up, diagnosis, and appropriate treatment regimen.

Classic Rheumatoid Nodules

The CRN is skin colored, firm, movable, and non-tender subcutaneous nodule with genetic predisposition in patients with severe, seropositive RA. It is the most common extra-articular manifestation in RA, particularly in white male patients with active disease [29, 30]. They present in approximately 25–30% of patients with RA and 40% of all RF seropositive patients, yet even more frequently (up to 75%) in RA-associated Felty syndrome [25, 29–31]. Rarely, in about 6% of those with CRN, patients are RF seronegative, however, high RF factor levels correlate with an increased frequency of RA nodules [32]. Genetics affect the role of the appearance of CRN, with HLA-DR4 haplotype most commonly observed in RA patients [33].

Classic RA nodules usually present as a later manifestation of active arthritic disease, although occasionally is the initial manifestation. They are usually located on the extensor surfaces of the arms as multiple or single lesions, as large as 5–6 cm to as small as 2 mm in diameter [25, 32] (Fig. 17a). Rheumatoid nodules have a predilection for the elbows and fingers and also occur on the palms and soles (uncomfortable but generally painless) [25] (Fig. 17b). They can become attached to tendons, bursa and periosteum, causing tenderness and discomfort in these regions [25]. The nodules have a tendency to occur in areas of trauma (possibly the inciting event) such as the forearms, fingers, occiput, back, interphalangeal joints, and heel [34]. Other involved areas include the sacral prominences, skull, ischial tuberosities, foot joints, ears, penis, and vulva. Rheumatoid nodules are not exclusive

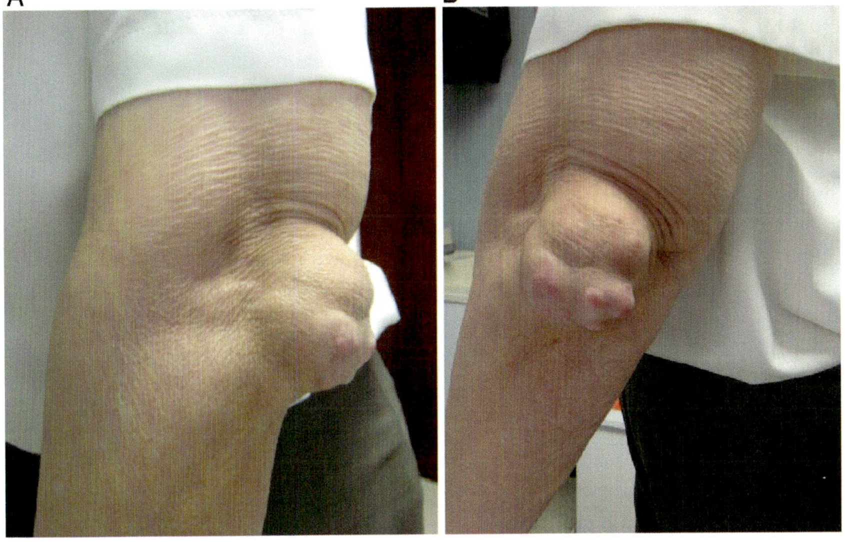

Fig. 17 (**a**, **b**) Rheumatoid nodules. Rheumatoid nodules have a predilection for the elbows and appear as skin colored, firm, and movable subcutaneous nodules

to the skin or to RA, but have also been described in such organs as the lung, sclera, pericardium, peritoneum, tendons, synovium, bones, heart, pharynx, vocal cords, kidney, breasts, and the nervous system and in other conditions such as lupus erythematosus, ankylosing spondylitis, and chronic active hepatitis, to name a few [35, 36].

Histopathologically RA nodules show distinct granulomas separated by scar tissue, each granuloma in different stages of maturity. The three characteristic stages include the acute inflammatory, granulomatous, and necrotic stage. The initial stage is characterized by the inflammation and proliferation of capillaries surrounded by undifferentiated mononuclear cells and fibroblasts [37]. Following, the second stage has the hallmark palisading granulomatous infiltrates of mononuclear cells and macrophages at the periphery of the initial focus of granulation tissue. Finally, the third stage is characterized by a large central focus of fibrin and necrotic collagen with fibrinoid material, fragments of cellular organelles, lymphocytes, and deposited hemoglobin. This inner necrotic zone is intensely eosinophilic, granular or fibrillary and surrounded by elongated histiocytes [38–40].

The exact pathogenesis of the rheumatoid nodules is not well understood, but it is probably due to a Th1-mediated mechanism [41]. Trauma has been implicated to play a role due to the neoangiogenesis and granulation tissue that it causes. Diagnosis is usually based on clinical findings of symmetric inflammatory polyarthritis, seropositive for RF, and extra-articular manifestations are highly suggestive. Diagnosis of the RA nodules is challenging, as the histological appearance is often confused for necrobiosis lipoidica and granuloma annulare due to the necrobiotic granulomas. Clinically, these nodules are included in the differential diagnosis with gouty tophi, fibromas, subcutaneous sarcoidosis, subcutaneous granuloma annulare, lupus panniculitis, metastatic tumors, amyloidosis, histoplasmosis, and epidermoid cysts [25]. The rheumatoid nodules are usually benign and may regress or persist indefinitely, but occasionally complications occur. Infection, fistula formation, ulceration, and gangrene are the most frequent complications after rupture of the skin overlying the subcutaneous nodules, requiring surgical excision [32]. Nodules are usually asymptomatic and more of a cosmetic problem than a medical necessity of treatment. Lesions should be left alone if asymptomatic and drained, injected or excised when symptomatic due to the high rates of recurrence [42]. Therapy by surgical excision is the treatment of choice when large nodules cause significant pain, show ulcerations, or are associated with bursitis or damage to underlying structures [43].

Accelerated Rheumatoid Nodulosis

ARN is the recognized complication of Methotrexate (MTX) therapy in patients with RA. It was first described in 1986 by Kramer and Lee during a long-term study of MTX [44]. It is characterized by the new presence of numerous, small, and tender nodules on the hands, feet, and ears in patients with chronic RA undergoing treatment with MTX, even despite good clinical response to the treatment [45]. Recently, ARN has also been reported with the use of other drugs of the TNF-alpha inhibitor profiles such as etanercept (Enbrel) and infliximab (brand name Remicade) [46, 47]. The incidence is approximately 8% of adult patients, whereas only 1.5% in Juvenile RA, on long-term treatment with MTX protocols for arthritis [48, 49]. It is most commonly found in males and in the areas such as the metacarpophalangeal and proximal interphalangeal joints. It does not require the presence of previous classic rheumatoid nodules, although histologically, these lesions are the same as the classical rheumatoid nodules [32]. Although the lesions are tender and multiple, 80% are not associated with significant discomfort or morbidity thus allowing for the treatment regimen to persist in hopes of improved arthritis [33, 49].

It has been postulated that the progression of ARN is caused by adenosine A1 receptor promotion of multinucleated cell formation by human monocytes. The lesions may resolve once MTX is stopped and recur after rechallenged. The addition to other anti-inflammatory drugs such as hydroxychloroquine, D-penicillamine, colchicines, or sulfasalazine to MTX may decrease the cases of ARN or improve the already present lesions. These lesions tend to last an average of 3 years [49].

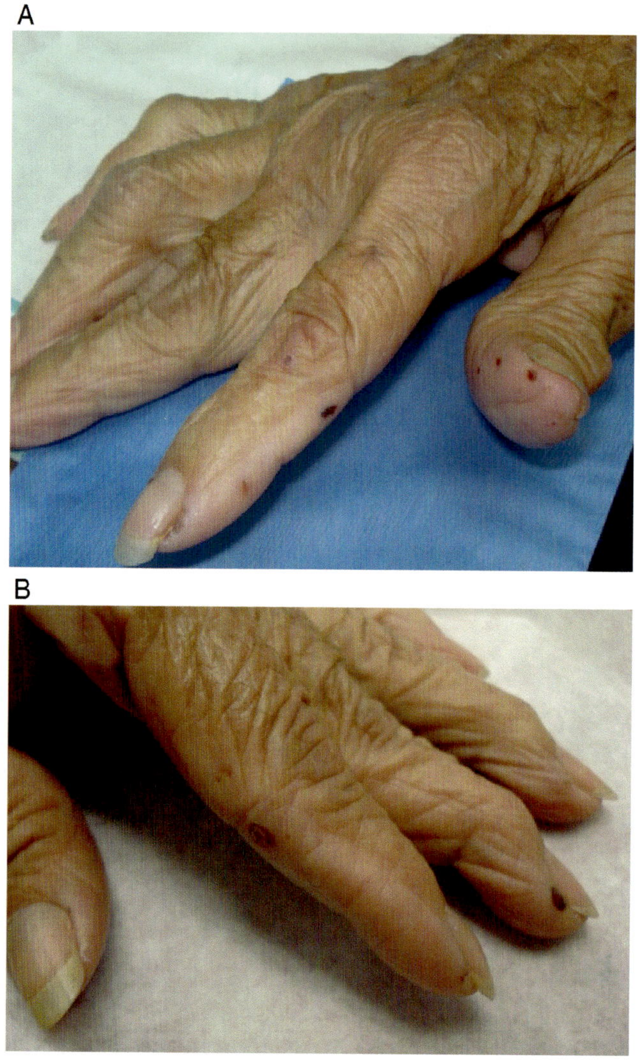

Fig. 18 (**a**, **b**) Bywater lesions on the nail fold, nail edge, and digital bulb

Rheumatoid Nodulosis

Rheumatoid nodulosis (RN) is the condition that describes a specific variant of polyarthritis associated with severe seropositive RA, radiological subchondral bone cysts, and subcutaneous rheumatoid nodules. In some instances, skin nodules are the predominant sign with minor or even absent joint symptoms. RN was first described in 1949 by Bywaters and later Ginsberg and coworkers received credit for the term RN for an intermittent arthritis associated with multiple rheumatoid nodules usually involving the hands and feet with intraosseous cystic changes [50, 51]. Couret and coworkers were the first to compile the subsequent diagnostic criteria for RN: (1) multiple subcutaneous rheumatoid nodules confirmed by biopsy, (2) recurrent joint symptoms with minimal clinical or radiological involvement, (3) a benign clinical course, and (4) mild or no systemic manifestations of RA [52]. It is important to recognize that the cystic lesions in RN do not result in erosive arthritis [53]. RN patients are commonly males, 80% of the time, in the third to fifth decades of life. It is not frequently associated with HLA-DRB1 allele as in classical rheumatoid nodules and despite the almost exact histological presentation as rheumatoid nodules, the clinical course is benign and does not lead to the progression of classic erosive RA with systemic manifestations [49, 53]. RN is usually a self-limited and symptomatically controlled with non-steroidal anti-inflammatory drugs (NSAIDs) or with slow acting anti-RA drugs. Complete resolution with hydrochloroquine is recorded in the literature [54]. Surgical removal of the nodules may be considered, whether they limit joint motion [49].

Rheumatoid Vasculitis

Rheumatoid vasculitis is an inflammatory condition of the small, medium, and large vessels that affect a sector of patients with RA. There are diverse cutaneous vasculitic manifestations clinically such as palpable and non-palpable purpura, erythematous nodules, ulcerations, livedo reticularis, digital infacts and gangrene, atrophie blanche (AB), and nail fold telangiectasias. Rheumatoid vasculitis (RV) affects as many as 5% of RA patients [20, 55]. Despite a low prevalence rate, the systemic form of RV occurs more often than Wegener granulomatosis or polyarterits nodosa [20, 56].

Cutaneous manifestations are the most frequent and often presenting extra-articular manifestation of RV, present in approximately 75–90% of RV patients [49, 56]. In about 10% of RA patients, RV can appear as an acute painful punched-out leg ulcer along the lateral malleolus and pretibial regions, attributable to vasculitis or the combination of both vasculitis and venous insufficiency [57]. Small vessel disease is characterized by periungual infarctions, localized petechiae or purpura and splinter hemorrhages. Splinter hemorrhages, also called Bywater lesions, are small, brown, purpuric and painless lesions on the nail fold, nail edge, or digital bulb [20] (Fig. 18). Medium vessel disease can present with nodules, ulcers, livedo reticularis, or systemic symptoms. AB is classified as a primary (occlusive process) or secondary, the latter of which can be related to connective tissue diseases such as RA, due to inflammation within the superficial blood vessels. AB appears as smooth, scar-like, slightly depressed ivory-white patches with telangiectasia and hyperpigmention along the borders [58]. The systemic signs of RV are common and include sensory and motor neuropathy in 50% of patients, hepatomegaly, splenomegaly, scleritis, pericarditis, arrhythmia, carditis, pleuritis, proteinuria, bowel ulcers, alveolitis, hematuria, pleuritis, cerebral infarction, and an acute abdomen [55, 59].

RV frequently occurs in seropositive RA patients, and rarely in RF seronegative patients, who have a protracted disease. The factors associated with RV include high titer of RF, joint erosions, male gender, and the presence of other extra-articular manifestations, particularly rheumatoid nodules [55]. RV can be present before or at the time of RA diagnosis, although it is usually seen late in the course of the disease (an average of 10–14 years after the onset of arthritis). It is more common in men suffering from RA, with a 10–15% incidence in such cases [56].

The variety of significant skin manifestations and the lack of specific signs and symptoms make the diagnosis dependent upon ruling out systemic conditions and on histological evidence of necrotizing vasculitis [60]. Biopies should be taken from the center of the lesions, except when the lesion is an ulcer, for which the biopsy should be taken from the border. The clinical diagnosis is established by the presence of RA plus one or more of the following: (1) mononeuritis multiplex, (2) peripheral gangrene, (3) presence of vasculitis in skin pathology, and (4) evidence of systemic involvement by RV [61]. Peripheral neuropathy, often seen as mononeuritis multiplex, affects up to 40% of patients with RA and medium sized vasculitis, therefore, nerve conduction and sural nerve biopsies should be carried out.

Histopathologically there is a spectrum of continuous vascular involvement. RA vasculitis is an immune complex disease characterized by the presence IgG RF complex-mediated vasculitis with high titers of C-reactive proteins and immunofluorescence revealing C3 and IgM deposits in small and medium-sized vessel walls. When the vasculitis affects medium-sized vessel walls, it can resemble polyarteritis nodosa histologically by the inflammatory necrotizing obliterative arteritis with focal panniculitis [20, 62]. Leukocytoclastic vasculitis, or dermal venulitis, is the most common presentation and shows a dense vascular infiltration of neutrophils with the formation of nuclear dust (leukocytoclasis), red blood cell extravasation, and fibrinoid necrosis of vessel walls [62].

Considerable morbidity and mortality arise in patients with RV, particularly those with a wide spectrum of cutaneous and systemic manifestations [20, 61]. The level of RF is often very high, reported to be greater than 1:2,560 in 38% of cases, and higher RF levels are associated with a higher mortality, as high as 43% [63]. The association with mononeuritis multiplex or bowel involvement has shown a fatal prognosis [62]. Due to this high mortality rate, aggressive therapeutic modalities should be administered without delay.

Treatment usually consists of the combination of oral prednisone, intravenous methylprednisolone, and cyclophosphamide for systemic RV and is effective, fast acting and associated with a lower relapse rates and mortality. Other treatments options for mild to moderate disease include NSAID's, azathioprine, mycophenolate mofetil, and cyclosporine [64].

Pyoderma Gangrenosum

Pyoderma Gangrenosum (PG) has four clinical variants: (1) ulcerative, (2) bullous, (3) pustular, and (4) vegetative. PG occurs more frequently in patients with RA and is associated with the ulcerative form, most often with a seronegative polyarthritis [65]. Seropositive RA occurs with pyoderma gangrenosum in only 4–50% of patients [66, 67]. It is reported that more than a fourth of PG cases have an arthritic component, although associated PG lesions do not worsen the severity of the arthritis and is considered an independent disease process [68]. It occurs most often in women [66]. The pathogenesis is not well understood because PG is also seen in other immunologic conditions such as inflammatory bowel disease and hematologic diseases.

The lesion of PG is usually solitary and on the lower extremities (especially sites of trauma or irritation). It progresses from a tender, erythematous, or violaceous papule to a rapidly expanding ulcerative lesion with purulence, necrosis, and violaceous undermining ragged borders [20]. 20% of cases affect areas other than the lower extremities such as the face, arms, and trunk [66, 68]. The ulcerations can last for months to years and leave a resultant scar. Lesions can be as large as 10 cm in diameter [20].

There is no characteristic morphology. Histopathology changes show a deep neutrophilic infiltrate at the border of the ulcers with proliferation of vessels but no evidence of leukocytoclastic or non-thrombotic vasculitis [62, 68]. The differential diagnosis includes other vasculitis, mycobacterial infections, halogenodermas (skin eruptions after exposure to iodide, bromide, and fluoride), deep fungal infections, facticial diseases, and syphilis [20].

Small lesions may be treated conservatively with intralesional steroids, topical antibiotics, and avoidance of trauma, although some may even resolve spontaneously [65]. Larger lesions should be treated with high-dose systemic prednisone to induce remission and/or with minocycline, cyclophosphamide, tacrolimus, clofazimine, chlorambucil infliximab, cyclosporine, azathioprine, and dapsone [65, 69].

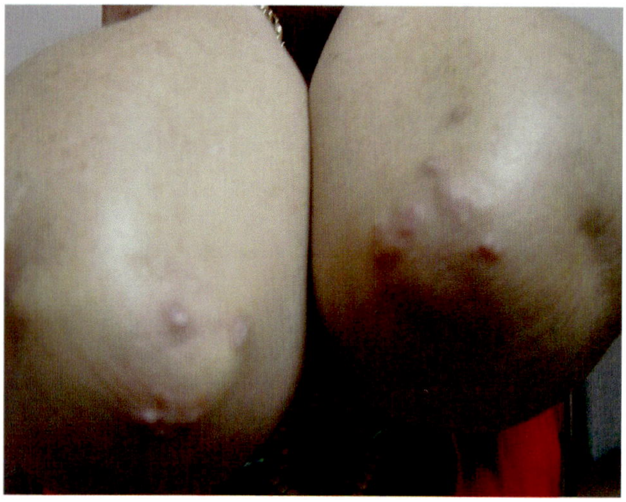

Fig. 19 Interstitial granulomatous dermatitis. Presenting with papules and nodules with a slight linear distribution

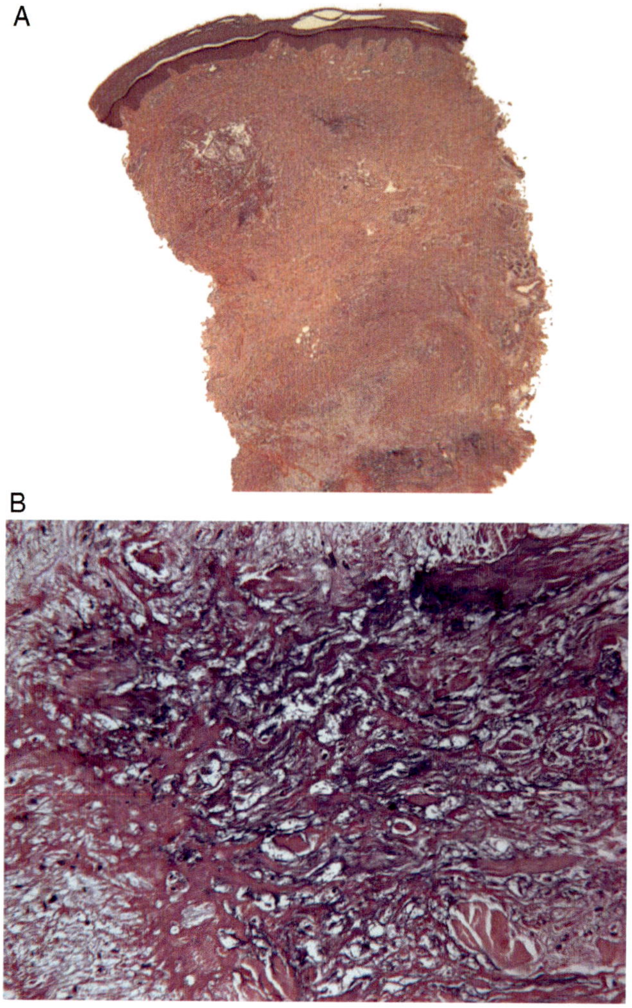

Fig. 20 (**a**, **b**) Histopathology of interstitial granulomatous dermatitis. Diffuse interstitial and focal palisading infiltrates of lymphocytes, histiocytes, eosinophils, and neutrophils and with the degeneration of collagen found in the reticular dermis

Interstitial Granulomatous Dermatitis with Arthritis

IGDA was first described by Dykman et al. in 1965 for a linear palpable area extending from the axilla to the abdomen in RA patients; however, it was Ackerman who is responsible for the name IGDA [70, 71]. Although the etiology is unknown, the relationship between the granulomatous dermatitis and arthritis is thought to be related to autoimmunity; it has been associated with autoimmune thyroiditis, SLE, and lymphoproliferative disorders [72].

The clinical setup of this condition is most often characterized by a middle-aged woman with high RF titers and severe RA with fluctuations between remission and flares. Interstitial granulomatous dermatitis can occur prior, during, or after the arthritis presents [72]. These patients usually have elevated ESR [73].

The clinical findings are linear, indurated, and subcutaneous cord such as lesions of the axilla and trunk which are often reported as painful and burning, thus also referred to as the "rope sign" [72, 74]. Occasionally, the lesions are papules, nodules, or plaques ranging from erythematous to violaceous color in the similar linear distribution [72, 73] (Fig. 19).

Histologically, the lesion shows diffuse interstitial and focal palisaded infiltrates of lymphocytes, histiocytes, eosinophils, and neutrophils and with the degeneration of collagen found in the reticular dermis. The eruptions appear as an interstitial infiltrate of histiocytes with neutrophils also described as leukocytoclastic vasculitis and histiocytic palisaded granulomas surrounding altered collagen and fibrin [62, 71, 72] (Fig. 20). The differential diagnosis includes other palisading granulomas such as granuloma annulare, granulomatous slack skin, necrobiosis lipoidica, Blau syndrome, and interstitial granulomatous drug reactions [75]. Treatment options of IGDA include prednisone and NSAID's, for which the results have been variable.

Palisaded Neutrophilic Granulomatous Dermatitis

Rheumatoid palisaded neutrophilic granulomatous dermatitis (PDGD), characterized by papules, plaques, nodules, and urticarial wheals over the extensor surface of the upper extremities and trunk and was first described by Sangueza et al. [76]. These lesions are usually grouped, non-tender and non-pruritic and associated with severe and disabling RA. Similar to IGDA, RA can occur prior to, during, or after this dermatologic manifestation. This entity has been poorly defined and been given many different names. Histologically, there are extensive neutrophilic infiltrates and occasional scant lymphocytes, eosinophils, and histiocytes without the evidence of leukocytoclastic vasculitis [77]. The differential diagnosis includes PG, Behcet syndrome, Sweet syndrome, and bowel-bypass syndrome [78]. The treatment is dapsone (or low-dose prednisone if allergic), and the clinical course may be protracted if therapy is not initiated.

Conclusion

Connective tissue diseases present a diagnostic challenge to physicians given the wide range of cutaneous manifestations and the fact that they are diagnosed by fulfillment of specific criteria that encompass different organ systems. Therefore, it is important to consider these diseases and the constellation of clinical findings with which they may present every time we see a patient with a skin rash to direct history and physical examination towards obtaining the appropriate diagnosis. By instituting early and adequate therapy, the serious complications of these diseases can be avoided.

References

1. Sontheimer RD. Dermatomyositis: an overview of recent progress with emphasis on dermatologic aspects. Dermatol Clin. 2002;20: 387–408.
2. Ostezan LB, Callen JP. Cutaneous manifestations of selected rheumatologic diseases. Am Fam Physician. 1996;53:1625–36.
3. Fabbri P, Cardinali C, Giomi B, Caproni M. Cutaneous lupus erythematosus: diagnosis and management. Am J Clin Dermatol. 2003;4:449–65.
4. Laman SD, Provost TT. Cutaneous manifestations of lupus erythematosus. Rheum Dis Clin North Am. 1994;20:195–212.
5. Akbarian M, Faezi ST, Gharibdoost F, et al. Systemic lupus erythematosus in Iran: a study of 2280 patients over 33 years. Int J Rheum Dis. 2010;13:374–9.
6. Farley-Loftus R, Elmariah SB, Ralston J, et al. Hypertrophic discoid lupus erythematosus. Dermatol Online J. 2010;16:1.
7. Tan EM, Cohen AS, Fries JF, et al. The 1982 revised criteria for the classification of systemic lupus erythematosus. Arthritis Rheum. 1982;25:1271–7.
8. Kuhn A, Gensch K, Haust M, et al. Photoprotective effects of a broad-spectrum sunscreen in ultraviolet-induced cutaneous lupus erythematosus: a randomized, vehicle-controlled, double-blind study. J Am Acad Dermatol. 2011;64:37–48.
9. Mastalgia FL, Garlepp MJ, Phillips BA, Zilko PJ. Inflammatory myopathies: Clinical, diagnostic and therapeutic aspects. Muscle Nerv. 2003;27:407–25.
10. Koler RA, Montemarano A. Dermatomyositis. Am Fam Physician. 2001;64:1565–72.
11. Hochberg MC, Silman AJ, Smolen JS, Weinblatt ME, Weisman MH. Practical rheumatology. 3rd ed. London: Mosby; 2004.
12. Rider LG, Miller FW. Deciphering the clinical presentations, pathogenesis, and treatment of the idiopathic inflammatory myopathies. JAMA. 2011;305:183–90.
13. Distad BJ, Amato AA, Weiss MD. Inflammatory myopathies. Curr Treat Options Neurol. 2011;13(2):119–30.
14. Olsen NJ. Scleroderma: the need for extreme remedies. Am J Med Sci. 2011. (Epub ahead of print).
15. Black CM. Scleroderma, clinical aspects. J Intern Med. 1993;234: 115–8.
16. Hassoun PM. Lung involvement in systemic sclerosis. Presse Med. 2011;40(1 Pt 2):e3–17.
17. Masi AT, Rodnan GP, et al. Preliminary criteria for the classification of systemic sclerosis (scleroderma). Arthritis Rheum. 1980;23: 581–90.
18. Clements PJ. Systemic sclerosis. 2nd ed. Philadelphia: Lippincott Williams & Wilkins; 2004. p. 129–35.
19. Mahoney Jr WM, Fleming JN, Schwartz SM. A unifying hypothesis for scleroderma: identifying a target cell for scleroderma. Curr Rheumatol Rep. 2011;13:28–36.
20. Sehgal VN, Srivastava G, et al. Localized scleroderma/morphea. In J Dermatol. 2002;41:467–75.
21. Nakamura T, Higashi S, Tomoda K, et al. Cutaneous nodules in patients with rheumatoid arthritis: a case report and review of literatures. Clin Rheumatol. 2011;30(5):719–22.
22. Lee DM, Weinblatt ME. Rheumatoid arthritis [comment]. Lancet. 2001;358:903–11.
23. Gabriel SE. The epidemiology of rheumatoid arthritis. Rheum Dis Clin North Am. 2001;27:269–81.
24. Symmons D, Turner G, Webb R, Asten P, Barrett E, Lunt M, et al. The prevalence of rheumatoid arthritis in the United Kingdom: new estimates for a new century. Rheumatology. 2002;41:793–800.
25. Sayah A, English JC. Rheumatoid arthritis: A review of the cutaneous manifestations. J Am Acad Dermatol. 2005;53:191–209.
26. Ergun T, Inanc N, Tuney D, Kotiloglu EK, Seckin D, Direskeneli H. Skin manifestations of rheumatoid arthritis: a study of 215 Turkish patients. Int J Dermatol. 2008;47(9):894–902.
27. Ruddy S, Harris ED, Sledge CB. Kelley's textbook of rheumatology. 6th ed. Philadelphia: WB Saunders; 2001.
28. Jorizzo JL, Gonzalez EB, Daniels JC. Red lunulae in a patient with rheumatoid arthritis. J Am Acad Dermatol. 1983;8:711–4.
29. Ziff M. The Rheumatoid nodule. Arthritis Rheum. 1990;33:761–7.
30. Magro CM, Crowson AN. The spectrum of cutaneous lesions in rheumatoid arthritis. A clinical and pathological study of 43 patients. J Cutan Pathol. 2003;30:1–10.
31. Young A, Koduri G. Extra-articular manifestations and complications of rheumatoid arthritis. Best Pract Res Clin Rheumatol. 2007;21(5):907–27.
32. Kaye BR, Kaye RL, Bobrove A. Rheumatoid nodules. Review of the spectrum of associated conditions and proposal of a new classification, with a report of four seronegative cases. Am J Med. 1984;76:279–92.
33. Ahmed SS, Arnett FC, Smith CA, et al. The HLA-DRB1*0401 allele and the development of methotrexate-induced accelerated rheumatoid nodulosis: a follow-up study of 79 Caucasian patients with rheumatoid arthritis. Medicine. 2001;80:271–8.
34. Lems WF, Dijkmans BA. Rheumatoid arthritis: clinical picture and its variants. In: Firestein GS, Panayi GS, Wollheim FA, editors. Rheumatoid arthritis: frontiers in pathogenesis and treatment. New York: Oxford University Press; 2000. p. 219.
35. Higaki Y, Kim KJ, Kawashima M. Rheumatoid nodules on the distal region of the sole. J Dermatol. 1997;24:798.
36. Appleton MA, Ismail SM. Ulcerating rheumatoid nodule of the vulva. J Clin Pathol. 1996;49:85–7.
37. Sokoloff L, McCluskey RT, Bunim JJ. Vascularity of the early subcutaneous nodules of RA. Arch Pathol. 1953;55:475–95.
38. Aherne MJ, Bacon PA, Blake DR, et al. Immunohistochemical findings in rheumatoid nodules. Virchows Arch A Pathol Anat Histopathol. 1985;407:191–202.
39. Miyasaka N, Sato K, Yamamoto K, et al. Immunological and immunohistochemical analysis of rheumatoid nodules. Ann Rheum Dis. 1989;48:220–6.
40. Palmer DG, Hogg N, Highton J, et al. Macrophage migration and maturation within rheumatoid nodules. Arthritis Rheum. 1987;30:728–36.
41. Hessian P, Highton J, Kean A, et al. Cytokine profile of the rheumatoid nodule suggests that it is a Th1 granuloma. Arthritis Rheum. 2003;48:334–8.

42. Gall EP. General features. In: Schumacher HR, Gall EP, editors. Rheumatoid arthritis: an illustrated guide to pathology, diagnosis, and management, vol. 1. Philadelphia: JB Lippincott; 1988. p. 28.
43. Sibbitt WL, Williams RC. Cutaneous manifestations of rheumatoid arthritis. Int J Dermatol. 1982;21:563–72.
44. Kremer JM, Lee JK. The safety and efficacy of the use of methotrexate in long-term therapy for rheumatoid arthritis. Arthritis Rheum. 1986;29:822–31.
45. Segal R, Caspi D, Tishler M, et al. Accelerated nodulosis and vasculitis during methotrexate therapy for rheumatoid arthritis. Arthritis Rheum. 1988;31:1182–5.
46. Cunnane G, Warnock M, Fye KH, Daikh DI. Accelerated nodulosis and vasculitis following etanercept therapy for rheumatoid arthritis. Arthritis Rheum. 2002;47:445–9.
47. Kekow J, Welte T, Kellner U, et al. Development of rheumatoid nodules during anti-tumor necrosis factor alpha therapy with etanercept. Arthritis Rheum. 2002;46:843–4.
48. Kernstens PJ, Boerbooms AM, Jeurissen ME, Fast JH, Assmann KJ, van de Putte LB. Accelerated nodulosis during low dose methotrexate therapy for rheumatoid arthritis. An analysis of ten cases [comment]. J Rheumatol. 1992;19:867–71.
49. Garcia-Patos V. Rheumatoid nodule. Semin Cutan Med Surg. 2007;26:100–7.
50. Bywaters EG. A variant of rheumatoid arthritis characterized by recurrent digital pad nodules and palmar fasciitis, closely resembling palindromic rheumatism. Ann Rheum Dis. 1949;8:2–30.
51. Ginsberg MH, Genant HK, Yu TF, et al. Rheumatoid nodulosis: an unusual variant of rheumatoid arthritis. Arthritis Rheum. 1975;18: 49–58.
52. Couret M, Combe B, Chuong VT, et al. Rheumatoid nodulosis: report of two new cases and discussion of diagnostic criteria. J Rheumatol. 1988;15:1427–30.
53. Toussirot E, Tiberghien P, Balblanc JC, Kremer P, Despaux J, Dupond JL, et al. HLA DRB1* alleles in rheumatoid nodulosis: a comparative study with rheumatoid arthritis with and without nodules. Rheumatol Int. 1998;17:233–6.
54. Kai Y, Anzai S, Shibuya H, et al. A case of rheumatoid nodulosis successfully treated with surgery. J Dermatol. 2004;31:910–5.
55. Voskuyl AE, Zwinderman AH, Westedt ML, Vandenbroucke JP, Breedveld FC, Hazes JM. Factors associated with the development of vasculitis in rheumatoid arthritis: results of a case-control study. Ann Rheum Dis. 1996;55:190–2.
56. Watts RA, Carruthers DM, Symmons DP, Scott DG. The incidence of rheumatoid vasculitis in the Norwich Health Authority. Br J Rheumatol. 1994;33:832–3.
57. Tuveri M, Genenni S, Matucci-Cerinic M, Aloe L. NGF, a useful tool in the treatment of chronic vasculitic ulcers in rheumatoid arthritis. Lancet. 2000;356:1739–40.
58. Sommer S, Sheehan-Dare RA. Atrophie blanche-like scarring after pulsed dye laser treatment. J Am Acad Dermatol. 1999;41(1): 100–2.
59. Chen KR, Toyohara A, Suzuki A, Miyakawa S. Clinical and histopathological spectrum of cutaneous vasculitis in rheumatoid arthritis. Br J Dermatol. 2002;147:903–13.
60. Genta MS, Genta RM, Gabay C. Systemic rheumatoid vasculitis: a review. Semin Arthritis Rheum. 2006;36(2):88–98.
61. Scott DG, Bacon PA. Intravenous cyclophosphamide plus methylprednisolone in treatment of systemic rheumatoid vasculitis. Am J Med. 1984;76:377–84.
62. Chen KR, Toyohara A, Suzuki A, Miyakawa S. Clinical and histopathological spectrum of cutaneous vasculitis in rheumatoid arthritis. Br J Dermatol. 2002;147(5):905–13.
63. Geirsson AJ, Sturfelt G, Truedsson L. Clinical and serological features of severe vasculitis in rheumatoid arthritis: prognostic implications. Ann Rheum Dis. 1987;46:727–33.
64. O'Gradaugh D, Watts RA, Scott DG. Extra-articular features of rheumatoid arthritis. In: Firestein GS, Panayi GS, Wollheim FA, editors. Rheumatoid arthritis: frontiers in pathogenesis and treatment. New York: Oxford University Press; 2000. p. 229–32.
65. Powell FC, Su WP, Perry HO. Pyoderma gangrenosum: classification and management. J Am Acad Dermatol. 1996;34:395–409.
66. von den Driesh P. Pyoderma gangrenosum: a report of 44 cases with follow-up. Br J Dermatol. 1997;137:1000–5.
67. Hickman JG, Lazarus GS. Pyoderma gangrenosum: a reappraisal of associated systemic diseases. Br J Dermatol. 1980;102:235–7.
68. Holt PJ, Davies MG, Saunders KC, Nuki G. Pyoderma gangrenosum: clinical and laboratory findings in 15 patients with special reference to polyarthritis. Medicine. 1980;59:114–33.
69. Reynolds NJ, Peachey RD. Response of atypical bullous pyoderma gangrenosum to oral monocycline, hydrochloride, and topical steroids. Acta Derm Venereol. 1990;70:538–9.
70. Dykman CJ, Galens GJ, Good AE. Linear subcutaneous bands in rheumatoid arthritis: an unusual form of rheumatoid granuloma. Ann Intern Med. 1965;63:134–40.
71. Ackerman AB, White WL, Guo Y. Differential diagnosis in dermatopathology, vol. 4. Philadelphia: Lea & Febiger; 1994. p. 34–7.
72. Long D, Thiboutot DM, Majeski JT, Vasily DB, Helm KF. Interstitial granulomatous dermatitis with arthritis. J Am Acad Dermatol. 1996;34:957–61.
73. Vemeuil L, Dompmartin A, Comoz F, Pasquier CJ, Leroy D. Interstitial granulomatous dermatitis with cutaneous cords and arthritis: a disorder associated with autoantibodies. J Am Acad Dermatol. 2001;45:286–91.
74. Wollina U, Schoniebe J, Unger L, Weigel K, Kostler E, Nusslein H. Interstitial granulomatous dermatitis with plaques and arthritis. Clin Rheumatol. 2003;22:347–9.
75. Magro CM, Crowson AN, Schapiro BL. The interstitial granulomatous drug reaction: a distinctive clinical and pathological entity. J Cutan Pathol. 1998;25:72–8.
76. Sangueza OP, Caudell MD, Mengesha TM, Davis LS, Barnes CJ, Griffen JE, et al. Palisaded neutrophilic granulomatous dermatitis in rheumatoid arthritis. J Am Acad Dermatol. 2002;47:251–7.
77. Scherbenske JM, Benson PM, Lupton GP, Samlaska CP. Rheumatoid neutrophilic dermatitis. Arch Dermatol. 1989;125:1105–8.
78. Brown TS, Fearyhough PK, Burruss JB, Callen JP. Rheumatoid neutrophilic dermatitis in a woman with sero-negative rheumatoid arthritis. J Am Acad Dermatol. 2001;45:596–600.

Cutaneous Manifestations of Pulmonary Disease

Jennifer Rullán, Rachelle E. Seijo-Montes, Annie Vaillant, and Néstor P. Sánchez

The recognition and correct elucidation of the cutaneous signs of diseases that primarily affect the pulmonary system may assist the clinician in diagnosis and estimation of prognosis. This chapter describes selected pulmonary diseases with distinctive cutaneous findings. Often times in medicine, findings on the skin may prove very helpful in exposing an underlying systemic condition. Pulmonary conditions can be particularly life threatening, and early detection and treatment may impact the course of a patient's life. In all fields of medicine, especially internal medicine, pneumology, nephrology, pediatrics, and dermatology, physicians can enhance their clinical proficiency by better understanding the rare and common cutaneous manifestations of pulmonary diseases such as sarcoidosis, tuberculosis, Birt–Hogg–Dubé syndrome (BHDS), and cystic fibrosis.

Sarcoidosis

The variable, multi-systemic disease of sarcoidosis was first described by Jonathan Hutchinson from England in 1875. Shortly after, in 1877, he described a patient with cutaneous sarcoidosis [1–3]. In 1899, the Norwegian dermatologist Caesar Boeck from Norway was accredited for the word "sarcoidosis" and the histopathologic description of skin nodules characterized by "epithelioid cells with large pale nuclei and also a few giant cells" which he called "multiple benign sarcoid of the skin" [4, 5]. The etiology remains uncertain; however, several genetic polymorphisms are associated with an increased risk of developing sarcoidosis, suggesting that genetic susceptibility to sarcoidosis is probably polygenic [6]. Environmental factors may also modify the susceptibility to sarcoidosis. The pathogenesis of this condition involves a T-helper-1-mediated immune response to environmental antigens in a genetically susceptible host [6]. The characteristic histologic feature of the non-infectious, non-caseating granulomas of sarcoidosis are the epithelioid tubercles (macrophages faced with chronic cytokine stimulation differentiate into epithelioid cells) that are "naked," in other words, there are few to no plasma cells or lymphocytes associated with the granuloma [5, 7].

Pulmonary disease occurs in up to 90% of sarcoid patients, of which 90% are associated with hilar and/or paratracheal lymphadenopathy. Fibrosis with bronchiolectasis (dilatation of the bronchioles) and honeycombing of the lung parenchyma occurs in 25% of patients and is the most common mechanism responsible for pulmonary hypertension in these patients [5, 7]. Although the lung is the most common organ affected by the disease, there have been reports of skin involvement in approximately 25–35% of the patients [5, 8, 9]. Cutaneous sarcoidosis can represent a diagnostic challenge due to its widely variable morphologies; hence, it is often known as one of the great imitators in dermatology [10]. The presence of cutaneous manifestations in sarcoidosis has shown significantly decreased time to diagnosis and can provide relevant prognostic implications. The importance of taking into account cutaneous sarcoidosis in the clinical differential diagnosis of a given skin lesion depends on the systemic involvement and the convenience of the skin as a tissue source for histologic analysis [9, 11].

The cutaneous lesions of sarcoidosis are classified in one of two ways: either specific, because of the presence of the hallmark naked sarcoid granulomas upon histologic evaluation, or nonspecific, because of the absence of such granulomas [9]. Specific lesions occur in 16% of patients and are associated with a poor prognosis or a chronic form of the disease [3, 12]. The most common specific lesions of cutaneous sarcoidosis include lupus pernio, infiltrated plaques, macular and papular lesions, and subcutaneous nodules [13]. Other such lesions include scar sarcoidosis, alopecia, ulcerative lesions, and

J. Rullán (✉) • R.E. Seijo-Montes • N.P. Sánchez
Department of Dermatology, University of Puerto Rico School of Medicine, Medical Sciences Campus, San Juan, Puerto Rico
e-mail: rullanmed@yahoo.com

A. Vaillant
Department of Obstetrics and Gynecology, San Juan City Hospital, Medical Sciences Campus, San Juan, Puerto Rico

N.P. Sánchez (ed.), *Atlas of Dermatology in Internal Medicine*,
DOI 10.1007/978-1-4614-0688-4_2,

hypopigmented patches. Patients with nonspecific lesions tend to have a good prognosis since these are mostly associated with an acute form of sarcoidosis. The most common nonspecific lesion is erythema nodosum. Other forms include nail, mucosal, and childhood sarcoidosis [9].

Specific Sarcoidosis

Lupus Pernio (Besnier–Boeck–Schaumann Disease)

The classic specific lesion of sarcoidosis is lupus pernio, first described in 1889 by Besnier [14]. It is characterized by relatively symmetric, violaceous, shiny, indurated, smooth, and doughy plaques and papules. The term "lupus" was used originally to describe lesions with an eroded appearance and the term "pernio" is used to describe the inflammation caused upon exposure to the cold [14]. The violaceous color has often been described as having a cyanotic hue as that seen in frostbite. It is frequently found on the nose (especially the alar rim), earlobes, cheeks, and sometimes the fingers, areas primarily affected by cold weather (Fig. 1). It occurs more commonly in women and in patients with black skin [3, 11, 12, 15]. This persistent lesion is not painful and does not disturb the epidermis causing ulceration; however, the lesions are disfiguring and may erode into the underlying cartilage and bone. Even a small amount of little papules on the nose may be associated with granulomatous dissemination into the nasal mucosa and upper respiratory tract, resulting in ulcerations, masses, or even serious airway obstruction [16]. Lupus pernio is associated with the chronic form of sarcoidosis and extra-pulmonary involvement [5, 9, 12, 16, 17].

Lupus Pernio patients have lung involvement in 75% of the cases and upper respiratory tract involvement 50% of the time [7]. In addition, patients with lupus pernio have increased occurrence of lytic and cystic bone lesions underlying affected skin areas, especially the hands and feet, chronic uveitis, and fibrotic sarcoid in the kidneys and lacrimal glands [7, 18].

Papules, Macules, Nodules, and Plaques

Granulomatous infiltrates of the skin most commonly present as persistent papules, nodules, or plaques. Papules, nodules, and maculopapular eruptions, as a group, are the most common cutaneous manifestations of sarcoidosis (Fig. 2) [3]. They may be red-brown or yellow-brown with an erythematous base, or violaceous in color and the surface is smooth due to the lack of epidermal involvement [1, 12]. They are most commonly found on the face, specifically the eyelids, periorbital area, and nasolabial folds, but are also common in other areas of the body such as the trunk, extremities, nape of the neck, and upper back [5, 9, 19]. Diascopy, a procedure used to study the lesions by compressing a slide against them, reveals blanching, and a yellowish brown or "apple-jelly" color, which is characteristic of sarcoidal skin [9, 13].

Papules can evolve into plaques. Some plaques may show hyperpigmentation with scales and they commonly form an annular configuration with central clearing (Figs. 3 and 4). When the plaques contain telangiectasias, or dilated blood vessels near the surface of the skin, it is called angiolupoid sarcoidosis [7, 19]. Sarcoid plaques are usually distributed symmetrically and bilaterally [8, 9]. It is important for a physician to be able to distinguish the presence of plaques because they are more likely to be associated with a chronic form of the disease [9, 13]. Since these lesions are often elevated and crusted, they are more likely than papules to resolve with scarring [9, 13, 19]. A rare variant of the sarcoid plaques that

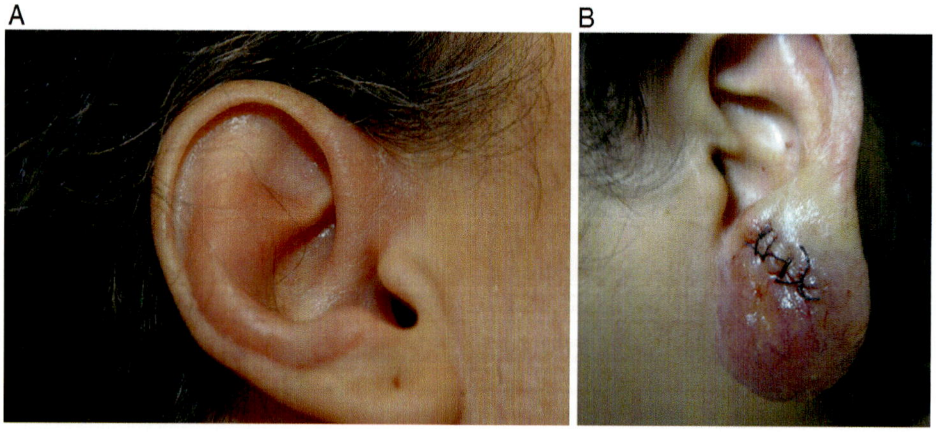

Fig. 1 (a, b) Lupus pernio. The cyanotic hue is characteristic. The earlobes, nose, and cheeks are affected areas most prone to perniosis. It may be disfiguring and destructive (origin of name lupus)

presents with scaly lesions on the knees and elbows is called psoriasiform plaques. It can be distinguished from true psoriasis by the fact that they heal with scarring [9, 13].

Subcutaneous Nodules (Darier–Roussy)

The first documented case of subcutaneous sarcoidosis was in 1904 by Darrier and Roussy [20, 21]. It encompasses 12.0% of the specific lesions of sarcoidosis and it occurs in 1.4–6.0% of patients who have systemic disease [9, 13, 22]. The peak incidence occurs during the fourth decade of age. The pathology of subcutaneous nodules are restricted to the subcutaneous tissue and does not affect the epidermis. These lesions can be painless or tender, firm, mobile, and the nodules vary from about 0.5 to 2.0 cm in diameter (Fig. 5) [19]. They are mostly found on the extremities, specifically the forearms, but may also be found on the trunk and face with a symmetric distribution. When the forearms are affected, the dorsum of the hand and the fingers tend to swell in a fusiform pattern [13, 20–22].

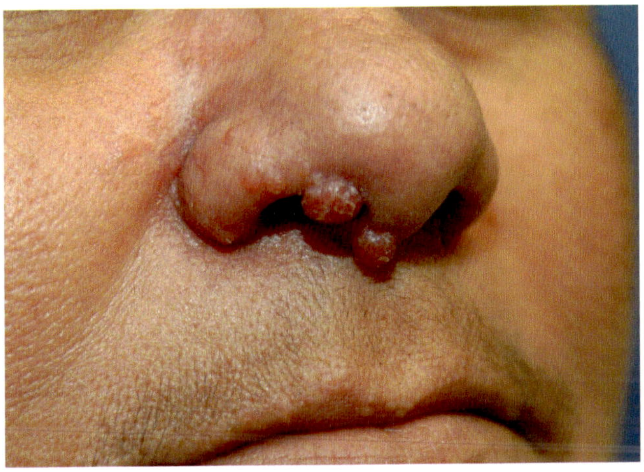

Fig. 2 Sarcoidosis: papules and nodules. *Red-brown* nodules occur predominantly around the nose

These skin lesions are the only subset of sarcoidosis frequently (80%) associated with systemic disease, particularly bilateral hilar adenopathy. Despite the associated systemic disease, it usually resolves within several months and is not associated with a chronic fibrotic disease [3, 9, 13, 21, 23, 24]. Subcutaneous sarcoidosis has a consistent clinicopathologic presentation and usually appears at the beginning of the disease. The confirmatory diagnosis requires the detection of pannicular (fat lobules) sarcoid or epitheliod granulomas with minimal lymphocytic inflammation and minimal septal involvement (Fig. 6) [21, 24, 25].

Scar Sarcoidosis

Scar sarcoidosis was first described in 1899 by Caesar Boeck. It frequently presents in West Africans [26, 27]. Scar sarcoidosis shows characteristic granulomatous invasion of previously traumatized skin or areas with imbedded foreign material, such as tattoos [3, 5, 23]. It often occurs with other cutaneous manifestations; however, it tends to occur near the beginning of the onset of sarcoidosis when the presence of pulmonary involvement may have not yet begun [13, 26]. Particular attention should be given to sites on the body such as areas for venipuncture access, previous Mantoux test sites,

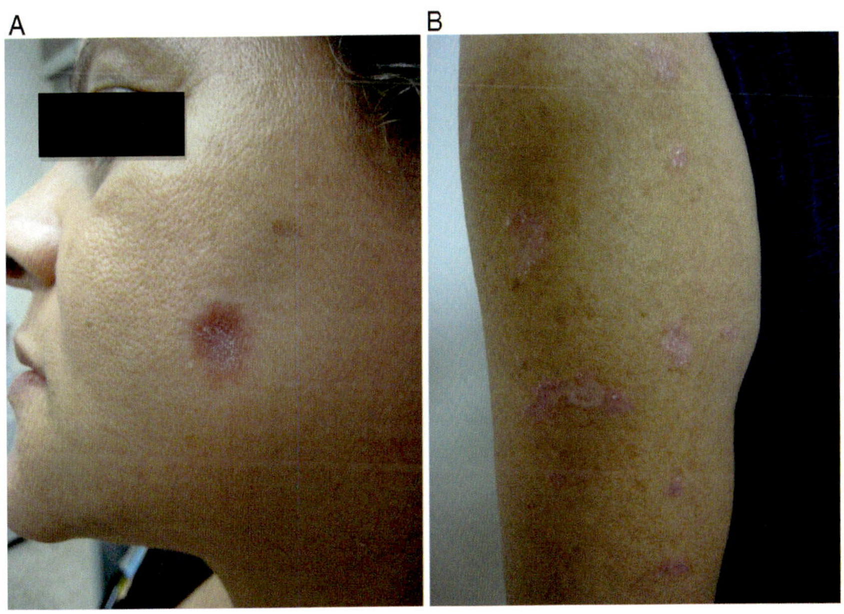

Fig. 3 (**a**, **b**) Sarcoidosis: annular plaques. Plaques with an annular configuration and central clearing affecting the face and arms

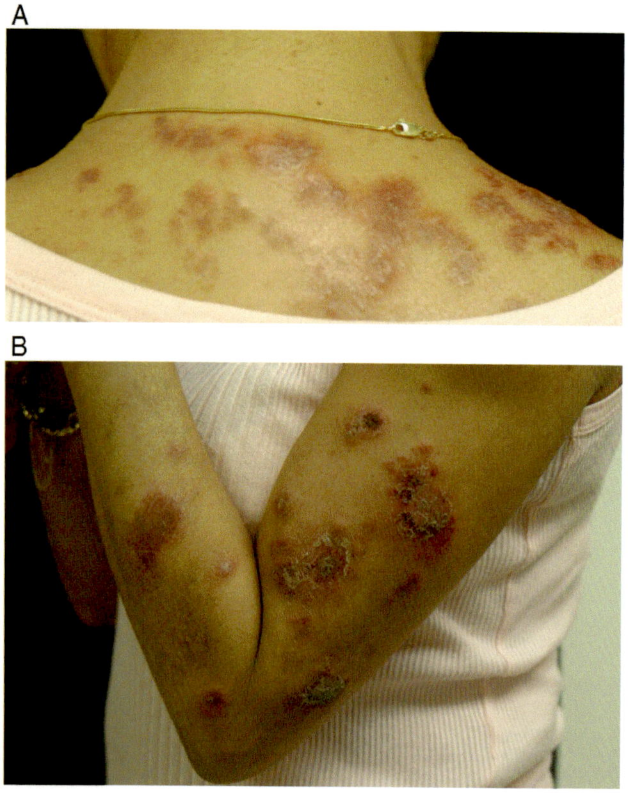

Fig. 4 (**a**, **b**) Sarcoidosis: plaques. A patient presenting with widespread *red-brown* plaques occurring on the bilateral extremities. The trunk is a common site. Most of these patients have pulmonary involvement, lymphadenopathy, and splenomegaly

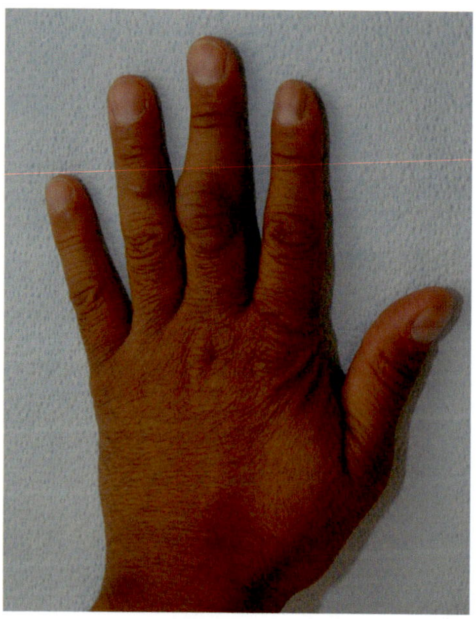

Fig. 5 Sarcoidosis: subcutaneous nodules (Darier–Roussy)

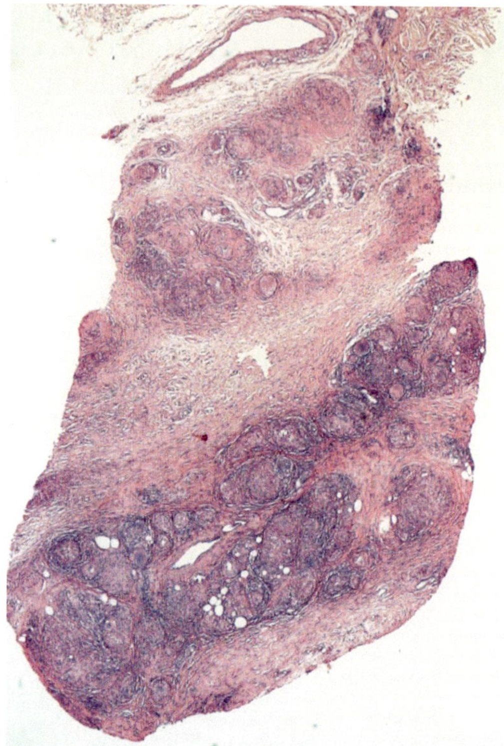

Fig. 6 Histopathology of Darier–Roussy. Sarcoid granulomas in the inferior dermis and subcutaneous tissue

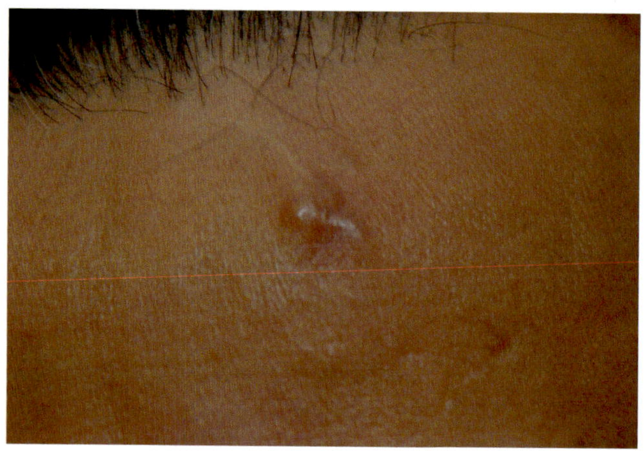

Fig. 7 Sarcoidosis associated with a scar. Granulomatous invasion of old scar tissue is particularly characteristic

healed herpes zoster dermatomes, tattoos, post-cutaneous laser surgery areas, post-consecutive botox injection areas, and injury scars [26, 28, 29]. The old scars, often atrophic and hypopigmented, evolve into elevated, purple or red lesions with associated new nodules or plaques (Fig. 7) [3, 9, 13, 19, 23].

Alopecia

Sarcoidal alopecia is a type of secondary scarring alopecia [30]. It tends to commence on the fronto-parietal area and progress into the scalp as an atrophic, red, and scaly plaque of alopecia. It can easily be confused with cutaneous discoid lupus erythematosus because it also presents as an erythematous, scaly, and atrophic plaque of alopecia [30, 31]. A biopsy is needed in such situations to differentiate between these two conditions histopathologically. These lesions present in various morphologies including macular lesions, scaly plaques, and infiltrated nodules [9]. The few cases reported mostly involve African-American women, of which, also tend to have other cutaneous manifestations. Physicians should carefully evaluate the patient to rule out systemic sarcoidosis after the diagnosis of scalp sarcoidosis is established [30, 32].

Ichthyosiform Sarcoidosis

An acquired ichthyosis secondary to sarcoidosis was first described by Braverman in 1981 [33]. Ichthyosis refers to dry and scaly skin due to a defect in keratinization. The classic presentation of this rare manifestation of sarcoidosis is nontender, adherent, pigmented, polygonal scales on the anterior lower limbs [33, 34]. Histopathology reveals the specific naked granuloma and ichthyosis vulgaris changes of the epidermis, such as compact orthokeratosis and a decrease or absence of the granular layer [34]. This subtype of sarcoidosis is significant due to its high association with systemic disease, where over 95% of reported cases have systemic involvement [33, 34].

Hypopigmentation

The first report of sarcoidosis hypopigmented macules was in 1963 by Thomas et al. [35, 36]. Oftentimes, sarcoidosis on black or dark skin only presents with hypopigmented papules, macules, or dermal nodules. They are most often found on the extremities. Since it may be the presenting sign of the disease, it is important to recognize these lesions and rule out similar clinical presentations seen in vitiligo, pinta, post-inflammatory changes, and pityriasis versicolor [35, 36]. A biopsy showing dermal sarcoid granulomas is always confirmatory [9, 36]. The mechanism of action remains controversial; however, a nutritional deficiency in melanocytes, a fixation artifact, or an increased susceptibility to damage of the mitochondria of melanocytes are postulated hypotheses [36–38].

Nonspecific Sarcoidosis

Erythema Nodosum

Erythema nodosum (EN) is the most common nonspecific cutaneous eruption of sarcoidosis [18]. It occurs in about 10% of patients with sarcoidosis and usually resolves spontaneously within 6 weeks [5, 9, 39]. It is a painful disorder of the subcutaneous fat. The characteristic lesion is a tender, erythematous, poorly delineated subcutaneous nodule usually distributed in a symmetric pattern. The main causes of EN include idiopathic (55%), streptococcal pharyngitis (48%), sarcoidosis (25%), drugs (10%), pregnancy (5%), and enteropathies (4%) [40]. EN lesions typically occur on the anterior tibial surface, but can also be present on the extensor surface of the forearms, the thighs, and the trunk [3, 8, 40]. The nodules can vary from 1 to 10 cm in diameter. The essential histologic features are those of a septal panniculitis where there is intense inflammation of the deep dermis and fibrous septum with relative sparing of the fat lobules, without evidence of vasculitis [9, 40].

In the 1950s, Lofgren and Lundback discovered the association between EN and bilateral hilar lymphadenopathy, now referred to as Löfgren's syndrome [3]. Löfgren's syndrome encompasses sarcoidosis with hilar adenopathy, polyarthritis, and EN. Other symptoms may include fever or ocular involvement. This syndrome, similar to the EN sarcoid patients, has a good prognosis due to the association with an acute or transient form of the disease [3, 8, 9, 13, 40].

Other

Nail, Mucosal, and Childhood Sarcoidosis

Some of the most unusual manifestations of sarcoidosis are those lesions involving in the nails or mucosa, as well as presenting with disease manifestations as a child. Nail sarcoidosis findings include clubbing, subungual hyperkeratosis, brittleness, pitting, discoloration, and onycholysis. Nail involvement is indicative of the chronic form of the disease and is considered a specific lesion because of the presence of the hallmark non-caseating granulomas upon histologic examination [2, 7, 9].

Mucosal sarcoidosis presents as granulomatous lesions affecting the oral, nasal, anal, and, less frequently, the genital mucosa. The most common presentation is nodules of the buccal mucosa, gingival tissue, tongue, lips, hard palate, and salivary glands [7, 9].

Sarcoidosis is uncommon in adolescents and children. In the case of children ranging from 9 to 15 years, the disease presents with the same lesions adults exhibit, except erythema nodosum and lupus pernio. In children younger than 6 years, sarcoidosis has the characteristic triad presentation of skin lesions, arthritis, and uveitis. The first manifestation is cutaneous: erythematous maculopapular rash on the extremities which later becomes generalized. The pulmonary manifestations are rare, but when present, include stage one changes on chest radiographs (bilateral hilar lymphadenopathy without infiltration). Childhood sarcoidosis can be easily confused with polyarticular rheumatoid juvenile arthritis and Blau's syndrome (however Blau's syndrome does not involve the lung), so it is important for the physician to carefully distinguish between the three [7, 9].

Treatment

The first-line treatment of choice is corticosteroids, either in the topical, intralesional, or oral from. The cutaneous lesions in sarcoidosis are not life threatening and the therapeutic regimen should be dependent and adjusted according to the progression and severity of the disease. The most mutilated skin lesions should be injected with triamcinolone acetonide weekly. The traditional treatment of systemic disease is oral prednisone at a dose of 1 mg/kg/day for 4–6 weeks, usually 20–40 mg in daily divided doses, followed by tapering of the dose over the following months. The alternate day use of prednisone for maintenance therapy has proven to be just as effective as the daily dose regimen [9, 12, 21].

Chronic skin lesions tend to respond well to chloroquine (250–500 mg/day) and hydroxychloroquine (200–400 mg/day) antimalarial drugs, but one must be cautious for serious side effects such as retinopathy and blindness. Chloroquine can also be used intralesionally once a month. Other treatment options include the following: methotrexate (15 mg/week), thalidomide (50–300 mg/day), infliximab and allopurinol (100–300 mg/day), to mention a few [9, 12, 21].

Lupus pernio and disfiguring skin plaques have been treated successfully in some patients with laser treatments such as pulsed-dye and the CO_2 laser, however, as with all medications, not all patients respond the same. Cosmetic options should be taken into consideration due to the social and psychological impact such cutaneous lesions can have on a patient [16, 41].

Tuberculosis

Théophile Laennec, from France, especially known for his invention of the stethoscope, can also be recognized for his elucidation of the pathogenesis and the description of the physical findings in pulmonary disease of tuberculosis at the beginning of the nineteenth century (1819). Laennec described a "prosecutor wart" in 1826, the first reported example of cutaneous tuberculosis [42, 43]. The German physician and scientist, Dr. Robert Koch, discovered the etiology of tuberculosis, the infectious bacillus bacteria. He was awarded a Nobel Prize for his discovery in 1905 and became known as the "father of bacteriology" [44].

Tuberculosis presents a significant public health issue with 8–9 million new infections annually. The World Health Organization estimates that approximately one-third of the world's population is affected, and claims about 3 million lives a year [45]. TB has become the most common cause of death in AIDS-infected patients and is considered a true AIDS-defining illness in patients infected with human immunodeficiency virus (HIV) by the Center for Disease Control (CDC) [46, 47]. An estimated 15 million people are co-infected with HIV and *Mycobacterium tuberculosis*, and 6,00,000 of the 3 million HIV deaths in 2003 were specifically ascribed to TB [45, 48].

Tuberculosis was a major problem in the late nineteenth century but declined due to improved hygiene, improved living standards, use of BCG immunization, and the introduction of chemotherapy [49]. However, there has been a resurgence of TB since the 1980s, for which, the Centers for Disease Control and Prevention attributes to several factors, including HIV infection, TB among foreign-born immigrants, the rise of drug-resistant TB, and the decline of TB control programs [48, 50]. In developing countries, contributing issues include shortages of healthcare facilities with appropriate diagnostic equipment, reduced access to treatment, and poor treatment compliance among patients who often resort to traditional medicine [51]. The global incidence of TB is increasing at a rate of 1.1% per year, fueled primarily by countries in sub-Saharan Africa and the former Soviet Union [52]. In addition, the recent FDA approval of biologic therapies for plaque psoriasis and other autoimmune diseases has introduced dermatologists into the management and screening of TB infections. Biologic agents, especially etanercept, infliximab, alefacept, efalizumab, and adalimumab, are known to cause reactivation TB due to the suppression of the cell-mediated immune response [48]. The ability to detect tuberculosis of the skin will serve as a valuable skill in the rapid detection and realization of therapy for physicians of the twenty-first century.

The disease primarily affects the lungs due to the transmission via droplets of respiratory secretions. Since TB-causing bacteria are obligate aerobes, they are able to remain suspended in the air for hours (droplet nuclei) and survive in well-ventilated alveoli [53]. Pulmonary macrophages swallow up the TB organisms in the alveolar spaces and then migrate to draining regional lymph nodes to initiate a cell-mediated immune response to contain the infection. The introduction of TB into the lungs is asymptomatic in the majority of patients and without radiographic changes, but later develops into a chronic non-productive cough. The primary disease may also present with constitutional symptoms such as fever, weight loss, night sweats, anorexia, and malaise

Table 1 Cutaneous manifestations of tuberculosis

Disease	Infection	Clinical presentation	Dermatopathology	Culture
True cutaneous TB				
Lupus vulgaris	H,L,C, BCG vaccine, direct	Types: Plaque, hypertrophic, ulcerative, or painless papulonodule that ulcerates with adenopathy	+/– Tuberculoid granuloma	+/– (Direct+)
Scrofuloderma	C	Nodule over affected lymph node, ulcerates	Necrosis, abscess, bacilli	+
Miliary TB	H	Copious discrete pinpoint papules	Microabscesses, many bacilli	+
Orificial TB	Auto-inoculation	Nodules, painful punched-out ulcers	Tuberculoid granuloma, many bacilli	+
TB chancre	D (exogenous)	Painless papulonodule, ulcerates, adenopathy	Acute inflammation, reaction granuloma, many bacilli	+
TB verrucosa cutis	D (exogenous)	Papule, verrucous plaque with soft center	Tuberculoid granuloma	+/–
Tuberculids				
Lichen scrofulosorum	H	Perifollicular lichenoid papules in clusters on the trunk, heals without scarring	Tuberculoid granuloma in papillary dermis	–
Erythema induratum of Bazin	H	Indurated, ulcerated erythematous nodules of calf veins healing with atrophic scars	Tuberculoid granuloma, lobular panniculitis	–
Papulonecrotic tuberculid	H	Small papules, crust, ulcerates	Wedge-shaped necrosis	–
Nodular tuberculid	H	1–2 cm nodules, non-ulcerating, red-blue in color, lower extremities	Granulomatous vasculitis at the junction of the dermis and subcutaneous fat	–

Derived from Tables I, II, and III in Cutaneous tuberculosis diagnosis and treatment. Am J Clin Dermatol 2002;3:319–28
H Hematogenous, *L* lymphatic, *C* contiguous, *D* direct, + positive, – negative, +/– may or may not be present

[54, 55]. Primary infections are traditionally characterized by any pneumonic infiltrate (granuloma) in the middle or lower lung zones (Ghon focus), especially a circular shape, associated with an ipsilateral hilar or mediastinal adenopathy, together known as the primary complex. A reactivation of TB, in contrast, classically has cavitary lesions in the upper lobes of the lung [48].

Systemic involvement in tuberculosis is commonly associated with cutaneous TB. The incidence of skin tuberculosis is gradually rising in both developing and developed countries parallel to systemic TB. It remains to be one of the most elusive and more difficult diseases to diagnose [56]. The incidence of systemic tuberculosis in children is around 26% and up to 35% in adults [57, 58]. Extra-pulmonary manifestations of TB account for approximately 13.7% of cases, and this percent may be much higher in patients co-infected with HIV [47]. Cutaneous manifestations of TB are very rare and only represent 1.5% of all extra-pulmonary forms of TB [42, 59, 60]. Several published studies have revealed that cutaneous TB is best diagnosed using a comprehensive work up of the patient in which histologic study of the skin biopsy specimen is most essential [61]. Skin lesions are distinguished by whether *M. tuberculosis* is revealed upon acid-fast bacilli (AFB) stains, culture, or polymerase chain reaction (PCR). Lesions that in fact demonstrate the presence of *M. tuberculosis* are classified as true cutaneous tuberculosis. True cutaneous tuberculosis can be acquired exogenously or endogenously and includes such lesions as tuberculous chancre, tuberculosis verrucosa cutis (TVC), lupus vulgaris (LV), scrofuloderma, miliary tuberculosis, orificial tuberculosis, and gummatous tuberculosis. Tuberculids, on the other hand, do not reveal *M. tuberculosis* on AFB stains, culture, or PCR and are defined as cutaneous hypersensitivity reactions to an underlying focus of tuberculosis [42]. The tuberculids include lichen scrofulosorum, erythema induratum of Bazin (EIB), tuberculonecrotic tuberculid, and nodular tuberculid [49, 59].

Cutaneous lesions of tuberculosis can also be attributed to another strain of bacteria, specifically *M. bovis*, or even by the BCG vaccine which is an attenuated form of the former [49]. The major difference is that *M. bovis* infection is spread from animals to humans, most frequently through infected milk products [62] (Table 1).

True Cutaneous Tuberculosis

Endogenously Acquired Disease

Lupus Vulgaris

LV is the most common form of cutaneous tuberculosis in most countries, especially in India and Africa [63–66]. Up to 40% of LV cases are associated with lymphadenitis and up to 20% involve the lungs and bones [65]. Its pathogenesis is multifactorial: direct inoculation, BCG vaccination, contiguous, lymphatic, and hematogenous route of infection [49, 65].

The lesions may present in a variety of morphologies including the classic plaque or keratotic type (gelatinous), the hypertrophic form (tumor-like soft nodule), the ulcerative form (necrosis), and the vegetative form (papule with ulceration and necrosis). The plaque form is the most common form of LV, accounting for 32% of cases [42, 57]. It initially presents as asymptomatic, flat, red-brown papules and plaques. It progresses into slowly expanding skin-colored or erythematous plaques with deep tiny nodules arising near the margins of the plaque. On diascopy, the nodules are seen as yellow-brown macules (the characteristic "apple-jelly" color). The expanding plaque has an atrophic center with a raised red-brown border, occasionally with scaling [67]. The ulcerative form is the most destructive and deforming of all LV lesions because the underlying tissue becomes ulcerated and necrotic, leaving behind an atrophic scar. It can be especially destructive, if the auricular or nasal cartilage is involved. Finally, the vegetative form is similar to the ulcerative form in that it is characterized by necrosis and ulceration; however, there is minimal scarring left behind [49, 59]. After many decades with the disease, squamous cell carcinoma may develop in the lupus vulgaris lesion [67, 68].

The areas in the body where these lesions appear vary among different places in the world. In Western countries, LV is most commonly seen on the neck and face, especially the nose and cheeks, and rarely involves the mucous membranes [69]. In the tropics and developing countries, on the other hand, where kids play without protective clothing, it occurs most often on the lower extremities and buttocks [42, 49].

As a consequence of the developed antibodies due to previous exposure to the organism, LV is exceptionally chronic with a slow and destructive progression. It occurs in patients with moderate to high immunity against *M. tuberculosis*, as evidenced by a strongly positive tuberculin test [70]. Since lupus vulgaris is a paucibacillary form of tuberculous infection, the culture is often negative and the diagnosis is mainly based on the histopathological appearance and the response to chemotherapy [59].

The histopathologic examination shows the hallmark tubercles, which consist of accumulations of epithelioid histiocytes with Langerhans giant cells and varying amount of caseation necrosis in the center [71]. A significant finding also includes fibrosis of the dermis due to the chronic long-standing course with intermittent episodes of healing. Neither caseation necrosis nor tuberculoid granulomas are pathognomonic because deep fungal infections, syphilis, and leprosy can show similar histological features. It is the additional clinical criteria that is helpful in the differential diagnosis, such as the soft texture of the lesions, the brownish-red color, the slow progression, and the apple-jelly nodules revealed by diascopy [71].

Scrofuloderma

Scrofuloderma, also known as tuberculosis cutis colliquativa, arises from the extension of underlying tubercle bacilli from an infected lymph node, bone, joint, or epididymis to the overlying skin in patients with a weak immune response [69, 72, 73]. This is the most common cutaneous TB in children and it is more common in girls than in boys [42, 57, 66, 69]. It has been postulated that the consumption of unboiled/unpasteurized milk is a common occurrence around the world that leads to the *M. bovis* infestation of the cervical lymph nodes [49, 66, 69, 72, 73].

Scrofuloderma initially presents as a red-brown profound nodule overlying the site of the deeper infection. The nodule becomes indurated and forms an abscess. Over a period of months, it begins to ulcerate, eventually forming the hallmark sinus tracts that drain watery, purulent, or caseous material [49, 60, 72].The ulcers are shallow with undermined blue-colored borders. Healing forms an elongated scar or keloid, the characteristic puckered scar [49, 59, 60].

The presence of scrofuloderma suggests a systemic TB infection, especially pulmonary involvement [49, 59, 66, 69]. The incidence of systemic involvement in adults with scrofuloderma is 35% [58].The most commonly affected area is the neck, but may also occur on the axillae, chest, or groin [66, 69, 72–74]. At times, lupus vulgaris may arise from scrofuloderma. This form of cutaneous TB may take several years to spontaneously heal [49, 59, 71].

Gummatous TB is another cutaneous tuberculosis lesion, indistinguishable from scrofuloderma. It is also referred to as metastatic tuberculous abscesses that arise on the trunk, extremities, or head [46, 47, 49, 54, 59, 74]. It occurs after dissemination of an active infection, usually in seasons of low immunologic resistance, as occurs with undernourished children or immunosuppressed patients.

Acute Miliary Tuberculosis

Acute miliary tuberculosis is the extensive dissemination of *M. tuberculosis* due to hematogenous spread. It is a rare presentation encompassing 1–3% of all TB cases. The internal focus of the active disease most commonly originates from the lungs. This rare form of TB has become increasingly common among HIV-infected patients. The first documented case that presented with cutaneous findings was reported in 1990 in an AIDS patient [75]. Patients with acute miliary TB usually have a serious systemic infection, especially those with AIDS because of their extreme $CD4^+$ T cell depletion. As a result, they have a poor prognosis, with many cases leading to death [49, 59].

The cutaneous manifestations consists of widespread discrete blue-red to brown-colored papules, pustules, purpura, and uncommonly, umbilicated vesicles [49, 60, 71–73]. The vesicles may either rupture or dry with a crust that later develops into an ulcer. By the fourth week, the lesions are usually healed with remaining white atrophic scars that have a surrounding brown halo [49, 71, 72]. Histology confirms the diagnosis, revealing multiple microabscesses with neutrophils and numerous AFB organisms surrounded by macrophages and giant cells [49, 60].

Orificial Tuberculosis

Orificial tuberculosis, also known as tuberculosis cutis orificialis, is an atypical manifestation of TB that usually occurs in patients with advanced infection of the lungs, intestine, or genito-urinary tract. Recognizing this cutaneous lesion is significant because it indicates advanced internal disease and poor prognosis. It presents as red- or yellow-colored nodules that ulcerate around the mucosal orifices, such as on the lips, inside the mouth, or on the anogenital region. These painful ulcers have an irregular circular shape, with an undermined border and a shallow, punched-out, and granulomatous appearance. It spreads to infect the mucosa or orificial skin by means of autoinoculation, where an active infection drains to the nearest orifice [49, 59]. An active TB infection of the lungs and pharynx tends to manifest in the mouth, whereas infection of the intestines manifests in the anus orifice [49, 59, 60, 74]. Perianal tuberculosis is believed to be a consequence of auto-inoculation from swallowed bacilli-containing sputum through defects in the perianal mucosa [71].

Exogenously Acquired Disease

Tuberculous Chancre

The tuberculous chancre, also known as the primary inoculation tuberculosis, is seen following primary infection with *M. tuberculosis*, in other words, the patient is nonsensitized or non-immune (initially negative purified protein derivative test) [49, 59, 60]. It accounts for 1–2% of cutaneous TB [46, 47, 49, 54, 59]. The tubercle bacilli cannot penetrate intact skin, thus only after the patient suffers some sort of skin trauma or minor abrasion can the organism infiltrate and cause infection. It has also been reported to occur post-mouth-to-mouth resuscitation, jail-house tattooing, circumcision, piercings, and in health care workers [49, 72].

The chancre appears 2–4 weeks after inoculation as a reddish-brown papulonodular lesion, which quickly grows and erodes [49, 59]. The resultant shallow ulcer is painless, with an indurated granular base. The borders of the ulcer are well defined, blue-red in color, and have an undermined appearance. Sometimes the border has scattered pustules and the edge may have an adherent crust on the surface [68, 71, 72, 76]. When the chancre is coupled with regional lymphadenopathy, usually 3–8 weeks after inoculation, it accounts for what is known as primary tuberculous complex [71]. These lesions appear primarily on the face and extremities and are able to heal without treatment after several months, but may leave an atrophic scar. Treating this condition with anti-tuberculous medications can not only prevent scarring, but can also avoid the evolution of these lesions into Tuberculosis Verrucosa Cutis (TVC), lupus vulgaris, or scrofuloderma [49, 59, 72, 73]. Histologically, it initially reveals nonspecific inflammation and later, after the development of adenopathy, a granulomatous pattern with scattered bacilli can be seen [62, 72].

After the bacilli Calmette-Guerin (BCG) vaccination, a sore may persist, on the upper outer arm, which imitates the TB chancre, but is referred to as a BCG granuloma. It tends to occur 2–6 weeks after vaccination. It appears as a small solitary brown nodule or papule that ulcerates, scabs, and heals as a scar [62, 72].

Tuberculosis Verrucosa Cutis

TVC results from a reinfection with *M. tuberculosis* or *M. bovis* by direct inoculation (through abrasions or wounds). Unlike the chancre, these patients are previously sensitized and have strongly positive PPD's; therefore, BCG vaccination would be futile [49, 74, 77]. Since this cutaneous manifestation entails reinfection, it occurs most often in those who have occupational exposure, such as physicians (especially pathologists or forensic scientists), other medical personnel, or butchers [49, 62, 68]. This cutaneous variant of TB occurs in patients with strong cell-mediated immunity.

The lesion first appears as a small, solitary, asymptomatic, and reddish-brown papule that progresses into a large, irregular verrucous plaque [49, 60]. The margins are firm while the center is soft, and there is a surrounding erythematous border. There are deep fissures on the surface which often expel pus [49, 59]. TVC is found most commonly on the lower limbs and buttocks in eastern countries and on the dorsal hands in western countries [77]. There have been cases where it appears on the face or around the anus [74]. They persist for several years (slow growing and chronic in nature), but they eventually heal spontaneously with an atrophic scar [49, 77].

Histology reveals hyperkeratosis and papillomatosis of the epidermis. The dermis contains tuberculoid granulomas with necrosis and occasional acid-fast bacilli [49, 60].

Tuberculids

Tuberculids are due to an immune response to the antigenic component of *M. tuberculosis*, often described as a hypersensitivity reaction. They are characterized by negative smears and cultures, but strong positive PPD reactivity. No bacilli are seen in the lesions due to the rapid destruction in the skin by the high immune system of the patient [49, 78, 79]. The skin lesions are numerous and distributed symmetrically. In 1896, Jean Darier introduced the term tuberculid to designate papular and nodular skin outbreaks that spontaneously involute and recur in individuals with a previous history of active TB [49, 79]. Histologically, all tuberculids share a granulomatous inflammation, necrosis, and vasculitis [49].

Lichen Scrofulosorum

Lichen scrofulosorum (LS) has been reported as the most common form of tuberculids and the most common cutaneous manifestation of TB in children. It was first described by Hebra in 1868 and it accounts for about 8% of all patients with cutaneous tuberculosis. This form of cutaneous TB is associated with the infection of the lungs, lymph nodes, or bones [42, 49, 74, 80, 81]. The lesions of LS usually appear on the trunk and proximal extremities as asymptomatic, lichenoid, firm follicular, and parafollicular papules. Micropustules and central adherent crust may also be present, but scaling is minimal or absent. Lesions may coalesce to form annular or discoid plaques [82]. The papules have a yellow-brown or pink color [7, 42, 49, 60, 78]. Upon histologic evaluation, there is evidence of dermal non-caseating granulomas around the hair follicles and sweat ducts. These lesions heal spontaneously without scarring after several months [49, 59, 74]. Lichen scrofulosorum needs to be differentiated from similar follicular disorders such as keratosis pilaris, lichen spinulosus, lichen nitidus, pityriasis rubra pilaris, and lichenoid sarcoidosis [42].

Erythema Induratum of Bazin

EIB, also known as nodular vasculitis, was first described in 1861 by Ernest Bazin [83, 84]. About 15% of EIB cases are associated with lung disease [85]. This form of cutaneous TB is one of the most common types of tuberculids among patients, the typical patient being a middle-aged woman with fatty or heavy legs characterized by some degree of venous insufficiency [65, 79, 86, 87]. It describes a tuberculid response manifesting with flares of indurated violaceous nodules of the calves that tend to ulcerate and then recur every 3–4 months [79, 88, 89]. The lesions appear bilaterally on the posterior calves, or, in rare occasions on the thighs or arms [49, 59]. There are four common histologic findings involving the deep subcutaneous fat including septal panniculitis, fat tissue necrosis, vasculitis, and caseating granulomas [74, 89]. Healing usually occurs spontaneously after several months with postinflammatory hyperpigmentation and atrophic scarring. The differential diagnosis for such lesions includes nodular vasculitis, perniosis, polyarteritis nodosa, and erythema nodosum [88].

Papulonecrotic Tuberculid

Papulonecrotic tuberculid presents as multiple, painless, and scattered pustular or necrotizing papules on the extensor aspects of the extremities and buttocks of children or adolescents. These dusky-red papules become necrotic and leave behind a hyperpigmented atrophic scar or may even progress to lupus vulgaris [89]. These lesions occasionally coexist with EIB [79]. Histologic examination reveals the presence of vasculitis and wedge-shaped areas of necrosis or infarction [59, 71].

Nodular Tuberculid

Nodular tuberculid, the fourth and most recent adoption to the tuberculid family, was described in 1997 in Japan by Hara as a nodular thickening along the course of the veins [89–91]. The nodules are 1 and 2 cm in diameter, non-ulcerating, red-blue in color, and predominately occur on the lower extremities [89]. Nodular tuberculid has a characteristic histological pattern: a granulomatous vasculitis at the junction of the dermis and subcutaneous fat, between the superficial papulonecrotic tuberculid (papillary dermis) and the deep EIB (subcutaneous fat) [89, 91]. It has been previously called "nodular granulomatous phlebitis" and has remarkable similarities with superficial migratory thrombophlebitis.

Treatment

The treatment regimens used for pulmonary tuberculosis are sufficient for treating cutaneous tuberculosis because the bacillary load is much smaller in cutaneous tuberculosis than in pulmonary tuberculosis [49]. The Centers for Disease Control and Prevention recommends a two phase treatment schedule: an intense initial phase with isoniazid, rifampin, pyrazinamide and either ethambutol or streptomycin for 8 weeks and a final continuation stage of isoniazid and rifampin for 16 weeks. The initial phase is meant to quickly destroy a large number of living organisms and the second maintenance phase is meant to kill the remaining persistent organisms [60, 71]. The treatment should be continued for at least 2 months after the cutaneous lesions have entirely regressed due to the fact that viable organisms can be cultured from clinically healed lesions. Surgical excision is a useful adjunct to the management in scrofuloderma and the localized lesions of verrucosa cutis and lupus vulgaris [71, 81]. Lupoid nodules in areas of scar tissue can be eliminated with electrocautery or cryotherapy [49, 73].

Birt–Hogg–Dubé Syndrome

BHDS was first described in 1977 by the Canadian physicians Birt, Hogg, and Dubé [92, 93]. BHDS is a rare, autosomal dominant predisposition to the development of benign skin tumors, lung cysts, and spontaneous pneumothorax. Also, there is a strong association with renal cancers, often multiple and bilateral, and detected at a median age of 51 [94]. BHDS is caused by a mutation of the folliculin gene (FLCN) whose product is a novel protein with tumor suppressor effects [94]. The folliculin gene lies within the chromosome band 17p11.2. This genodermatosis is characterized by a large spectrum of mutations and clinical heterogeneity. It is thought to be associated with colonic neoplastic polyps, medullary carcinoma of the thyroid, and connective tissue nevi. Eighty-four percent of BHDS patients have lung cysts on CT imaging and 38% of patients have a history of pneumothorax. The skin lesions usually develop during the third or fourth decades of life. The three skin lesions originally described in the BHDS include fibrofolliculomas, trichodiscomas, and acrochordons (skin tags). Ninety percent of families with BHDS had individuals with multiple histologically confirmed fibrofolliculomas [95]. All these three associated skin lesions are small, firm, papular, and painless. There can be several to over a hundred papules that develop gradually over the scalp, face, neck, upper chest, back, popliteal fossa, and antecubital fossa. It is important to be able to recognize these three benign skin lesions associated with this syndrome as it may aid in a more rapid detection of renal carcinoma or a spontaneous pneumothorax, ensuing in possible better prognosis and decreased mortality [92, 93, 95].

Fibrofolliculoma

A fibrofolliculoma is a benign tumor developing from the hair follicle. They are small, flesh, or pale yellow-colored papules measuring 2–4 mm in diameter. Histologically, they are circumscribed proliferations of collagen and fibroblasts that surround the distorted hair follicles. The inside of the hair follicle is packed with keratinous debris or a hair shaft, appearing as a dilated cyst. This is surrounded by abundant loose connective tissue full of elastic fibers, fine collagen, and numerous vessels [7, 19, 96].

Trichodiscomas

Trichodiscomas cannot be distinguished from fibrofolliculomas based on clinical inspection. Both are 2–4 mm, white or flesh colored, smooth, and dome-shaped papules. A trichodiscoma, however, is a benign tumor or hamartoma of the hair disk, which is now considered a non-existent structure. Trichodiscomas are today considered to be fibrofolliculomas or perifollicular fibromas. In the superficial dermis there is a loose myxoid stroma and spindle cell proliferation [93, 95, 96].

Acrochordons

Acrochordons are also known as skin tags, cutaneous papilloma, soft fibromas, and fibroepithelial polyps. Acrochordons are tiny raised or pedunculated pigmented soft papules, with a tan or brown color. Most acrochordons in BHDS are smaller than usual, about 1–2 mm in diameter. The polyps are histologically characterized by mature keratinizing squamous epithelium overlying a fibrovascular core with papillomatosis and hyperkeratosis [93, 95, 96].

Cystic Fibrosis

Cystic fibrosis is an autosomal recessive disorder reported in 1/1,500 live births in Northern American and Northern European Caucasian populations [97]. The mutated gene, called the cystic fibrosis transmembrane conductance regulator (CFTR), is the reason for the abnormal ion transport. Approximately 90% of children with cystic fibrosis present with classic pulmonary or gastrointestinal symptoms, such as cough, dyspnea, or steatorrhea [98]. The cutaneous manifestations that have been reported are nonspecific, yet may be important initial presentations which include: wrinkling, cutaneous vasculitis, and cystic fibrosis nutrient deficiency dermatitis (CFNDD) or an acrodermatitis enteropathica-like eruption.

Premature skin wrinkling subsequent to water exposure is a primary consequence of cystic fibrosis. It is due to the increased concentration of electrolytes in the sweat, creating an aquagenic skin wrinkling effect [97, 99–101]. It presents clinically as poorly demarcated edematous white papules and plaques of the palms and soles that develop after exposure to water.

The vasculitis, a secondary sequela, most commonly presents with a recurrent macular purpura that progresses to palpable purpura on the lower extremities [97, 102–105]. Urticarial vasculitis and bullae secondary to vasculitis have also been reported [102, 103, 106, 107]. Intermittent arthralgias have been associated with such skin lesions [102, 105, 108]. In these patients, vasculitic dermatoses are associated with exacerbations of pulmonary symptoms [23]. The mechanism of action of such vasculitic lesions has been shown to be due to antigens from bacteria, antibiotics, and from pancreatic enzyme supplements because they lead to increased circulating immune complexes [102, 104, 107, 109–111].

Rarely, cystic fibrosis may present with CFNDD, a primary and secondary sequela, presenting at 2 weeks to 6 months of age. The skin involvement commences in the perineum, perioral, and periorbital regions as erythematous papules that subsequently spread to the extremities over weeks to months and progress to desquamating plaques [97, 98, 112–116]. This cutaneous manifestation is typically coexistent with failure to thrive, hypoproteinemia, and edema prior to any pulmonary manifestations [117–120]. It can be differentiated from acrodermatitis enteropathica due to the normal mucous membranes and nails, and the lack of involvement of the skin folds [97, 112–114].

References

1. Sharma OP. Sarcoidosis: a historical perspective. Clin Dermatol. 2007;25:232–41.
2. Hutchison J. Case of a livid papillary psoriasis. In: Hutchison J, editor. Illustrations of clinical surgery. London: J & A Churchill; 1877. p. 42.
3. Rose A, Tielker M, Knox K. Hepatic, ocular, and cutaneous sarcoidosis. Clin Chest Med. 2008;29:509–24.
4. Boeck C. Multiple benign sarcoid of the skin. J Cutan Genitourin Dis. 1899;17:543–50.
5. Iannuzzi M, Rybicki B, Teirstein A. Medical progress sarcoidosis. N Engl J Med. 2007;357:2153–65.
6. Ali MM, Atwan AA, González ML. Cutaneous sarcoidosis: updates in the pathogenesis. Eur Acad Dermatol Venereol. 2010;24:747–55.
7. Howard A, White CR. Non-infectious granulomas. In: Bolognia JL, Jorizzo JL, Rapini RP, et al., editors. Dermatology. Philadelphia: Elsevier; 2003. p. 1455–60.
8. Katta R. Cutaneous sarcoidosis: a dermatologic masquerader. Am Fam Physician. 2002;65:1581–4.
9. Fernandez-Faith E, McDonnell J. Cutaneous sarcoidosis: differential diagnosis. Clin Dermatol. 2007;25:276–87.
10. Kannan S, Simpson GL, Sheehan DJ, et al. Giant verrucous nodules in a patient with tuberculosis. Am J Dermatopathol. 2009;31:591–3.
11. Judson M, Thompson B, Rabin D, et al. The diagnostic pathway to sarcoidosis. Chest. 2003;123:406–12.
12. Marchell R, Judson M. Chronic cutaneous lesions of sarcoidosis. Clin Dermatol. 2007;25:295–302.
13. Rosenberg B. Ichthyosiform sarcoidosis. Dermatology Online Journal. http://dermatology.cdlib.org. Accessed 3 Nov 2008.
14. Stedman TL. Stedman's medical dictionary. 24th ed. Baltimore: Williams & Wilkins; 1982. p. 813.
15. Edmondstone W, Wilson A. Sarcoidosis in Caucasians, Blacks and Asians in London. Br J Dis Chest. 1985;79:27–36.
16. Yanardag H, Pamuk O, Pamuk G. Lupus pernio in sarcoidosis: clinical features and treatment outcomes of 14 patients. J Clin Rheumatol. 2003;9:72–6.
17. Judson M, Thompson B, Rabin D, et al. The diagnostic pathway to sarcoidosis. Chest. 2003;123(2):406–12.
18. Lodha S, Sanchez M, Prystowsky S. Sarcoidosis of the skin: a review for the pulmonologist. Chest. 2009;136:583–96.
19. English J, Patel P, Greer K. Sarcoidosis. J Am Acad Dermatol. 2001;44:725–43.
20. Darier J, Roussy G. Un cas de tumeurs benignes multiples (Sarcoidessouscutanées ou tuberculides nodulaires hypodermique). Ann Dermatol Syphiligr. 1904;5:144–9.
21. Marcoval J, Moreno A, Mana J, Peyri J. Subcutaneous sarcoidosis. Dermatol Clin. 2008;26:553–6.
22. Vainsencher D, Winkelmann R. Subcutaneous sarcoidosis. Arch Dermatol. 1984;120:1029–31.
23. Mana J, Marcoval J, Graells J, et al. Cutaneous involvement in sarcoidosis. Relationship to systemic disease. Arch Dermatol. 1997;122:882–8.
24. Ahmed L, Harshad S. Subcutaneous sarcoidosis: is it a specific subset of cutaneous sarcoidosis frequently associated with systemic disease? J Am Acad Dermatol. 2006;54:55–60.
25. Requena L, Sanchez Y. Panniculitis. Part II. Mostly lobular panniculitis. J Am Acad Dermatol. 2001;45:325–61.
26. Mehta V, Balachandran C, Mathew M. Scar sarcoidosis sparing a surgical scar. Dermatology Online Journal. http://dermatology.cdlib.org. Accessed 10 Nov 2008.
27. Minus H, Grimes P. Cutaneous manifestations of sarcoidosis in blacks. Cutis. 1983;32:361–3.
28. Selim A, Ehrsam E, Atassi M, Khachemoune A. Scar sarcoidosis: a case report and brief review. Cutis. 2006;78:418–22.
29. Ahbib S, Lachapelle J, Marot L. Sarcoidal granulomas following injections of botulic toxin A (Botox) for corrections of wrinkles. Ann Dermatol Venereol. 2006;133:43–5.
30. Henderson C, Lafleur L, Sontheimer R. Sarcoidal alopecia as a mimic of discoid lupus erythematous. J Am Acad Dermatol. 2008;59:143–5.
31. Douri R, Chawaf A, Alreface B. Cicatricial alopecia due to sarcoidosis. Dermatology Online Journal. http://dermatology.cdlib.org. Accessed 10 Nov 2008.
32. Katta R, Nelson B, Chen D, Roenigk H. Sarcoidosis of the scalp: A case series and review of the literature. J Am Acad Dermatol. 2000;42:690–2.
33. Cather J, Cohen P. Ichthyosiform sarcoidosis. J Am Acad Dermatol. 1999;40:862–5.
34. Rosenberg B. Ichthyosiform sarcoisis. Dermatology Online Journal. http://dermatology.cdlib.org. Accessed 10 Nov 2008.
35. Patterson J, Fitzwater J. Case report. Hypopigmented sarcoidosis. J Tenn Med Assoc. 1978;71:662–4.
36. Thomas RH, McKee P, Black M. Hypopigmented sarcoidosis. J R Soc Med. 1981;72:921–3.
37. Breathmach A. Branched cells in the epidermis: an overview. J Invest Dermatol. 1980;75:6–11.
38. Clayton R, Breathnach A, Martin B, Feiwel M. Hypopigmented sarcoidosis in the negro. Report of eight cases with ultrastructural observations. Br J Dermatol. 1977;96:118–27.
39. James D. Erythema nodosum. Br Med J. 1961;1:853–7.
40. Schwartz R, Nervi S. Erythema nodosum: a sign of systemic disease. Am Fam Physician. 2007;75:695–700.
41. Rosell A, Garcia-Arranz G, Romero N, et al. Lupus pernio with involvement of nasal cavity and maxillary sinus. ORL J Otorhinolaryngol Relat Spec. 1998;60:236–9.
42. Vashisht P, Sahoo B, Khurana N, Reddy B. Cutaneous tuberculosis in children and adolescents: a clinicohistological study. J Eur Acad Dermatol Venereol. 2007;21:40–7.
43. Marmelzat W. Laennac and the 'prosecutor's wart'. Arch Dermatol. 1962;86:546–51.
44. Daniel TM. The history of tuberculosis. Respir Med. 2006;100: 1862–70.
45. World Health Organization. Global tuberculosis control – surveillance, planning, financing. WHO report 2005. Geneva: World Health Organization; 2005. p. 1–247.
46. Valadas E, Antunes F. Tuberculosis, a re-emergent disease. Eur J Radiol. 2005;55:154–7.
47. Aaron L, Saadoun D, Calatroni I, et al. Tuberculosis in HIV-infected patients: a comprehensive review. Clin Microbiol Infect. 2004;10:388–98.
48. Hernandez C, Cetner A, Jordan J, et al. Tuberculosis in the age of biologic therapy. J Am Acad Dermatol. 2008;59:363–80.
49. Barbagallo J, Tager P, Ingleton R, et al. Cutaneous tuberculosis: diagnosis and treatment. Am J Clin Dermatol. 2002;3:319–28.
50. McKenna MT, McCray E, Onorato I. The epidemiology of tuberculosis among foreign-born persons in the United States, 1986 to 1993. N Engl J Med. 1995;332:1071–6.
51. Morrone A, Dassoni F, Pajno MC, et al. Ulcers of the face and neck in a woman with pulmonary tuberculosis: presentation of a clinical case. Rural Remote Health. 2010;10:1485.
52. Kaufmann SH. New issues in tuberculosis. Ann Rheum Dis. 2004;63:50–6.
53. American Thoracic Society. Diagnostic standards and classification of tuberculosis in adults and children. Am J Respir Crit Care Med. 2000;161:1376–95.
54. Harries A, Dye C. Tuberculosis. Ann Trop Med Parasitol. 2006;100:415–41.

55. Chesnutt MS, Prendergast TJ. Pulmonary tuberculosis. In: McPhee SJ, Papadakis MA, Tierney LM, editors. Current medical diagnosis and treatment 2007. New York: McGraw-Hill; 2007. p. 260–8.
56. Sahin N, Aydin NE, Senol M, et al. Longstanding skin ulcers due to Mycobacterium tuberculosis in a healthy man. Trop Biomed. 2010;27:120–4.
57. Pandhi D, Reddy B, Chowdhary S, Khurana N. Cutaneous tuberculosis in Indian children: the importance of screening for involvement of internal organs. J Eur Acad Dermatol Venereol. 2004;18:546–51.
58. Yates V, Pormedero L. Cutaneous tuberculosis in Blackburn district (UK): a 15-year prospective series. Br J Dermatol. 1996;136:483–9.
59. MacGregor R. Cutaneous tuberculosis. Clin Dermatol. 1995; 13:245–55.
60. Sethuraman G, Ramesh V, Raman M, Sharma V. Skin tuberculosis in children: learning from India. Dermatol Clin. 2008;26:285–94.
61. Ranawaka RR, Abeygunasekara PH, Perera E, et al. Letter: Clinico-histopathological correlation and the treatment response of 20 patients with cutaneous tuberculosis. Dermatol Online J. 2010;16:13.
62. Ara M, Pharm C, Baselga C, et al. Primary tuberculous chancre caused by Mycobacterium bovis after goring with a bull's horn. J Am Acad Dermatol. 2000;43:535–7.
63. Ramesh V, Misra R, Beena K, Mukherjee A. A study of cutaneous tuberculosis in children. Pediatr Dermatol. 1999;16:262–9.
64. Terranova M, Padovese V, Fornari U, Morrone A. Clinical and epidemiological study of cutaneous tuberculosis in Northern Ethiopia. Dermatology. 2008;217:89–93.
65. Ho CK, Ho MH, Chong LY. Cutaneous tuberculosis in Hong Kong: an update. Hong Kong Med J. 2006;12:272–7.
66. Kumar B, Muralidhar S. Cutaneous tuberculosis: A twenty-year prospective study. Int J Tuberc Lung Dis. 1999;3:494–500.
67. Lipsker D, Grosshans E. What is Lupus vulgaris in 2005? Dermatology. 2005;211:189–90.
68. Du Vivier A. Atlas of clinical dermatology: the skin and systemic disease. 3rd ed. Boston: Churchill Livingstone; 2002. p. 264–8, 391,509–13.
69. Kumar B, Rai R, Kaur I, et al. Childhood cutaneous tuberculosis: a study over 25 years from northern India. Int J Dermatol. 2001;40:26–32.
70. Morais P, Ferreira O, Nogueira A, et al. A nodulo-ulcerative lesion on the nose. Dermatol Online J. 2010;16:11.
71. Tappeiner G, Wolff K. Tuberculosis and other mycobacterial infections. In: Fitzpatrick TB, Freedberg IM, Eisen AZ, Wolff K, Austen KF, editors. Dermatology in general medicine. 5th ed. New York: McGraw-Hill; 2003. p. 1933–50.
72. Sehgal V, Wagh S. Cutaneous tuberculosis: current concepts. Int J Dermatol. 1990;28:355–62.
73. Sehgal V. Cutaneous tuberculosis. Dermatol Clin. 1994;12:645–53.
74. Bravo F, Gotuzzo E. Cutaneous tuberculosis. Clin Dermatol. 2007;25:173–80.
75. Stack R, Bickley L, Coppel I. Miliary tuberculosis presenting as skin lesions in a patient with acquired immunodeficiency syndrome. J Am Acad Dermatol. 1990;23:1031–5.
76. Sehgal VN, Wagh SA. Cutaneous tuberculosis. Current concepts. Int J Dermatol. 1990;29:237–52.
77. Erbagci S, Almila T, Nazan B, Erkilic S, Bayram A. Tuberculosis verrucosa cutis in a patient with long-standing generalized lichen planus: Improvement of lichen after antitubercular polychemotherapy. J Dermatolog Treat. 2006;17:314–8.
78. Sehgal V. Lichen scrofulosorum: current status. Int J Dermatol. 2005;44:521–3.
79. Mascaró J, Baselga E. Erythema induratum of Bazin. Dermatol Clin. 2008;26:439–45.
80. Hebra F. Lichen scrofulosorum. In: Fagge CH, Pye Smith PH, editors. Diseases of the skin. London: New Syndenham Society; 1868. p. 52.
81. Singal A. Lichen scrofulosorum: A prospective study of 39 patients. Int J Dermatol. 2005;44:489–93.
82. Kumar U, Sethuraman G, Verma P, et al. Psoriasiform type of lichen scrofulosorum. Pediatr Dermatol 2010. Dec 7. doi:10.1111/j.1525-1470.2010.01304X.
83. Bazin E. Leçons théoriques et cliniques sur la scrofule. 2nd ed. Paris: Delahaye; 1861.
84. Schneider J, Jordaan H, Geiger D, et al. Erythema induratum of Bazin. Am J Dermatopathol. 1995;17:350–6.
85. Shimizu A, Takahashi A, Negishi I, et al. The close association of lymphadenitis tuberculosa and erythema induratum of Bazin in Japanese patients. Dermatology. 2003;207:426–7.
86. Garcia-Rodriguez J, Monteagudo-Sanchez B, Marino-Callejo A. Cutaneous tuberculosis: a 15-year descriptive study. Enferm Infect Microbiol Clin. 2008;26:205–11.
87. Segura S, Pujol R, Trindade F, et al. Vasculitis in erythema induratum of Bazin: a histopathologic study of 101 biopsy specimens from 86 patients. J Am Acad Dermatol. 2008;59:839–51.
88. Heinemann C, Kaatz M, Elsner P. Erythema induratum of Bazin and Poncet's disease–successful treatment with antitubercular drugs. Eur Acad Dermatol Venereol. 2003;17:334–6.
89. Freidman P, Husain S, Grossman M. Nodular tuberculid in a patient with HIV. J Am Acad Dermatol. 2005;53:S154–6.
90. Hara K, Tsuzuki T, Takagi N, et al. Nodular granulomatous phlebitis of the skin: a fourth type of tuberculid. Histopathology. 1997;30:129–34.
91. Motswaledi H, Schulz E. Superficial thrombophlebitic tuberculide. Inter J Dermatol. 2006;45:1337–40.
92. Birt A, Hogg G, Dubé W. Hereditary multiple fibrofolliculomas with trichodiscomas and acrochordons. Arch Dermatol. 1977;113:1674–777.
93. Vincent A, Farley M, Chan E, James WD. Birt-Hogg-Dube syndrome: a review of the literature and the differential diagnosis of firm facial papules. J Am Acad Dermatol. 2003;49:698.
94. Stavrakoglou A, Dubrey SW, Dorkins H, et al. The Birt–Hogg–Dubé syndrome: dermatological features and internal malignancies. Q J Med. 2010;103:987–90.
95. Toro J, Wei M-H, Glenn G, Weinreich M, et al. BHD mutations, clinical and molecular genetic investigations of Birt-Hogg-Dubé syndrome: a new series of 50 families and a review of published reports. J Med Genet. 2008;45:321–31.
96. Gruson L. Birt-Hogg-Dube syndrome. Dermatol Online J. 2004;10(3):15–16. http://dermatology.cdlib.org. Accessed 10 Nov 2008.
97. Bernstein M, McCusker M, Grant-Kels J. Cutaneous manifestations of cystic fibrosis. Pediatr Dermatol. 2008;25:150–7.
98. Zedek D, Morrell D, Graham M, et al. Acrodermatitis enteropathica-like eruption and failure to thrive as presenting signs of cystic fibrosis. J Am Acad Dermatol. 2008;58:S5–8.
99. Franks A, Werth V. Cutaneous aspects of cardiopulmonary disease. In: Fitzpatrick TB, Freedberg IM, Eisen AZ, Wolff K, Austen KF, editors. Dermatology in general medicine. 5th ed. New York: McGraw-Hill; 2003. p. 1625–34.
100. Johns M. Skin wrinkling in cystic fibrosis. Med Biol Illus. 1975;25:205–10.
101. Katz K, Yan A, Turner M. Aquagenic wrinkling of the palms in patients with cystic fibrosis homozygous for the delta F508 CFTR mutation. Arch Dermatol. 2005;141:621–4.
102. Fradin M, Kalb R, Grossman M. Recurrent cutaneous vasculitis in cystic fibrosis. Pediatr Dermatol. 1987;4:108–11.
103. Garty B, Scanlin T, Goldsmith D, et al. Cutaneous manifestations of cystic fibrosis: possible role of cryoglobulins. Br J Dermatol. 1989;121:655–8.

104. Soter N, Mihm M, Colten H. Cutaneous necrotizing venulitis in patients with cystic fibrosis. J Pediatr Scand. 1979; 95:197–201.
105. Schidlow D, Goldsmith D, Palmer J, et al. Arthritis in cystic fibrosis. Arch Dis Child. 1984;59:377–9.
106. John E, Medenis R, Rao S. Cutaneous necrotizing venulitis in patients with cystic fibrosis. J Pediatr. 1980;97:505.
107. Finnegan M, Hinchcliffe J, Russel-Jones D, et al. Vasculitis complicating cystic fibrosis. Q J Med. 1989;72:609–21.
108. Schidlow D, Panitch H, Saeri N, et al. Purpuric rashes in cystic fibrosis. Am J Dis Child. 1989;143:1030–2.
109. Abman S, Ogle J, Harbeck R, et al. Early bacteriologic, immunologic, and clinical course of young infants with cystic fibrosis identified by neonatal screening. J Pediatr. 1991;119:211–7.
110. Disis M, McDonald T, Colombo J, et al. Circulating immune complexes in cystic fibrosis and their correlation to clinical parameters. Pediatr Res. 1986;20:385–90.
111. Hodson M, Beldon I, Batten J. Circulating immune complexes in patients with cystic fibrosis in relation to clinical features. Clin Allergy. 1985;15:363–70.
112. Crone J, Huber W, Eichler I, Granditsch G. Acrodermatitis enteropathica-like eruption as the presenting sign of cystic fibrosis-case report and review of literature. Eur J Pediatr. 2002;161: 475–8.
113. Patrizi A, Bianchi F, Neri I, Specchia F. Acrodermatitis enteropathica-like eruption as the presenting sign of cystic fibrosis. Pediatr Dermatol. 2003;20:187–8.
114. Hansen R, Lemen R, Revsin B. Cystic fibrosis manifesting with acrodermatitis enteropathica-like eruption. Association with essential fatty acids and zinc deficiencies. Arch Dermatol. 1983;119:51–5.
115. Darmstadt G, McGuire J, Ziboh V. Malnutrition-associated rash of cystic fibrosis. Pediatr Dermatol. 2000;17:337–47.
116. Darmstadt GL, Schmidt CP, Wechsler DS, et al. Dermatitis as a presenting sign of cystic fibrosis [comment]. Arch Dermatol. 1992;128:1358–64.
117. Lovett A, Kokta V, Maari C. Diffuse dermatitis: An unexpected initial presentation of cystic fibrosis. J Am Acad Dermatol. 2008;58:S1–4.
118. Darmstadt GL, Schmidt CP, Wechslet DS, Tunnessen WW, Rosenstein BJ. Dermatitis as a presenting sign of cystic fibrosis. Arch Dermatol. 1992;128:1389–90.
119. Abman S, Accurso F, Bowman C. Persistent morbidity and mortality of protein calorie malnutrition in young infants with cystic fibrosis. J Pediatr Gastroenterol Nutr. 1975;5:393–6.
120. Muñiz A, Bartle S, Foster R. Edema, anemia, hypoproteinemia, and acrodermatitis enteropathica: an uncommon initial presentation of cystic fibrosis. Pediatr Emerg Care. 2004;20:112–4.

Cutaneous Manifestations of Renal Disease

Lilliam S. Chiqués Colón and Rosbel González Rivera

Chronic kidney disease (CKD) is very common among internal medicine patients. In the majority of cases, the skin is affected in some way. In this chapter, we discuss some of the cutaneous signs and symptoms associated with CKD, as well as some of the cutaneous syndromes. The clinical and histological features, pathogenesis, diagnostic evaluation, and management of uremic pruritus, calciphylaxis, benign nodular calcification, nephrogenic systemic fibrosis, and bullous disease of hemodialysis are also discussed.

Introduction

Renal insufficiency is a commonly encountered problem in internal medicine patients. A large proportion of patients with kidney disease frequently report cutaneous signs and symptoms. In patients with acute renal failure, only edema and uremic frost are seen. Uremic frost results in cases of extreme uremia from the deposition on the skin of urea crystals excreted from sweat, and has the appearance of crystalline white powder. With the widespread availability of hemodialysis (HD), it is now rare. In chronic kidney disease (CKD), however, there are a wide variety of cutaneous manifestations.

General Changes

General changes in the skin of patients with CKD include xerosis, nail changes and pigmentation changes. The cause of the xerosis has been thought to be from a combination of sweat gland atrophy [1, 2], fluid shifts during dialysis, and altered vitamin A metabolism [3]. Nail changes include thinness, subungal hemorrhages, Lindsey's or half-and-half nails (normal in distal 50% and white in the proximal 50%), and Terry's nails (only the distal 20% is normal). The skin in patients with CKD is often pale, secondary to anemia. It may also take on a grayish yellow discoloration because of accumulated carotenoid and nitrogenous pigments in the dermis. A brown-gray discoloration can result from hemosiderin deposition secondary to iron overload from repeated blood transfusions, and hyperpigmentation can result from an increase in beta-melanocyte stimulating hormone, which is difficult to dialyse [4–6]. In the rest of this chapter, we will be discussing some of the other manifestations and clinical syndromes that can be found on the skin of renal patients.

Uremic Pruritus

Pruritus is a very common and frustrating complaint among patients with CKD, affecting up to 60% of hemodialysis patients [7–11]. It is associated with a higher mortality in patients with end stage renal disease (ESRD) [11]. Clinically these patients present with autoinduced excoriations on the trunk and extremities (Fig. 1). Typical lesions associated with scratching that are observed in these patients include: lichen simplex (localized lichenification, plaques of varying size often appearing at the extensor surface of forearms, inguinal, scrotal, and anogenital areas), prurigo nodularis (brown nodules covered by crusts, scales and abrasions), and keratotic papules (red or violaceous lesions with central plug often appearing on extensor surface of limbs) [12]. Histopathological examination of tissue is usually not helpful in these cases to determine the cause of the pruritus or for diagnosis.

The etiology of pruritus in ESRD is still unclear, but multiple factors have been identified as possible culprits, so it is suspected that the etiology of uremic pruritus is multifactorial. How each factor contributes to the symptom of pruritus is still unclear. The release of histamine from skin

L.S. Chiqués Colón (✉)
Department of Medicine, University of Puerto Rico School of Medicine, Medical Sciences Campus, San Juan, Puerto Rico
e-mail: lchiques@gmail.com

R. González Rivera
Department of Dermatology, University of Puerto Rico School of Medicine, Medical Sciences Campus, San Juan, Puerto Rico

N.P. Sánchez (ed.), *Atlas of Dermatology in Internal Medicine*,
DOI 10.1007/978-1-4614-0688-4_3, © Springer Science+Business Media, LLC 2012

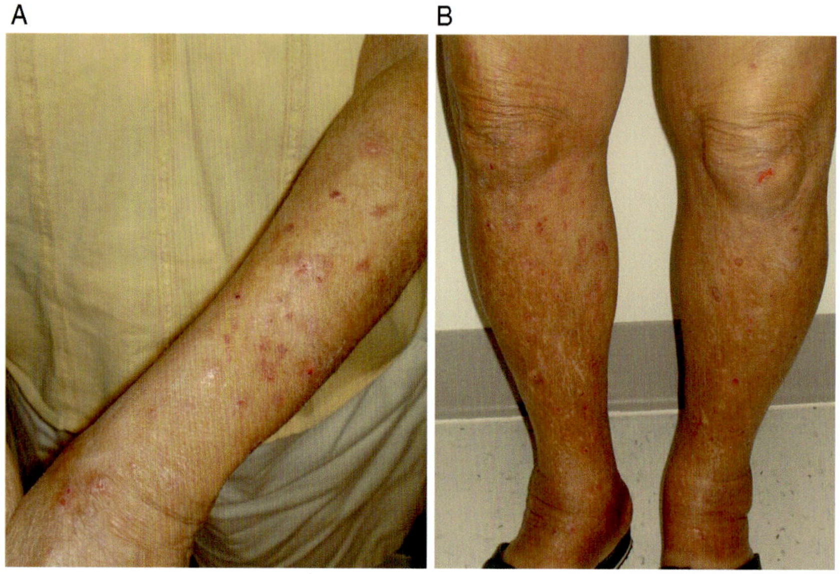

Fig. 1 (**a**, **b**) Uremic pruritus. A renal insufficiency patient whose generalized itch manifested with multiple excoriations

mast cells causes the pruritus [13, 14]. It is suspected that ESRD patients are sensitized to antigens to which they are exposed during HD [15]. The perception of pruritus is thought to be controlled by neural pathways mediated by opioid receptors [16]. Strong correlations have been found between pruritus and secondary hyperparathyroidism, dry skin from sweat gland atrophy [17–19], elevated phosphate levels [20, 21], inadequate hemodialysis [22, 23], increased beta 2 microglobulin levels [22], anemia or decreased erythropoietin levels [13], increased aluminum levels [24], and immune dysfunction [25].

Ensuring adequate dialyzation and good control of plasma calcium and phosphate concentrations are a priority when monitoring ESRD patients [23, 26]. Symptom control can be attempted with antihistamines, ultraviolet B light [13], erythropoietin administration, opioid antagonists, topical capsaicin, oral evening primrose oil, gabapentin, oral granisetron, and polymethylmethacrylate dialysis membranes [14, 18, 27–37]. More research is needed to establish the relative efficacy of these treatments. Some experts recommend a combination of erythropoietin, UVB light, and antihistamines; however, an optimum regimen is yet to be determined [7].

Calcinosis Cutis

In chronic renal failure, there is impaired renal clearance of phosphate, vitamin D deficiency, and hyperparathyroidism, all of which lead to a high calcium phosphate solubility product, with the subsequent deposition of calcium salts in tissues [38]. When calcium deposits in small vessels, it can result in calciphylaxis via thrombosis of vessels. When it deposits in the dermis or subcutaneous tissues, calcinosis cutis (benign nodular calcification) can result.

The incidence and prevalence of calcinosis cutis in renal disease is not known. It is characterized by firm and whitish papules, plaques, and nodules. They can be tender and restrict joint mobility, and sometimes they can ulcerate and exude a chalky white material [38, 39].

There are several types of calcinosis cutis. The type most often associated with CKD is metastatic calcinosis cutis, which is characterized by the widespread, symmetrical deposition of calcium around large joints and fingertips [39]. Dystrophic calcification, which is characterized by calcium deposits at sites of tissue injury, has been described in at least one case report [40]. Iatrogenic calcinosis cutis can happen as a result of a medical treatment or procedure. It has been described in at least two case reports in renal patients using low molecular weight heparin, with lesions developing at the site of injection [41, 42]. It can also happen following parenteral administration of calcium or phosphate, and in the setting of tumor lysis syndrome (which leads to tissue damage from the chemotherapy, and the release of phosphate from tissues) [43].

Diagnosis is made with skin biopsy, which demonstrates calcium deposits in the dermis and sometimes in the subcutaneous tissue. Sometimes, associated foreign-body giant cell reaction can be observed [43]. There are several case reports of fine needle aspiration of nodules done when malignancy was suspected, in which calcinosis cutis was diagnosed instead [44–46]. Workup can include bone scan and plain radiography to evaluate the extent of involvement with calcinosis cutis. Calcium, phosphate, alkaline phosphatase, blood urea nitrogen, creatinine, albumin, parathyroid hormone (PTH) levels, and vitamin D levels should be obtained [43].

Treatment when the disease is associated with CKD revolves around normalizing the calcium phosphate product. This can be done with dietary restriction of phosphorus, phosphate binders, and parathyroidectomy [39]. Other treatments include the use of the calcium channel blocker diltiazem [47–49], intralesional corticosteroids, probenecid, colchicine, warfarin, sodium etidronate [43], and myo-inositol hexaphosphonate [50, 51]. Surgical removal of lesions can be performed when indicated for pain control, infection, ulceration, or functional impairment [43].

Calciphylaxis

Calciphylaxis, also known as "calcific uremic arteriolopathy," is characterized by medial calcification of arteries, leading to ischemia and skin necrosis [52]. Although still rare, it has been increasing in incidence, probably secondary to the use of calcium-based phosphate binders and vitamin D analogs in the treatment of associated hyperparathyroidism in renal patients [53]. A cross-sectional study of HD patients placed its prevalence at 4% [54]. It is most common among patients with ESRD or who have undergone renal transplant [53, 55–59], but has been described in patients with other conditions, including breast cancer, systemic lupus erythematosus, and liver cirrhosis [60–67].

The pathogenesis of calciphylaxis is poorly understood. Hyperphosphatemia, hypercalcemia, hyperparathyroidism, and vitamin D administration are thought to be implicated [52]. Additional suspects are obesity [58], hypercoagulable states [71–74], and deficiencies of inhibitors of vascular calcification such as fetuin-A and matrix Gla protein [75–81].

Calciphylaxis is characterized by the appearance of firm, bilateral, symmetric, painful violaceous plaques, and subcutaneous nodules, often with associated livedo reticularis. They are often preceded by flaccid or hemorrhagic bullae and can progress to necrotic ulcers with eschars (Fig. 2) [39]. Peripheral pulses are usually preserved distal to the areas of necrosis [39]. They tend to be located on the trunk, buttocks, and proximal extremities, and can also occur distally [58]. Myopathy, hypotension, fever, dementia, and infarction of the central nervous system, bowel or myocardium have also been observed as a result of systemic calciphylaxis [68].

Histological examination of affected dermal and subcutaneous tissue demonstrates medial calcification and intimal hyperplasia of small arteries and arterioles, as well as fibrin thrombi within the calcified vessels. Ischemic necrosis can be found in the overlying epidermis [39]. An acute and chronic calcifying septal panniculitis can also be seen (Fig. 3) [69]. Other modalities such as a bone scan study may aid in the diagnosis, but the sensitivity and specificity of this modality for diagnosis is unclear [52]. Radiography, specifically with the mammography technique, can also help confirm the diagnosis [70].

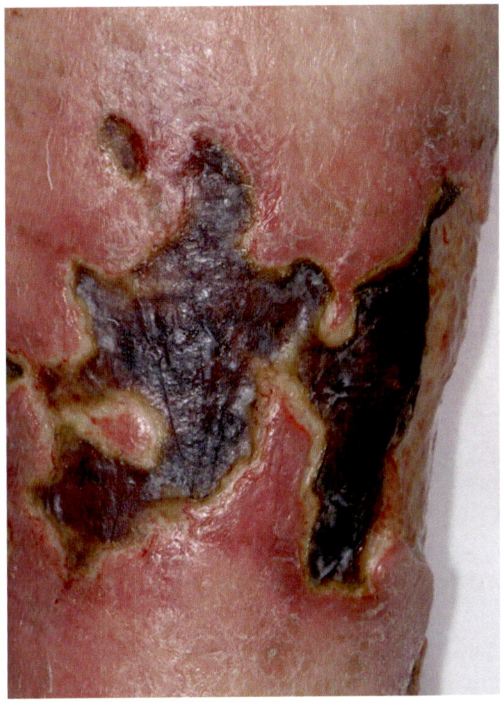

Fig. 2 Calciphylaxis lesions which have progressed to necrotic ulcers with eschar. *Picture courtesy of Mayo Clinic*

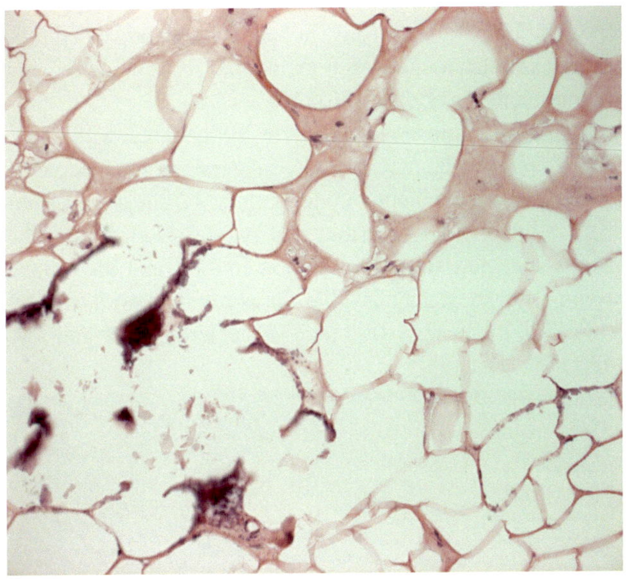

Fig. 3 Calciphylaxis affecting subcutaneous tissue: extravascular calcification with prominent fat necrosis can be seen in the panniculus

Calciphylaxis is associated with a high mortality, with estimates ranging from 58 to 80%, and is most commonly caused by superinfection of the lesions [39, 53, 55]. Negative prognostic features include proximal lesions and advanced disease at time of diagnosis. When the lesions occur distally, the patient has a better prognosis [82].

Management includes aggressive wound care, pain control, and avoidance of tissue trauma [52]. Control of plasma calcium and phosphate levels is also important [83]. Non-calcium-containing phosphate binders are preferred [84–86]. Cinacalcet (parathyroid gland calcimimetic) or parathyroidectomy is recommended for the normalization of PTH levels [87–92]. Other interventions may include increasing the number of sessions of renal replacement therapy [85], discontinuation of warfarin (the activity of matrix Gla protein depends on vitamin K carboxylation), and lowering the dose of immunosuppresion in renal transplant patients who are refractory to the above interventions [52]. New therapies being evaluated include intravenous sodium thiosulfate [93–97], biphosphonates [98], hyperbaric oxygen therapy [96, 97, 99, 100], and prednisone (for non-ulcerating plaques) [53].

Nephrogenic Systemic Fibrosis

In the late 1990s, a condition characterized by thickening and hardening of the skin was identified in patients with ESRD [101–103]. It was initially termed "nephrogenic fibrosing dermopathy," but the name was changed to "nephrogenic systemic fibrosis" (NSF) after fibrosis was identified in other organs [104]. By December 2006, the International NSF Registry at Yale University had 215 cases that had been reported [105]. It occurs only in patients with advanced kidney disease, has no gender or racial predilection, and occurs predominantly in adults [106–110].

Skin involvement is present in all patients with NSF. Lesions tend to be symmetrical, bilateral, fibrotic papules, plaques, or subcutaneous nodules (Fig. 4); they are sometimes erythematous, pruritic, and painful [111–113]. The lesions start peripherally in the extremities, and then move proximally. They may involve the abdominal wall and, in rare cases, the head [107, 114, 115]. Sclerodactyly and loss of skin appendages of the dorsum of hands and legs may occur. Joint mobility can be lost secondary to fibrosis of the overlying skin [104, 107, 111]. Systemic involvement occurs in some patients and may include fibrosis of muscles, lungs, diaphragm, myocardium, pericardium, pleura, and dura mater [108, 111, 116–119]. Yellow scleral plaques are a common finding [105, 109].

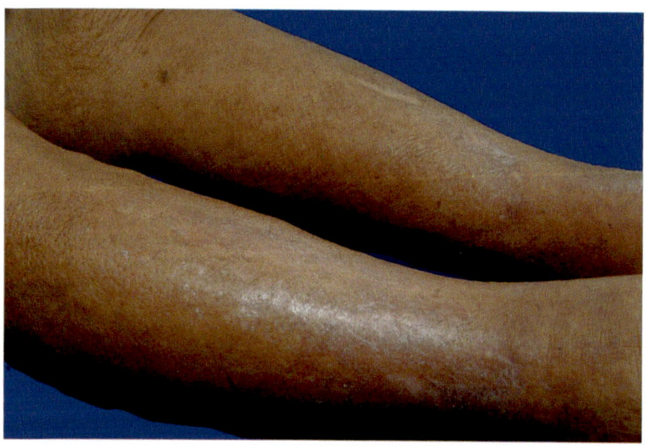

Fig. 4 Nephrogenic systemic fibrosis. Indurated and hyperpigmented plaques affecting the bilateral extremities in a patient with renal insufficiency

NSF appears to be a new disease, and its pathogenesis is still not well understood. Activation of the transforming growth factor-beta (TGF-β) pathway resulting in an increase in circulating fibrocytes is thought to contribute to the tissue fibrosis [109, 115, 120, 121]. These events might be initiated by an outside agent, such as a new toxin. Epidemiological evidence shows an association of NSF with exposure to gadolinium-containing contrast agents [122, 123]. Gadolinium (Gd) is used during magnetic resonance (MR) imaging studies as a contrast agent, and its half-life is markedly increased in ESRD. Evidence from observational studies points to a temporal relationship between NSF and Gd exposure [105, 122–127]. In addition, Gd deposits have been found in tissue from patients with NSF [128–131].

In a recent study, Altun et al. identified a significant decrease in the incidence of NSF in tertiary care centers of two universities following the switch from gadodiamine to gadobenate dimeglumine and gadopentetate dimeglumine, as well as the adoption of restrictive gadolinium-based contrast agent (GBCA) policies for patients who underwent gadolinium-enhanced studies. The absence of NSF cases in the postadoption period may reflect the effect of the use of different GBCAs on the incidence of NSF [132]. Given the association of Gd with NSF, the United States Food and Drug Administration issued a boxed warning on all Gd-based contrast agents warning about the risk for NSF recommending the avoidance of Gd in patients with advanced kidney disease, or prompt HD after the study if Gd must be used [151].

Other associations include proinflammatory events (e.g., major surgery, infection, etc.), elevated PTH levels, erythropoietin therapy, fistula reconstruction, dialysis catheter placement, and kidney or liver transplantation [109, 133–137].

The diagnosis is made by tissue biopsy. Light microscopy reveals proliferation of dermal fibrocytes in early cases, and marked thickening of the dermis and abundant proliferation of fibrocytes with long dendritic processes in advanced cases. Thick collagen bundles with clefts and increases in mucin and elastic fibers in the dermis are also seen. Immunohistochemical staining shows a proliferation of CD34+ cells in the dermis, and an increased number of CD68+ and factor XIII+ dendritic cells. The lesions may extend into the subcutaneous tissue [105, 108, 111, 138]. A deep incisional or punch biopsy is recommended as the changes may not only extend into the subcutaneous tissues, but also include the muscle [109, 139].

Pulmonary function tests, two-dimensional echocardiography, and muscle biopsy may be obtained to evaluate for systemic involvement [115, 140]. Differential diagnoses include systemic sclerosis, scleromyxedema, and eosinophilic fasciitis.

NSF appears to run a chronic course in most patients [109, 115, 120, 125, 138, 141]. A fulminant form has been described in 5% of patients. Remission of NSF has been seen in some patients who recovered renal function [109, 110, 115, 120].

Extracorporeal photopheresis, ultraviolet A phototherapy, plasmapheresis, photodynamic therapy, pentoxifylline, intravenous sodium thiosulfate, and high-dose intravenous immune globulin have all been used as therapy in small series or case reports with some promising results, but more information is needed to determine an appropriate therapy [103, 117, 125, 137, 142–150]. Intensive physical therapy is recommended to manage disability related to joint contractures [145]. Currently, the best recommendation is prevention.

Bullous Disease of Hemodialysis

Vesicles and bullae in patients on renal replacement therapy can occur in the setting of severe elevation of porphyrin levels (porphyria cutanea tarda), or when the levels are normal to minimally elevated (pseudoporphyria).

Porphyria Cutanea Tarda

The majority of the cases of porphyria cutanea tarda (PCT) are associated with acquired deficiencies in the hepatic enzyme uroporphyrinogen decarboxylase (URO-D), which leads to the accumulation of photosensitive porphyrins. However, it has also been documented in patients with ESRD on chronic hemodialysis, in which the following mechanisms for the development of PCT have been suggested: (1) decreased URO-D activity due to suppressive effects of hepatotoxins and iron and (2) inadequate porphyrin clearance by renal replacement therapies [152], as porphyrins are poorly dialyzable with either standard hemodialysis (HD) or peritoneal dialysis [153]. This can lead to very high levels of porphyrins, occasionally exceeding 200 μg/dl [154]. Likewise, the deposition of porphyrins in the skin can result in photosensitivity and subepidermal bullae (Fig. 5) [155, 157, 158].

On histopathology, one can see a characteristic subepidermal blister. A scant perivascular infiltrate and an edematous dermal papilla can be seen (Fig. 6). On direct immunofluorescence of the dermoepidermal junction, one can see immunoglobulin G, immunoglobulin A, immunoglobulin M, fibrin, and complement around the dermal venules [158, 159].

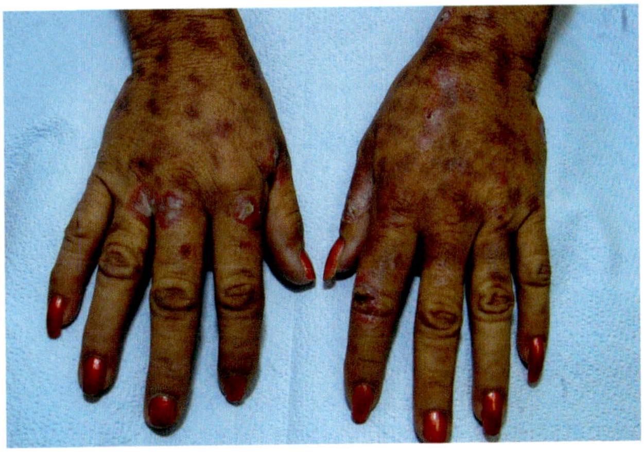

Fig. 5 Bullae, erosions, and scaring on the dorsum of the hands in a patient with porphyria

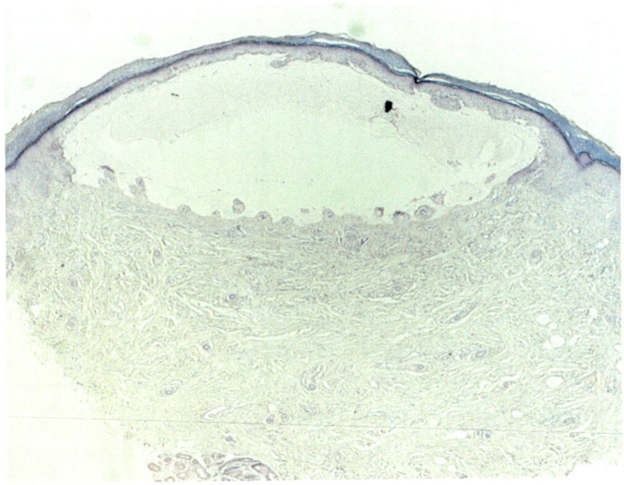

Fig. 6 A biopsy of a patient with porphyria cutanea tarda showing a characteristic subepidermal blister formation with the preservation of the papillary dermis accompanied by minimal perivascular infiltrate

Management involves administration of recombinant erythropoietin with or without phlebotomy [160–162]. High-flux HD can be effective in removing porphyrins [163]. Deferoxamine and plasma exchange have been used with success in some patients [164, 165]. Chloroquine is ineffective because renal failure precludes the excretion of excess porphyrins mobilized by chloroquine [156, 166].

Pseudoporphyria

Pseudoporphyria (bullous dermatosis of dialysis) is characterized by cutaneous fragility and blistering in sun-exposed areas in patients with renal insufficiency, in the setting of normal or mildly elevated porphyrin levels. Prevalence according to several European studies ranges from 1 to 16% [167–170].

In pseudoporphyria, vesicles or bullae are seen with clear or hemorrhagic fluid mostly in the dorsum of hands, and can also be seen in the scalp, face, and neck. Lesions develop in skin that is subjected to sunlight or incidental trauma and in patients who have been on HD for months to years [171]. Although the pathophysiology is not well understood, there are several theories as to the cause of pseudoporphyria. Porphyrin photosensitization may occur in those with mildly elevated porphyrin levels [172]. It has been postulated that patients may also become photosensitized by compounds encountered during HD, but this remains unproven [170]. Elevated aluminum concentration from therapeutic or environmental sources may lead to the overproduction of porphyrins, but this too remains unproven [173]. Finally, concomitant use of photosensitizing medications needs to be considered [174–178].

Histologic examination resembles that of PCT, described above.

Management centers on sunlight avoidance, use of sunscreen, and protecting skin from trauma. *N*-acetylcysteine was helpful in a small clinical trial [179] and several case reports [180, 181].

Conclusion

The cutaneous manifestations of CKD are diverse and range in severity from benign to life threatening. An awareness of these manifestations can bring about appropriate and prompt diagnosis and treatment, and in some cases, it can provide information about prognosis. Dermatologists as well as primary care and hospitalist physicians need to be familiarized with these manifestations.

References

1. Rosenthal SR. Uremic dermatitis. Arch Dermatol Syphil. 1931;23:934.
2. Cawley EP, Hoch-Ligeti C, Bond GM. The eccrine seat glands of patients in uremia. Arch Dermatol. 1961;84:51.
3. Sweeney S, Cropley TG. Cutaneous changes in renal disorders. Fitzpatrick's dermatology in general medicine, vol. 2. 6th ed. New York: McGraw-Hill; 2003.
4. Masmoudi A, Ben Hmida M, Mseddi M, Meziou TJ, Walha N, Hachicha J, et al. Cutaneous manifestations of chronic hemodialysis. Prospective study of 363 cases. Presse Med. 2006;35(3 Pt 1): 399–406.
5. Sweeney S, Cropley TG. Cutaneous changes in renal disorders. Fitzpatrick's dermatology in general medicine, vol. 2. 6th ed. New York: McGraw-Hill; 2003.
6. Nunley JR. Dermatologic manifestations of renal disease. Emedicine. http://www.emedicine.com. Accessed 16 Sept 2007.
7. Ponticelli C, Bencini PL. Pruritus in dialysis patients: a neglected problem [editorial]. Nephrol Dial Transplant. 1995;10:2174.
8. Stahle-Backdahl M. Uremic pruritus: clinical and experimental studies. Acta Derm Venereol Suppl (Stockh). 1989;145:1.
9. Mettang T, Fritz P, Weber J, et al. Uremic pruritus in patients on hemodialysis or continuous ambulatory peritoneal dialysis (CAPD): the role of plasma histamine and skin mast cells. Clin Nephrol. 1990;34:136.
10. Zucker I, Yosipovitch G, David M, Gafter U. Prevalence and characterization of uremic pruritus in patients undergoing hemodialysis: uremic pruritus is still a major problem for patients with end-stage renal disease. J Am Acad Dermatol. 2003;49:842.
11. Pisoni RL, Wikstrom B, Elder SJ, et al. Pruritus in haemodialysis patients: international results from the Dialysis Outcomes and Practice Patterns Study (DOPPS). Nephrol Dial Transplant. 2006;21:3495.
12. Narita I, Iguchi S, Omori K, Gejyo F. Uremic pruritus in chronic hemodialysis patients. J Nephrol. 2008;21:161–5.
13. De Marchi S, Cecchin E, Villalta D, et al. Relief of pruritus and decreases in plasma histamine concentrations during erythropoietin therapy in patients with uremia. N Engl J Med. 1992;326:969.
14. Cohen EP, Russell TJ, Garancis JC. Mast cells and calcium in severe uremic itching. Am J Med Sci. 1992;303:360.
15. Kessler M, Moneret-Vautrin DA, Cao-Huu T, et al. Dialysis pruritus and sensitization. Nephron. 1992;60:241.
16. Peer G, Kivity S, Agami O, et al. Randomised crossover trial of naltrexone in uraemic pruritus. Lancet. 1996;348:1552.
17. Hampers CL, Katz AI, Wilson RE, Merrill JP. Disappearance of "uremic" itching after subtotal parathyroidectomy. N Engl J Med. 1968;279:695.
18. Rosenthal SR. Uremic dermatitis. Arch Dermatol Syphil. 1931; 23:934.
19. Cawley EP, Hoch-Ligeti C, Bond GM. The eccrine sweat glands of patients in uremia. Arch Dermatol. 1961;84:51.
20. Massry SG, Popovtzer MM, Coburn JW, et al. Intractable pruritus as a manifestation of secondary hyperparathyroidism in uremia. Disappearance of itching after subtotal parathyroidectomy. N Engl J Med. 1968;279:697.
21. Duque MI, Thevarajah S, Chan YH, et al. Uremic pruritus is associated with higher kt/V and serum calcium concentration. Clin Nephrol. 2006;66:184.
22. Narita I, Alchi B, Ornori K, et al. Etiology and prognostic significance of severe uremic pruritus in chronic hemodialysis patients. Kidney Int. 2006;69:1626.
23. Hiroshige K, Kabashima N, Takasugi M, Kuroiwa A. Optimal dialysis improves uremic pruritus. Am J Kidney Dis. 1995;25:413.
24. Friga V, Linos A, Linos DA. Is aluminum toxicity responsible for uremic pruritus in chronic hemodialysis patients? Nephron. 1997;75:48.
25. Mettang T, Pauli-Magnus C, Kuhlmann U. "Sick-bag" syndrome [letter]. Perit Dial Int. 2000;20:243.
26. Noordzij M, Boeschoten EW, Bos WJ, for the NECOSAD Study Group, et al. Disturbed mineral metabolism is associated with muscle and skin complaints in a prospective cohort of dialysis patients. Nephrol Dial Transplant. 2007;22(10):2944–9.
27. Ada S, Seckin D, Budakoglu I, Ozdemir FN. Treatment of uremic pruritus with narrowband ultraviolet B phototherapy: an open pilot study. J Am Acad Dermatol. 2005;53:149.
28. Balaskas EV, Uldall RP. Erythropoietin treatment does not improve uremic pruritus. Perit Dial Int. 1992;12:330.
29. Pauli-Magnus C, Mikus G, Alscher DM, et al. Naltrexone does not relieve uremic pruritus: results of a randomized, double-blind, placebo-controlled crossover study. J Am Soc Nephrol. 2000;11:514.
30. Wikstrom B, Gellert R, Ladefoged SD, et al. {kappa}-Opioid system in uremic pruritus: multicenter, randomized, double-blind, placebo-controlled clinical studies. J Am Soc Nephrol. 2005; 16:3742.
31. Cho YL, Liu HN, Huang TP, Tarng DC. Uremic pruritus: role of parathyroid hormone and substance P. J Am Acad Dermatol. 1997;36:538.

32. Yoshimoto-Furuie K, Yoshimoto K, Tanaka T, et al. Effects of oral supplementation with evening primrose oil for six weeks on plasma essential fatty acids and uremic skin symptoms in hemodialysis patients. Nephron. 1999;81:151.
33. Gunal AI, Ozalp G, Yoldas TK, et al. Gabapentin therapy for pruritus in haemodialysis patients: a randomized, placebo-controlled, double-blind trial. Nephrol Dial Transplant. 2004;19:3137.
34. Layegh P, Mojahedi MJ, Malekshah PE, Pezeshkpour F, Vahedian M, Nazemian F, et al. Effect of oral granisetron in uremic pruritus. Indian J Dermatol Venereol Leprol. 2007;73(4):231–4.
35. Aucella F, Vigilante M, Gesuete A, Maruccio G, Specchio A, Gesualdo L. Uraemic itching: do polymethylmethacrylate dialysis membranes play a role? Nephrol Dial Transplant. 2007;22 Suppl 5:v8–12.
36. Aoike I. Clinical significance of protein adsorbable membranes – long-term clinical effects and analysis using a proteomic technique. Nephrol Dial Transplant. 2007;22 Suppl 5:v13–9.
37. Makhlough A. Topical capsaicin therapy for uremic pruritus in patients on hemodialysis. Iran J Kidney Dis. 2010;4:137–40.
38. Walsh JS, Fairley JA. Calcifying disorders of the skin. J Am Acad Dermatol. 1995;33:693–706.
39. Robinson-Bostom L, Digiovanna JJ. Cutaneous manifestations of end-stage renal disease. J Am Acad Dermatol. 2000;43(6):975.
40. Taylor EN, Henderson JM, Rennke HG, Magee CC. Traumatic calcinosis cutis in a dialysis patient. Am J Kidney Dis. 2004; 44(2):e18–21.
41. Van Haren FM, Ruiter DJ, Hillbrands LB. Nadroparin-induced calcinosis cutis in renal transplant recipients. Nephron. 2001;87(3):279–82.
42. Eich D, Scharffetter-Kochanek K, Weihrauch J, Krieg T, Hunzelmann N. Calcinosis of the cutis and subcutis: an unusual nonimmunologic adverse reaction to subcutaneous injections of low-molecular-weight calcium-containing heparins. J Am Acad Dermatol. 2004;50(2):210–4.
43. Nunley JR, Joness LM. Calcinosis cutis. http://www.emedicine.com.
44. Gupta RK, Naran S, Cheung YK. Fine-needle aspiration cytology of soft tissue calcinosis presenting as an enlarging mass in the chest wall. Diagn Cytopathol. 1998;19(6):465–7.
45. Solans EP, Bakhos R, Castelli MJ, Gattuso P. Fine needle aspiration biopsy of calcinosis cutis. A case report. Acta Cytol. 1997;41(2):590–2.
46. Deshpande A, Munshi M. Calcinosis cutis: diagnosis by aspiration cytology – a case report. Diagn Cytopathol. 1999;21(3):200–2.
47. Abdallah-Lotf M, Grasland A, Vinceneux P, Sigal-Grinberg M. Regression of cutis calcinosis with diltiazem in adult dermatomyositis. Eur J Dermatol. 2005;15(2):102–4.
48. Palamaras J, Kyriakis K. Calcium antagonists in dermatology: a review of the evidence and research-based studies. Dermatol Online J. 2005;11(2):8.
49. Palmieri GM, Sebes JL, Aelion JA, Moinuddin M, Ray MW, Wood GC, et al. Treatment of calcinosis with diltiazem. Arthritis Rheum. 1995;38(11):1646–54.
50. Grasses F, Perello J, Isern B, Prieto RM. Study of a myo-inositol hexaphosphate-based cream to prevent dystrophic calcinois cutis. Br J Dermatol. 2005;152(5):1022–5.
51. Grasses F, Perello J, Isern B, Prieto RM. Study of the absorption of myo-inositol hexakisphosphate (InsP6) through the skin. Biol Pharm Bull. 2005;28(4):764–7.
52. Santos PW, Hartle JE, Quarles LD. Calciphylaxis. http://www.UpToDate.com. Accessed 19 Aug 2007.
53. Fine A, Zacharias J. Calciphylaxis is usually non-ulcerating: risk factors, outcome and therapy. Kidney Int. 2002;61:2210.
54. Angelis M, Wong LL, Myers SA, Wong LM. Calciphylaxis in patients on hemodialysis: a prevalence study. Surgery. 1997; 122:1083.
55. Adrogue HJ, Frazier MR, Zeluff B, Suki WN. Systemic calciphylaxis revisited. Am J Nephrol. 1981;1:177.
56. Kent RB, Lylerly RT. Systemic calciphylaxis. South Med J. 1994;87:278.
57. Perloff LJ, Spence RK, Grossman RA, Barker CF. Lethal post-transplantation calcinosis. Transplantation. 1979;27:21.
58. Janigan DT, Hirsch DJ, Klassen GA, MacDonald AS. Calcified subcutaneous arterioles with infarcts of the subcutis and skin ("calciphylaxis") in chronic renal failure. Am J Kidney Dis. 2000;35:588.
59. Rezaie W, Overtoom HA, Flens M, Klaassen RJ. Calciphylaxis in chronic renal failure: an approach to risk factors. Indian J Nephrol. 2009;19:115–8.
60. Goyal S, Huhn KM, Provost TT. Calciphylaxis in a patient without renal failure or elevated parathyroid hormone: possible aetiological role of chemotherapy. Br J Dermatol. 2000;143:1087.
61. Riegert-Johnson DL, Kaur JS, Pfeifer EA. Calciphylaxis associated with cholangiocarcinoma treated with low-molecular-weight heparin and vitamin K. Mayo Clin Proc. 2001;76:749.
62. Barri YM, Graves GS, Knochel JP. Calciphylaxis in a patient with Crohn's disease in the absence of end-stage renal disease. Am J Kidney Dis. 1997;29:773.
63. Korkmaz C, Dundar E, Zubaroglu I. Calciphylaxis in a patient with rheumatoid arthritis without renal failure and hyperparathyroidism: the possible role of long-term steroid use and protein S deficiency. Clin Rheumatol. 2002;21:66.
64. Pollock B, Cunliffe WJ, Merchant WJ. Calciphylaxis in the absence of renal failure. Clin Exp Dermatol. 2000;25:389.
65. James LR, Lajoie G, Prajapati D, et al. Calciphylaxis precipitated by ultraviolet light in a patient with end-stage renal disease secondary to systemic lupus erythematosus. Am J Kidney Dis. 1999;34:932.
66. Igaki N, Moriguchi R, Hirota Y, et al. Calciphylaxis in a patient with end-stage renal disease secondary to systemic lupus erythematosus associated with acral gangrene and mesenteric ischemia. Intern Med. 2001;40:1232.
67. Sakr SH, Russell EB, Jasin HE. Systemic lupus erythematosus and calciphylaxis. J Rheumatol. 2004;31:1851.
68. Adrogue HJ, Frazier MR, Zeluff B, Suki WN. Systemic calciphylaxis revisited. Am J Nephrol. 1981;1:177–83.
69. Essary LR, Wick MR. Cutaneous calciphylaxis. An under recognized clinicopathologic entity. Am J Clin Pathol. 2000;113:280.
70. Bleibel W, Hazar B, Herman R. A case report comparing various radiological tests in the diagnosis of calcific uremic arteriolopathy. Am J Kidney Dis. 2006;48:659.
71. Wong JJ, Laumann A, Martinez M. Calciphylaxis and antiphospholipid antibody syndrome. J Am Acad Dermatol. 2000;42:849.
72. Fischer AH, Morris DJ. Pathogenesis of calciphylaxis: study of three cases with literature review. Hum Pathol. 1995;26:1055.
73. Rostaing L, el Feki S, Delisle MB, et al. Calciphylaxis in a chronic hemodialysis patient with protein S deficiency. Am J Nephrol. 1995;15:524.
74. Mehta RL, Scott G, Sloand JA, Francis CW. Skin necrosis associated with acquired protein C deficiency in patients with renal failure and calciphylaxis. Am J Med. 1990;88:252.
75. Heiss A, DuChesne A, Denecke B, et al. Structural basis of calcification inhibition by alpha 2-HS glycoprotein/fetuin-A. Formation of colloidal calciprotein particles. J Biol Chem. 2003;278:13333.
76. Schafer C, Heiss A, Schwarz A, et al. The serum protein alpha 2-Heremans-Schmid glycoprotein/fetuin-A is a systemically acting inhibitor of ectopic calcification. J Clin Invest. 2003;112:357.
77. Price PA, Williamson MK, Nguyen TM, Than TN. Serum levels of the fetuin-mineral complex correlate with artery calcification in the rat. J Biol Chem. 2004;279:1594.
78. Ketteler M, Bongartz P, Westenfeld R, et al. Association of low fetuin A (AHSG) concentrations in serum with cardiovascular

mortality in patients on dialysis: a cross-sectional study. Lancet. 2003;361:827.
79. Luo G, Ducy P, McKee MD, et al. Spontaneous calcification of arteries and cartilage in mice lacking matrix GLA protein. Nature. 1997;386:78.
80. Wallin R, Cain D, Sane DC. Matrix Gla protein synthesis and gamma-carboxylation in the aortic vessel wall and proliferating vascular smooth muscle cells – a cell system which resembles the system in bone cells. Thromb Haemost. 1999;82:1764.
81. Coates T, Kirkland GS, Dymock RB, et al. Cutaneous necrosis from calcific uremic arteriolopathy. Am J Kidney Dis. 1998;32:384.
82. Roe SM, Grahan LD, Brock WB, Barker DE. Calciphylaxis: early recognition and management. Am Surg. 1994;60:81.
83. Block GA. Prevalence and clinical consequences of elevated Ca x P product in hemodialysis patients. Clin Nephrol. 2000;54:318.
84. Bleyer AJ, White WL, Choi MJ. Calcific small vessel ischemic disease (calciphylaxis) in dialysis patients [editorial]. Int J Artif Organs. 2000;23:351.
85. Russell R, Brookshire MA, Zekonis M, Moe SM. Distal calcific uremic arteriolopathy in a hemodialysis patient responds to lowering of Ca x P product and aggressive wound care. Clin Nephrol. 2002;58:238.
86. Don BR, Chin AI. A strategy for the treatment of calcific uremic arteriolopathy (calciphylaxis) employing a combination of therapies. Clin Nephrol. 2003;59:463.
87. Velasco N, MacGregor MS, Innes A, MacKay IG. Successful treatment of calciphylaxis with cinacalcet – an alternative to parathyroidectomy? Nephrol Dial Transplant. 2006;21:1999.
88. Robinson MR, Augustine JJ, Korman NJ. Cinacalcet for the treatment of calciphylaxis. Arch Dermatol. 2007;143:152.
89. Sharma A, Burkitt-Wright E, Rustom R. Cinacalcet as an adjunct in the successful treatment of calciphylaxis. Br J Dermatol. 2006;155:1295.
90. Velasco N, MacGregor MS, Innes A, MacKay IG. Successful treatment of calciphylaxis with cinacalcet-an alternative to parathyroidectomy? Nephrol Dial Transplant. 2006;21:1999.
91. Kang AS, McCarthy JT, Rowland C, et al. Is calciphylaxis best treated surgically or medically? Surgery. 2000;128:967.
92. Girotto JA, Harmon JW, Ratner LE, et al. Parathyroidectomy promotes wound healing and prolongs survival in patients with calciphylaxis from secondary hyperparathyroidism. Surgery. 2001;130:645.
93. Cicone JS, Petronis JB, Embert CD, Spector DA. Successful treatment of calciphylaxis with intravenous sodium thiosulfate. Am J Kidney Dis. 2004;43:1104.
94. Brucculeri M, Cheigh J, Bauer G, Serur D. Long-term intravenous sodium thiosulfate in the treatment of a patient with calciphylaxis. Semin Dial. 2005;18:431.
95. Guerra G, Shah RC, Ross EA. Rapid resolution of calciphylaxis with intravenous sodium thiosulfate and continuous venovenous haemofiltration using low calcium replacement fluid: case report. Nephrol Dial Transplant. 2005;20:1260.
96. Aray CE, Fennell RS, Neiberger RE, Dharnidharka VR. Sodium thiosulfate treatment for calcific uremic arteriolopathy in children and young adults. Clin J Am Soc Nephrol. 2006;1:1161.
97. Meissner M, Kaufmann R, Gille J. Sodium thiosulfate: a new way of treatment for calciphylaxis? Dermatology. 2007;214:278–82.
98. Monney P, Nguyen QV, Perroud H, Descombes E. Rapid improvement of calciphylaxis after intravenous pamidronate therapy in a patient with chronic renal failure. Nephrol Dial Transplant. 2004;19:2130.
99. Podymow T, Wherrett C, Burns KD. Hyperbaric oxygen in the treatment of calciphylaxis: a case series. Nephrol Dial Transplant. 2001;16:2176.
100. Basile C, Montanaro A, Masi M, et al. Hyperbaric oxygen therapy for calcific uremic arteriolopathy: a case series. J Nephrol. 2002;15:676.
101. Centers for Disease Control and Prevention (CDC). Fibrosing skin condition among patients with renal disease – United States and Europe, 1997–2002. MMWR Morb Mortal Wkly Rep. 2002;51:25.
102. Cowper SE, Robin HS, Steinberg SM, et al. Scleromyxoedema-like cutaneous diseases in renal-dialysis patients. Lancet. 2000; 356:1000.
103. Hubbard V, Davenport A, Jarmulowicz M, Rustin M. Scleromyxoedema-like changes in four renal dialysis patients. Br J Dermatol. 2003;148:563.
104. Galan A, Cowper SE, Bucala R. Nephrogenic systemic fibrosis (nephrogenic fibrosing dermopathy). Curr Opin Rheumatol. 2006;18:614.
105. Cowper SE. Nephrogenic fibrosing dermopathy [NFD/NSF Website]. 2001–2007. http://www.icnfdr.org. Accessed 8 Sept 2007.
106. Auron A, Shao L, Warady BA. Nephrogenic fibrosing dermopathy in children. Pediatr Nephrol. 2006;21:1307.
107. Moschella SL, Kay J, Mackool BT, Liu V. Case records of the Massachusetts General Hospital. Weekly clinicopathologic exercises. Case 35-2004. A 68 year-old man with end-stage renal disease and thickening of the skin. N Eng J Med. 2004;351:2219.
108. Daram SR, Cortese CM, Bastani B. Nephrogenic fibrosing dermopathy/nephrogenic systemic fibrosis: report of a new case with literature review. Am J Kidney Dis. 2005;46:754.
109. Cowper SE. Nephrogenic fibrosing dermopathy: the first 6 years. Curr Opin Rheumatol. 2003;15:785.
110. Cowper SE, Bucala R, LeBoit PE. Case 35-2004: nephrogenic fibrosing dermopathy. N Engl J Med. 2005;352:1723.
111. Jimenez SA, Artlett CM, Sandorfi N, et al. Dialysis-associated systemic fibrosis (nephrogenic fibrosing dermopathy): study of inflammatory cells and transforming growth factor beta1 expression in affected skin. Arthritis Rheum. 2004;50:2660.
112. Marckmann P, Skov L, Rossen K, et al. Nephrogenic systemic fibrosis: suspected causative role of gadodiamide used for contrast-enhanced magnetic resonance imaging. J Am Soc Nephrol. 2006;17:2359.
113. Edsall LC, English 3rd JC, Teague MW, Patterson JW. Calciphylaxis and metastatic calcification associated with nephrogenic fibrosing dermopathy. J Cutan Pathol. 2004;31:247.
114. Samtleben W. Nephrogenic systemic fibrosis. Radiologe. 2007;47(9):778–84.
115. Mendoza FA, Artlett CM, Sandorfi N, et al. Description of 12 cases of nephrogenic fibrosing dermopathy and review of the literature. Semin Arthritis Rheum. 2006;35:238.
116. Levine JM, Taylor RA, Elman LB, et al. Involvement of skeletal muscle in dialysis-associated systemic fibrosis (nephrogenic fibrosing dermopathy). Muscle Nerve. 2004;30:569.
117. Ting WW, Stone MS, Madison KC, et al. Nephrogenic fibrosing dermopathy with systemic involvement. Arch Dermatol. 2003;139:903.
118. Kucher C, Steere J, Elenitsas R, et al. Nephrogenic fibrosing dermopathy/nephrogenic systemic fibrosis with diaphragmatic involvement in a patient with respiratory failure. J Am Acad Dermatol. 2006;54:S31.
119. Gibson SE, Farver CF, Prayson RA. Multiorgan involvement in nephrogenic fibrosing dermopathy: an autopsy case and review of the literature. Arch Pathol Lab Med. 2006;120:209.
120. Swartz RD, Crofford LJ, Phan SH, et al. Nephrogenic fibrosing dermopathy: a novel cutaneous fibrosing disorder in patients with renal failure. Am J Med. 2003;114:563.
121. Cowper SE, Bucala R, Leboit PE. Nephrogenic fibrosing dermopathy/nephrogenic systemic fibrosis- setting the record straight. Semin Arthritis Rheum. 2006;35:208.
122. Jennifer OB, Maize JC, Woolson RF, Bodisavljevic MN. Nephrogenic systemic fibrosis after exposure to gadolinium in patients with renal failure. Nephrol Dial Transplant. 2007; 22:3179–3185.

123. Deo A, Fogel M, Cowper SE. Nephrogenic systemic fibrosis: a population study examining the relationship of disease development to gadolinium exposure. Clin J Am Soc Nephrol. 2007;2(2):264–7.
124. Grobner T. Gadolinium – a specific trigger for the development of nephrogenic fibrosing dermopathy and nephrogenic systemic fibrosis? Nephrol Dial Transplant. 2006;21:1104.
125. Marckmann P, Skov L, Rossen K, et al. Nephrogenic systemic fibrosis: suspected causative role of gadodiamide used for contrast-enhanced magnetic resonance imaging. J Am Soc Nephrol. 2006;17:2359.
126. http://www.fda.gov/cder/drug/advisory/gadolinium_agents_20061222.htm.
127. Morcos SK, Haylor J. Pathophysiology of nephrogenic systemic fibrosis: a review of experimental data. World J Radiol. 2010; 2:427–33.
128. Thakral C, Alhariri J, Abraham JL. Long-term retention of gadolinium in tissues from nephrogenic systemic fibrosis patient after multiple gadolinium-enhanced MRI scans: case report and implications. Contrast Media Mol Imaging. 2007;2(4):199–205.
129. Sadowski EA, Bennett LK, Chan MR, et al. Nephrogenic systemic fibrosis: risk factors and incidence estimation. Radiology. 2007;243:148.
130. High WA, Ayers RA, Chandler J, et al. Gadolinium is detectable within the tissue of patients with nephrogenic systemic fibrosis. J Am Acad Dermatol. 2007;56:21.
131. Boyd AS, Zic JA, Abraham JL. Gadolinium deposition in nephrogenic fibrosing dermopathy. J Am Acad Dermatol. 2007;56:27.
132. Altun E, Martin DR, Wertman R, Lugo-Somolinos A, Fuller 3rd ER, Semelka RC. Nephrogenic systemic fibrosis: change in incidence following a switch in gadolinium agents and adoption of a gadolinium policy – report from two U.S. universities. Radiology. 2009;253:689–96.
133. Sadowski EA, Bennett LK, Chan MR, Wentland AL, Garrett AL, Garrett RW, et al. Nephrogenic systemic fibrosis: risk factors and incidence estimation. Radiology. 2007;243(1):148–57.
134. Swaminathan S, Shah SV. New insights into nephrogenic systemic fibrosis. J Am Soc Nephrol. 2007;18(10):2636–43.
135. Swaminathan S, Ahmed I, McCarthy JT, et al. Nephrogenic fibrosing dermopathy and high-dose erythropoietin therapy. Ann Intern Med. 2006;145:234.
136. Maloo M, Abt P, Kashyap R, et al. Nephrogenic systemic fibrosis among liver transplant recipients: a single institution experience and topic update. Am J Transplant. 2006;6:2212.
137. Baron PW, Cantos K, Hillebrand DJ, et al. Nephrogenic fibrosing dermopathy after liver transplantation successfully treated with plasmapheresis. Am J Dermatopathol. 2003;25:204.
138. Cowper SE, Su LD, Bhawan J, et al. Nephrogenic fibrosing dermopathy. Am J Dermatopathol. 2001;23:383.
139. Edsall LC, English 3rd JC, Teague MW, Patterson JW. Calciphylaxis and metastatic calcification associated with nephrogenic fibrosing dermopathy. J Cutan Pathol. 2004;31:247.
140. Miskulin D, Gul A, Rudnick M, Cowper S. Nephrogenic systemic fibrosis/nephrogenic fibrosing dermopathy in advanced renal failure. http://www.UpToDate.com. Accessed 22 Sept 2007.
141. Cowper SE, Bucala R. Nephrogenic fibrosing dermopathy: suspect identified, motive unclear. Am J Dermatopathol. 2003; 25:358.
142. Yerram P, Saab G, Karuparthi PR, Hayden MR, Khanna R. Nephrogenic systemic fibrosis: a mysterious disease in patients with renal failure – role of gadolinium-based contrast media in causation and the beneficial effect of intravenous sodium thiosulfate. Nephrogenic systemic fibrosis: relationship to gadolinium and response. Clin J Am Soc Nephrol. 2007;2(2):258–63.
143. Richmond H, Zwerner J, Kim Y, Fiorentino D. Nephrogenic systemic fibrosis: relationship to gadolinium and response to photopheresis. Arch Dermatol. 2007;143(8):1025–30.
144. Kafi R, Fisher GJ, Quqan T, et al. UV-A1 phototherapy improves nephrogenic fibrosing dermopathy. Arch Dermatol. 2004;140:1322.
145. Schmook T, Budde K, Ulrich C, et al. Successful treatment of nephrogenic fibrosing dermopathy in a kidney transplant recipient with photodynamic therapy. Nephrol Dial Transplant. 2005;20:220.
146. Gilliet M, Cozzio A, Burg G, Nestle FO. Successful treatment of three cases of nephrogenic fibrosing dermopathy with extracorporeal photopheresis. Br J Dermatol. 2005;152:531.
147. Lauchli S, Zortea-Caflisch C, Nestle FO, et al. Nephrogenic fibrosing dermopathy treated with extracorporeal photopheresis. Dermatology. 2004;208:278.
148. Fisher GJ, Datta S, Wang Z, et al. c-Jun-dependent inhibition of cutaneous procollagen transcription following ultraviolet irradiation is reversed by all-trans retinoic acid. J Clin Invest. 2000;106:663.
149. Yerram P, Saab G, Karuparthi PR, et al. Nephrogenic systemic fibrosis: a mysterious disease in patients with renal failure – role of gadolinium-based contrast media in causation and the beneficial effect of intravenous sodium thiosulfate. Clin J Am Soc Nephrol. 2007;2:258.
150. Chung HJ, Chung KY. Nephrogenic fibrosing dermopathy: response to high-dose intravenous immunoglobulin. Br J Dermatol. 2004;150:596.
151. http://www.fda.gov/cder/drug/advisory/gadolinum_agents.htm. Accessed 9 Sept 2007.
152. Ryali ME, Whittier WL. Bullous skin lesions in a patient undergoing chronic hemodialysis. Semin Dial. 2010;23:83–7.
153. Hebert AA, Farmer KL, Poh-Fitzpatrick MB. Peritoneal dialysis does not reduce serum porphyrin levels in porphyria cutanea tarda [letter]. Nephron. 1992;60:240.
154. Seubert S, Seubert A, Rumpf KW, Kiffe H. A porphyria cutanea tarda-like distribution pattern of porphyrins in plasma, hemodialysate, hemofiltrate, and urine of patients on chronic hemodialysis. J Invest Dermatol. 1985;85:107.
155. Kelly MA, O'Rourke KD. Treatment of porphyria cutanea tarda with phlebotomy in a patient on peritoneal dialysis. J Am Acad Dermatol. 2001;44:336.
156. Stevens BR et al. Porphyria cutanea tarda in the setting of renal failure. Arch Dermatol. 1993;129:337.
157. Sarkell B, Patterson JW. Treatment of porphyria cutanea tarda of end-stage renal disease with erythropoietin. J Am Acad Dermatol. 1993;29:499.
158. Gilchrest B, Rowe JW, Mihm Jr MC. Bullous dermatosis of hemodialysis. Ann Intern Med. 1975;83(4):480–3.
159. Griffon-Euvrard S, Thivolet J, Laurent G, et al. Detection of pseudo-porphyria cutanea tarda in 100 hemodialyzed patients (author's transl). Dermatologica. 1977;155(4):193–9.
160. Anderson KE, Goeger DE, Carson RW, et al. Erythropoietin for the treatment of porphyria cutanea tarda in a patient on long-term hemodialysis. N Engl J Med. 1990;322:315 [published erratum appears in N Engl J Med 1990; 322(22):1616.
161. Yaqoob M, Smyth J, Ahmad R, et al. Haemodialysis-related porphyria cutanea tarda and treatment by recombinant human erythropoietin. Nephron. 1992;60:428.
162. Peces R, Enriquez de Salamanca R, Fontanellas A, et al. Successful treatment of haemodialysis-related porphyria cutanea tarda with erythropoietin. Nephrol Dial Transplant. 1994;9:433.
163. Carson RW, Dunnigan EJ, DuBose Jr TD, et al. Removal of plasma porphyrins with high-flux hemodialysis in porphyria cutanea tarda associated with end-stage renal disease. J Am Soc Nephrol. 1992;2:1445.
164. Stockenhuber F, Kurz R, Grimm G, et al. Successful treatment of hemodialysis-related porphyria cutanea tarda with deferoxamine. Nephron. 1990;55:321.
165. Disler P, Day R, Burman N, et al. Treatment of hemodialysis-related Porphyria cutanea tarda with plasma exchange. Am J Med. 1982;72:989.

166. Anderson KE et al. Erythropoietin for the treatment of porphyria cutanea tarda in a patient on long-term hemodialysis. N Engl J Med. 1990;322:315.
167. Chazot C, Chazot I, Charra B, et al. Functional study of hands among patients dialysed for more than 10 years. Nephrol Dial Transplant. 1993;8(4):347–51.
168. Griffon-Euvrard S, Thivolet J, Laurent G, et al. Detection of pseudo-porphyria cutanea tarda in 100 hemodialyzed patients (author's transl). Dermatologica. 1977;155(4):193–9.
169. Amblard P, Cordonnier D, Reymond JL, et al. Pseudo-pseudo-porphyria tarda in hemodialyzed patients. Ann Dermatol Venereol. 1981;108(12):1019–20.
170. Gibson GE, McGinnity E, McGrath P, et al. Cutaneous abnormalities and metabolic disturbance of porphyrins in patients on maintenance haemodialysis. Clin Exp Dermatol. 1997;22(3):124–7.
171. Poh-Fitzpatricks MB. Bullous disease of dialysis. http://www.emedicine.com. Accessed 19 Sept 2007.
172. Poh-Fitzpatrick MB, Sosin AE, Bemis J. Porphyrin levels in plasma and erythrocytes of chronic hemodialysis patients. J Am Acad Dermatol. 1982;7(1):100–4.
173. Gafter U, Mamet R, Korzets A, et al. Bullous dermatosis of end-stage renal disease: a possible association between abnormal porphyrin metabolism and aluminium. Nephrol Dial Transplant. 1996;11(9):1787–91.
174. Schanbacher CF, Vanness ER, Daoud MS, et al. Pseudoporphyria: a clinical and biochemical study of 20 patients. Mayo Clin Proc. 2001;76:488–92.
175. Sharp MT, Horn TD. Pseudoporphyria induced by voriconazole. J Am Acad Dermatol. 2005;53:341.
176. Harvey E, Bell CH, Paller AS, et al. Pseudoporphyria cutanea tarda: two case reports on children receiving peritoneal dialysis and erythropoietin therapy. J Pediatr. 1992;121:749.
177. Lim CK, Rideout JM, Peters TJ. Pseudoporphyria associated with consumption of brewers' yeast. Br Med J (Clin Res Ed). 1984; 288:1640.
178. Poh-Fitzpatrick MB. Porphyria, pseudoporphyria, pseudopseudoporphyria...? [editorial]. Arch Dermatol. 1986;122:403.
179. Vadoud-Seyedi J, de Dobbeleer G, Simonart T. Treatment of haemodialysis-associated pseudoporphyria with N-acetylcysteine: report of two cases. Br J Dermatol. 2000;142(3):580–1.
180. Massone C, Ambros-Rudolph CM, Di Stefani A, Müllegger RR. Successful outcome of haemodialysis-induced pseudoporphyria after short-term oral N-acetylcysteine and switch to high-flux technique dialysis. Acta Derm Venereol. 2006; 86(6):538–40.
181. Cooke NS, McKenna K. A case of haemodialysis-associated pseudoporphyria successfully treated with oral N-acetylcysteine. Clin Exp Dermatol. 2007;32(1):64–6.

Cutaneous Manifestations of Gastrointestinal Diseases

María I. Vázquez-Roque and Wilfredo E. De Jesús-Monge

Many gastrointestinal diseases have a variety of cutaneous manifestations that may herald the start of the disease or correlate with disease activity. The gastrointestinal diseases and its cutaneous manifestations that will be discussed in this chapter are inflammatory bowel disease (Crohn's disease and ulcerative colitis), erythema nodosum, pyoderma gangrenosum, Sweet's syndrome, nutritional and metabolic disorders (dermatitis herpetiformis), lichen planus, gastrointestinal hemorrhage (Kaposi's sarcoma), and gastrointestinal neoplasias (necrolytic migratory erythema and Gardner's, Müir–Torre, Peutz–Jeghers, and Bazex's syndrome). Early recognition of the cutaneous manifestations associated with gastrointestinal diseases or neoplasia will lead to prompt referral of the patient (and relatives if indicated) for gastroenterological evaluation and successful prevention, diagnosis, or therapy of these illnesses. This, in turn, may guide to early intervention, management, and decrease the progression to advanced disease.

Inflammatory Bowel Disease

Inflammatory bowel disease (IBD) is a spectrum of diseases in the gastrointestinal tract that consists of immune activation and inflammation. The two major forms of IBD are Crohn's disease (CD) and ulcerative colitis (UC). Both illnesses may be accompanied by cutaneous manifestations. CD is a chronic, recurrent disease characterized by patchy transmural inflammation involving any segment of the gastrointestinal tract from the mouth to the anus [1]. Flares are often associated with abdominal pain and diarrhea. Nonspecific skin findings, such as fistulas and fissures, are found commonly in CD (Fig. 1). Painless anal fissures occur in 50–60% of patients. CD may have oral manifestations of cobblestoning, ulcerations, and nodules. CD activity is distinguished by metastatic sarcoidal-type granulomatous lesions in the skin or mucosa [2] (Figs. 2 and 3).

UC is a chronic inflammatory disease that affects the large bowel, particularly the mucosa and submucosa. The most common skin manifestations associated with UC are drug reactions related to sulfasalazine and mesalamine therapy, which can range from hypersensitivity to photosensitivity reactions. The most common dermatologic manifestations associated with IBD are erythema nodosum, pyoderma gangrenosum, and Sweet's syndrome, which will be discussed in further detail below.

Erythema Nodosum

Erythema nodosum (EN) is an inflammatory process of the subcutaneous fat, which presents with tender, deep subcutaneous nodules (Fig. 4). The distribution is most commonly on the pretibial areas bilaterally, but sometimes appear on the thighs and forearms [3]. EN can occur at any age, but there seems to be a sex predilection for women [3–5]. The proposed pathogenesis for EN is a delayed hypersensitivity reaction (type IV) to antigens such as bacteria, viruses, and drugs. EN develops in approximately 7% of patients with CD and in 4% of patients with UC, and typically follows the underlying bowel disease activity [4, 5]. In addition to IBD as causes of EN, infections commonly account for these lesions. The most common infections are streptococcal and mycobacterial infections, primary coccidioidomycosis, tuberculosis, *Yersinia pseudotuberculosis*, and *Yersinia enterocolitica* infections [6]. A case was reported of a 74-year-old woman who presented to hospital with fever, vomiting, diarrhea, and 2 weeks later developed erythema nodosum (EN) on the legs, and was diagnosed with *Y. enterocolitica* infection based on her clinical course and microbiological examination of the stool. We should suspect infection by *Y. enterocolitica* when diagnosing cases of EN with gastrointestinal symptoms. Based on this and other case reports, EN is likely to appear

M.I. Vázquez-Roque (✉) • W.E. De Jesús-Monge
Department of Medicine, University of Puerto Rico
School of Medicine, Medical Sciences Campus,
San Juan, Puerto Rico
e-mail: vazquezroque.maria@mayo.edu

N.P. Sánchez (ed.), *Atlas of Dermatology in Internal Medicine*,
DOI 10.1007/978-1-4614-0688-4_4, © Springer Science+Business Media, LLC 2012

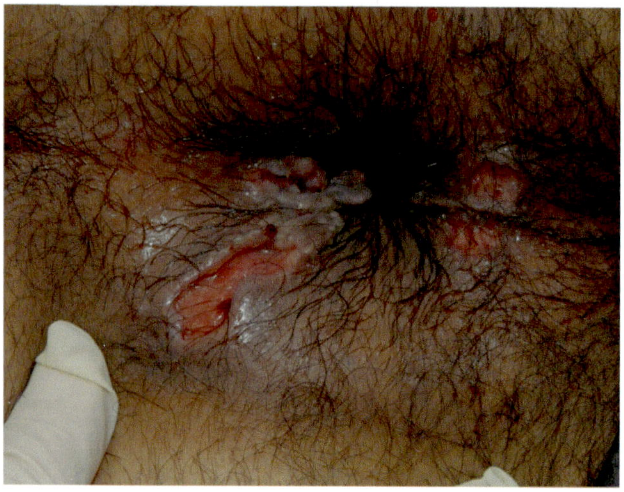

Fig. 1 Crohn's disease affecting perianal area

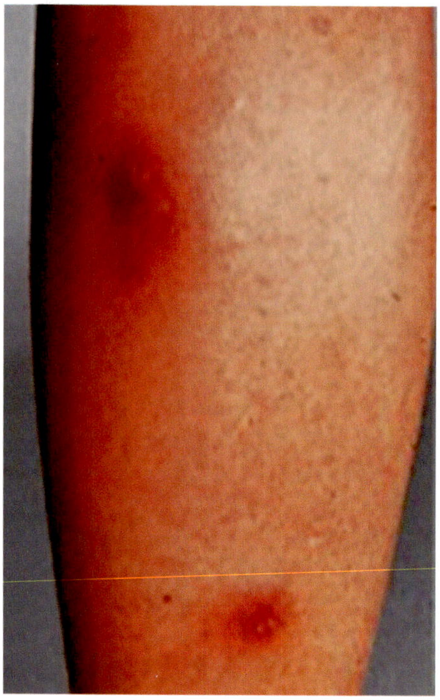

Fig. 2 Metastatic Crohn's disease may present as nodules with suppuration

2 weeks after the onset of gastrointestinal symptoms [7]. Medications have also been implicated as a causative agent, such as oral contraceptives and sulfasalazine. Histologically, EN is characterized as a panniculitis, with edematous septa and mild lymphocytic infiltrate. Early lesions may show a marked neutrophilic infiltrate and Miescher's microgranulomas, which are collections of macrophages within septa that are characteristic of EN [8].

The differential diagnosis of EN includes erythema induratum from tuberculosis, lupus panniculitis, and polyarteritis

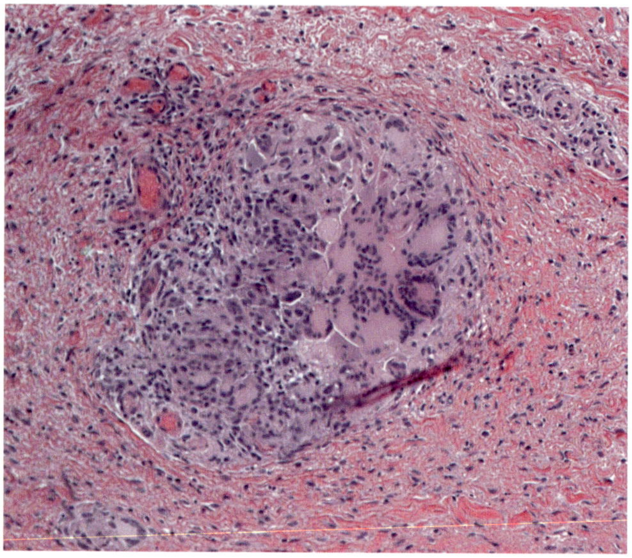

Fig. 3 Biopsy of a lesions of cutaneous Crohn's disease may demonstrate sarcoidal granulomas admixed with other inflammatory cells

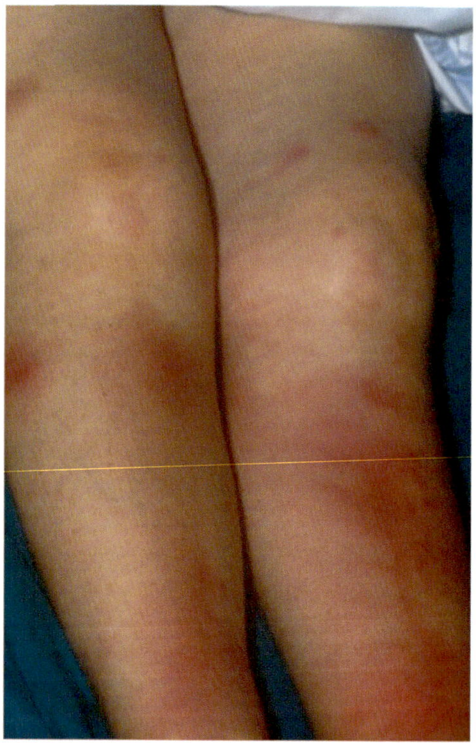

Fig. 4 Erythema nodosum: erythematous nodules localized on the pretibial areas bilaterally

nodosa. In the late stages, EN must be distinguished from simple bruises and contusions. The histologic finding of septal panniculitis is characteristic of EN. Evaluation should include a careful history and physical examination for prior upper respiratory infection, diarrheal illness, or deep fungal infection endemic to an area, and a chest X-ray, Mantoux

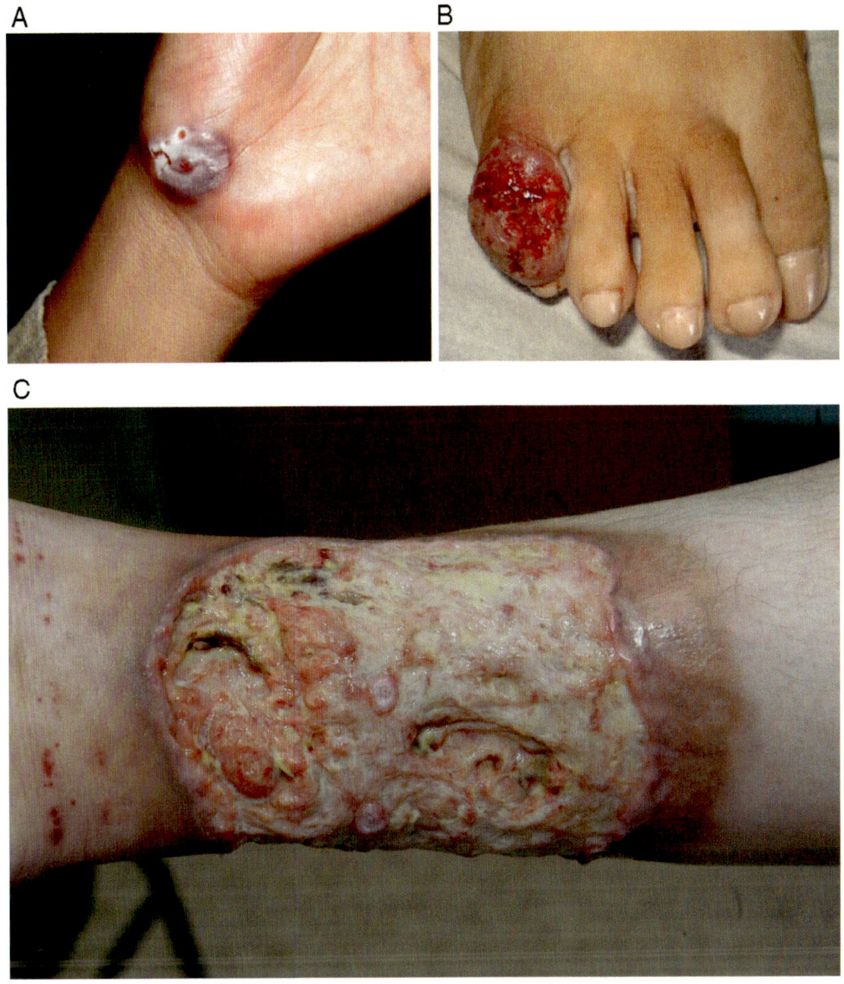

Fig. 5 (**a**–**c**) Pyoderma gangrenosum. (**a**, **b**) A painful violaceous plaque surrounded by a halo of erythema; (**c**) the ulcerative variant of pyoderma gangrenosum shows an undermined necrotic violaceous border and a purulent base

tuberculin (purified protein derivative, PPD) test, and two consecutive DNAseB titers at 2–4 week intervals [6].

Treatment of EN is mainly targeted at treating the underlying disease, bed rest, elevation of the legs, and anti-inflammatory agents, and/or potassium iodide for approximately 2 weeks [9–11]. A saturated solution of potassium iodide, 5–15 drops three times daily, results in prompt involution in many cases [6]. In severe and refractory cases systemic steroids and immunosuppressive therapy may be needed.

Pyoderma Gangrenosum

Pyoderma gangrenosum (PG) is an uncommon ulcerative disease strongly linked to systemic diseases, such as IBD, arthritis, and myeloproliferative disorders. While erythema nodosum represents the most common skin manifestation in IBD, affecting up to 15% of CD patients with a female predominance, pyoderma gangrenosum remains the most severe skin manifestation in IBD. In the Swiss Inflammatory Disease Cohort study, PG was identified in 2.2% of UC patients and 1.5% of CD patients [12]. The classic lesion is a painful ulcer with a necrotic, undermined border and a commonly purulent base (Fig. 5). The pathogenesis is thought to be due to a defect in cellular immunity and neutrophil function [13, 14]. Pathergy (an abnormal reaction to an allergen, either exaggerated and allergic or lessened and nonallergic) is always present, and not only initiates a lesion, but may aggravate it as well. These lesions are often misinterpreted as infected because of the purulence, but they are rarely associated with an infectious cause.

There are four different classifications for PG: ulcerative, bullous, pustular, and vegetative. Ulcerative PG presents as a painful necrotic ulcer with violaceous undermined borders. These ulcers are sterile and are specifically associated with IBD in approximately 5% of cases. The lesions in bullous PG progress from tense bullae to erosions to necrotic ulcers and have been described in patients with underlying hematologic disorders such as leukemia [15, 16]. Pustular PG is characterized by sterile painful pustules that can regress without scarring, but may progress to classical PG. These lesions are more commonly associated with IBD as well

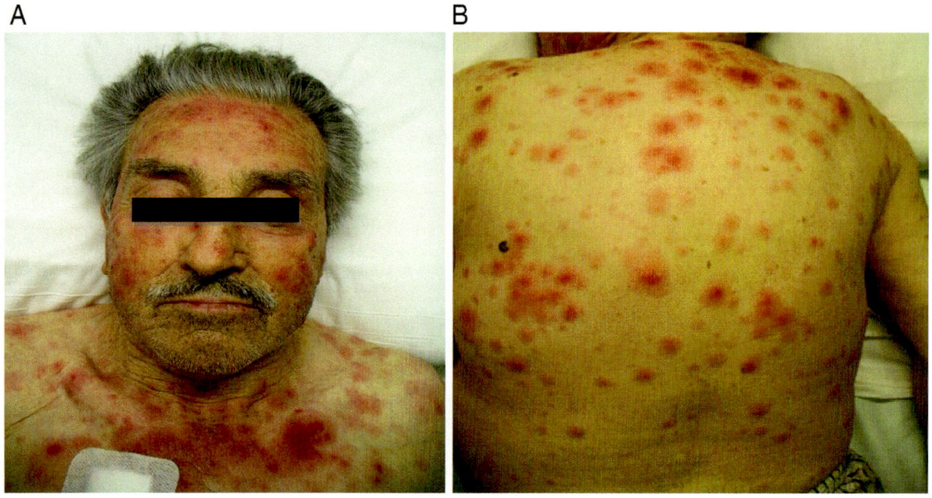

Fig. 6 (**a**, **b**) Sweet's syndrome: erythematous and edematous plaques affecting the face and trunk associated with fever and leukocytosis

[17]. Vegetative PG presents as a superficial ulcer without undermined borders and usually has a predilection for the trunk area. They often appear following trauma, such as surgery [18].

Early lesions of ulcerative PG are histologically characterized by mild-to-moderate perivascular lymphocytic infiltrates and endothelial swelling, and a dense neutrophilic infiltrate in the dermis [19]. Vegetative PG and late PG are characterized by granulomatous infiltrates of histiocytes, neutrophils, and giant cells. Bullous PG shows neutrophil-rich infiltrates and multilocular intraepidermal bullae [14].

The differential diagnosis of PG includes ulcers or pustules associated with CD, UC, diverticulitis, rheumatoid arthritis, systemic lupus erythematosus, lymphoma, leukemia, myeloproliferative disorders, carcinoma of breast, lung, colon, and prostate, Behçet's disease, and acquired immunodeficiency syndrome (AIDS) [2].

The evaluation of a patient with PG consists of a complete history and physical examination, followed by initial laboratory tests that include hematologic (complete blood count with differential, erythrocyte sedimentation rate by Westerngren, and peripheral smear), serum chemistries (kidney, liver, and bone), hormone (thyroid stimulating hormone and thyroxine levels), autoimmune (antinuclear antibody, antiphospholipid antibody, rheumatoid factor, antineutrophilic antibody, and cryoglobulins), and skin testing (biopsy and wound culture) [2].

The initial management of PG consists of local wound care with minimal or no debridement. It is important that debridement be avoided or kept at a minimum. The correct clinical diagnosis is of outmost importance because evaluation and treatment of the associated disease is imperative for management of skin involvement. The mainstay of therapy is systemic corticosteroids, with high doses often being necessary [2]. In severe disease, steroid sparing immunosuppressive agents may be of benefit such as azathioprine, cyclosporine, methotrexate, and mycophenolate mofetil [20–22]. PG associated with IBD has been shown to respond to sulfazalazine and dapsone, and recent reports have suggested that the use of anti-tumor necrosis factor-alpha agents such as infliximab and etanercept may be effective [23, 24]. Anti-TNFα therapy has shown effectiveness as a treatment option for PG in several clinical reports involving patients with PG or IBD with refractory PG. In a randomized, placebo-controlled trial, improvement in ulcer healing was observed as early as week 2 (primary endpoint) in 46% of patients versus placebo and, in a retrospective analysis, complete ulcer healing was observed in 72.7% (eight of 11 ulcers) after a mean of 12.5 weeks of anti-TNFα therapy [25]. Topical treatment with tacrolimus has also been reported in lesions that have a poor response to corticosteroids and peristomal PG [26].

Sweet's Syndrome

Sweet's syndrome is a febrile neutrophilic dermatosis that was first described in 1964 by Robert D. Sweet [27] and was originally named acute febrile neutrophilic dermatosis. It was renamed Sweet's syndrome in 1968 by C.H. Whittle [28]. It is a rare condition that occurs more frequently in women, has no racial predilection and may have pathergy as in PG. The clinical features include fever, peripheral neutrophilic leukocytosis, painful erythematous plaques and nodules on the extremities, head, and neck [2] (Fig. 6). A flu-like illness or upper respiratory tract infection may precede the skin lesions. Other systemic manifestations associated with Sweet's syndrome include neutrophilic pulmonary alveolitis, osteomyelitis, acute renal failure, transient involvement of the liver and pancreas, and aseptic meningitis [29].

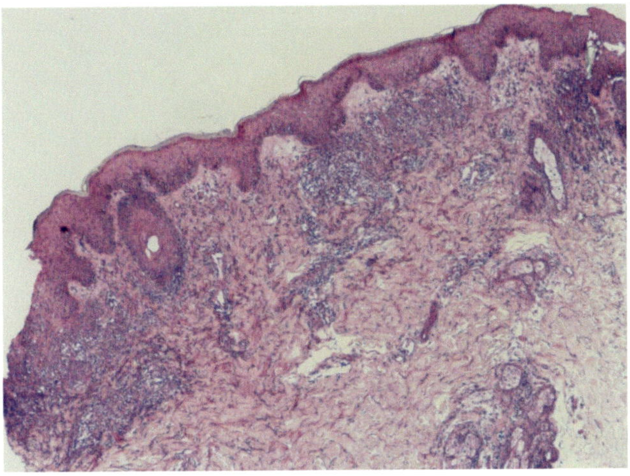

Fig. 7 Sweet's syndrome histopathology: edema of the papillary dermis accompanied with a dense nodular infiltrate composed primarily of neutrophils

Sweet's syndrome may be subdivided into three groups: classic, paraneoplastic or malignancy-associated, and drug-induced. Classic Sweet's syndrome is most commonly seen in IBD, and there are reports suggesting an association with *Helicobacter pylori* infection [30]. Malignancy-associated Sweet's syndrome occurs in approximately 10–15% of patients presenting with the characteristic lesions and is most often associated with lymphoproliferative disorders such as acute myelogenous leukemia and solid tumors of the gastrointestinal tract or breast [31–33]. The most common medications associated with drug-induced Sweet's syndrome are granulocyte colony-stimulating factor, all-trans retinoic acid, minocycline, trimethoprim–sulfamethoxazole, furosemide, hydralazine, and oral contraceptives, among others [34–36].

Histopathological examination of the lesions in Sweet's syndrome demonstrates numerous neutrophils infiltrating the superficial dermis, and significant edema of the papillary dermis [35] (Fig. 7). Direct immunofluorescence is negative.

The pathogenesis of Sweet's syndrome at present is unclear. Currently, it is thought to be secondary to an increased production of interleukin-1 and pro-inflammatory cytokines. This hypothesis is supported by the response of the disease to systemic corticosteroids [37, 38].

The differential diagnosis of Sweet's syndrome includes plaques and nodules associated with CD, UC, diverticulitis, rheumatoid arthritis, lymphoma, leukemia, myeloproliferative disorders, carcinoma of breast, lung, colon, kidney, ovaries, and prostate, Behçet's disease, AIDS, pregnancy, autoimmune disorders, and infections by *H. pylori* and *Y. enterocolitica* [2, 39].

The evaluation of a patient with Sweet's syndrome consists of a complete history and physical examination, followed by initial laboratory tests that include: hematologic (complete blood count with differential and erythrocyte sedimentation rate by Westerngren), serum chemistries (kidney, liver, pancreas, human immunodeficiency virus [HIV], beta-human chorionic gonadotropin, and alkaline phosphatase), autoimmune testing (antinuclear antibody, rheumatoid factor, and antineutrophilic antibody), and a skin biopsy.

The lesions in Sweet's syndrome may persist for weeks to months and usually resolve spontaneously, but recurrences are common. The simultaneous occurrence of Sweet's syndrome and erythema nodosum-like lesions in the same individual is not a rare entity; nevertheless, in only a limited number of cases in the literature have erythema nodosum-like lesions accompanying Sweet's syndrome have been biopsied, and reported as septal panniculitis without vasculitic features [40].

Treatment consists of systemic corticosteroid therapy, possibly for months, to suppress recurrences. Steroid-sparing agents are used in patients who have a potential systemic infection because corticosteroid use is contraindicated. Other alternative treatments include potassium iodide, colchicine, and dapsone [41]. Oral potassium iodide and colchicine may induce rapid resolution. Dapsone and cyclosporine may influence migration and other functions of neutrophils. There are reports of successful treatment of Sweet's syndrome with interferon-alpha but no controlled randomized clinical trials have been conducted to date [42].

Nutritional and Metabolic Disorders

Nutritional and metabolic disorders are usually associated with malabsorption because they are either a result of it, associated with it, caused by the disease process itself, or have a genetic susceptibility to it. Malabsorption results in the loss of vitamins and essential elements that result in eczematous eruptions, alterations in nails and hair, and changes in skin texture (specifically essential fatty acids, zinc, and vitamin B12). A common nutritional and metabolic disorder with cutaneous manifestations is dermatitis herpetiformis.

Dermatitis Herpetiformis

First described in 1884 by Dr. Louis Duhring, dermatitis herpetiformis (DH) is an extremely pruritic skin disorder characterized by vesicular or bullous lesions generally localized on the buttock and extensor areas, such as the elbows and knees [43] (Fig. 8). It has no association with herpes virus infection as the name suggests. This disease is most common in people from northern European ancestries and least common in African-Americans and Asians. It can appear in conjunction with gastrointestinal disease, usually celiac disease. Both of these disorders are associated with gluten (protein part of wheat, rye, barley, and other related grains)

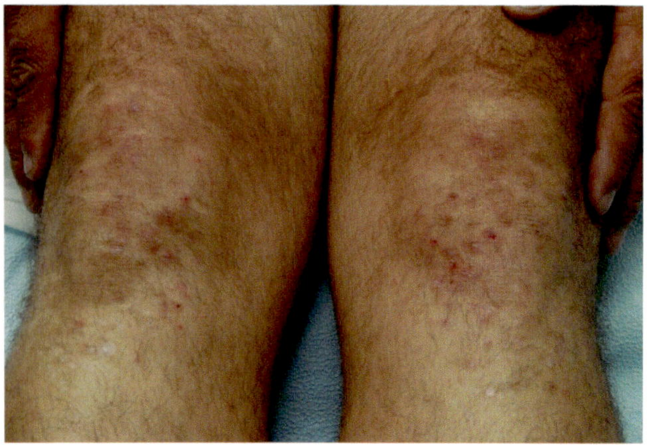

Fig. 8 Dermatitis herpetiformis: erythematous papules, vesicles, and erosions with crusts on the extensor areas

sensitivity as well as with the HLA haplotype DQ2 [44] and IgA anti-endomysial antibodies directed against tissue transglutaminase [45]. However, genetic and immune analysis is not needed for diagnosis.

Histological findings are consistent with neutrophilic infiltration of the dermal papillae and vesicle formation at the dermal–epidermal junction (Fig. 9). The hallmark of DH is the granular IgA deposition in the dermal papillae by direct immunofluorescence [6].

The differential diagnosis of DH includes the vesicular dermatoses: herpes simplex, herpes zoster, variola and vaccinia, vesiculobullous hand eczema, dermatophyte id reaction (allergy or sensitivity to fungi), and porphyria cutanea tarda [6].

The evaluation of a patient with DH starts with a complete history, especially directed towards malabsorption symptoms secondary to celiac sprue or gluten sensitive enteropathy with steatorrhea (passage of large amounts of fat in the feces). A complete physical examination and skin biopsy are of paramount importance. If appropriate, the diagnostic test is direct immunofluorescence analysis demonstrating granular deposits of IgA in the dermal papillae. The detection of IgA autoantibodies against epidermal transglutaminase is the most sensitive serological test in the diagnosis of dermatitis herpetiformis [46] .

Referral to a gastroenterologist is needed to evaluate for celiac sprue or gluten-sensitive enteropathy. Ingestion of gluten plays a role in the exacerbation of skin lesions, and strict long-term avoidance of dietary gluten has been shown to decrease the dose of dapsone (usually 100–200 mg daily) required to control the disease and may even eliminate the need for drug treatment [6]. A gluten-free diet may lead to clearing of vesicles, improvement in the intestinal mucosa, and disappearance of the IgA from the skin when reevaluated with immunofluorescence [42, 47].

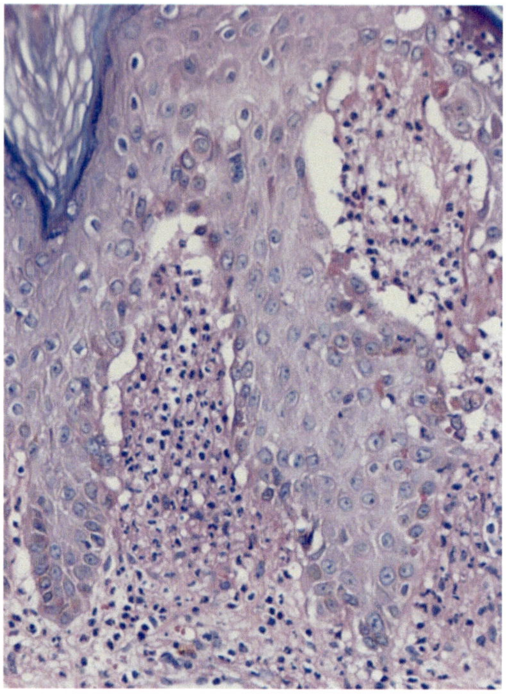

Fig. 9 Histopathological evaluation of the lesions in dermatitis herpetiformis reveals a neutrophilic infiltration in the tips of the dermal papillae and vesicle formation at the dermal–epidermal junction

Lichen Planus

Lichen planus is an inflammatory pruritic disease of the skin and mucous membranes characterized by papules especially in the bilateral flexor surfaces and trunk. Diagnostic findings are the skin lesions, mucosal lesions, and histopathology of band-like infiltration of lymphocytes and histiocytes with phagocytized melanin in the dermis [6]. Skin lesions are very pruritic, flat-topped, violaceous papules or plaques [2] (Fig. 10). Lacy white streaking or Wickham's striae may be on the penis, tongue, lips, buccal, and/or vaginal mucous membranes (Fig. 11). The nails are involved in 10% of patients with lichen planus (Fig. 12). The changes in the nails are secondary to damage to the nail matrix. A case was reported of a patient with LP limited to the toenails, which was successfully treated with etanercept monotherapy. The patient did not respond to previous treatment with potent corticosteroids and/or oral medication [48]. Lichen planus has been associated with viral hepatitis B and C, IBD, and primary biliary cirrhosis [2].

The differential diagnosis of lichen planus includes similar lesions produced by medications, psoriasis, lichen simplex chronicus, and syphilis. Diagnostic evaluation includes biopsy and often direct immunofluorescence for diagnosis. Topical corticosteroids are most helpful for localized disease in nonflexural areas. Psoralens plus long-wave ultraviolet light may be another effective treatment for lichen planus [6].

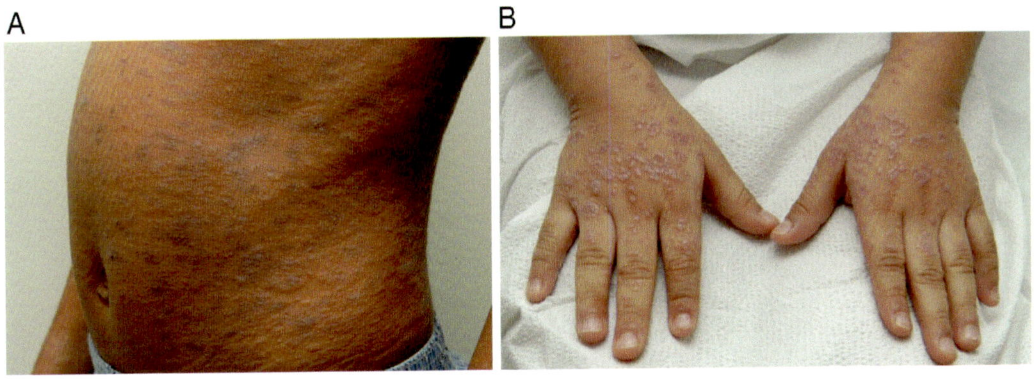

Fig. 10 (**a**, **b**) Lichen planus: flat-topped and violaceous papules and plaques affecting the trunk and the dorsum of the hands

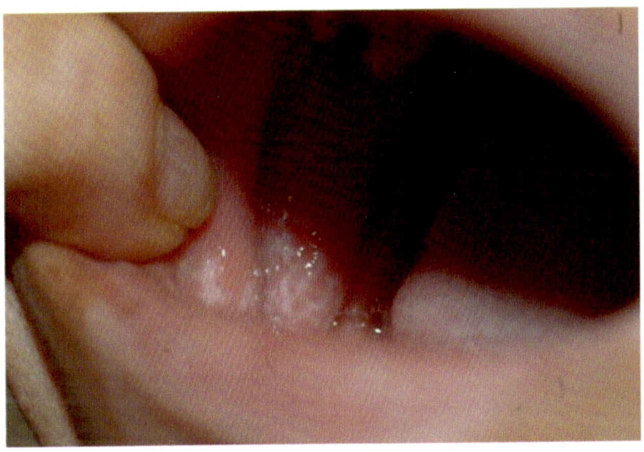

Fig. 11 Oral lichen planus: a whitish reticulated pattern of the buccal mucosa most commonly affecting this area of the mouth

Gastrointestinal Hemorrhage

Cutaneous syndromes are also associated with gastrointestinal hemorrhages. Vascular anomalies, connective tissue disorders, and vasculitis can lead to bleeding in the gastrointestinal tract [2]. Skin lesions could be premonitory of this deadly complication. In the following section, we will discuss Kaposi's sarcoma.

Kaposi's Sarcoma

Kaposi's sarcoma is a vascular neoplasm associated with HIV infection and elderly men of Mediterranean ancestry [2]. It is characterized by red or purple plaques or nodules on cutaneous or mucosal surfaces (Fig. 13). Kaposi's sarcoma involves the gastrointestinal tract in 50–80% of patients with skin involvement and virtually 100% of patients with oral lesions [2]. Human herpes virus 8 is present in all forms of Kaposi's sarcoma lesions and circulating B lymphocytes in patients [6]. Gastrointestinal bleeding may be significant but, when asymptomatic, these lesions often go undiagnosed [6].

The differential diagnosis of Kaposi's sarcoma includes pyogenic granuloma, hemangioma, lymphangioma, hemangioendothelioma, hemangiopericytoma, and bacillary angiomatosis.

Evaluation for Kaposi's sarcoma includes a complete physical examination, medical history, and a lesion biopsy [49]. Kaposi's sarcoma in the elderly is treated with intralesional chemotherapy or radiation. If the patient is on iatrogenic immunosuppression, therapy entails reducing the doses of the immunosuppressors. Kaposi's sarcoma in an HIV male who has sex with other males has been reported sporadically. It resembles classic Kaposi's sarcoma but occurring at a younger age, it is limited to the skin and has a good prognosis [50].

AIDS-associated Kaposi's sarcoma is first treated with antiretroviral therapy [6]. Once a cutaneous or mucosal Kaposi's sarcoma lesion is diagnosed, gastroenterology should be consulted for endoscopy and/or colonoscopy to look for Kaposi's sarcoma lesions in the gastrointestinal tract for early detection of a source of significant bleeding [49].

Gastrointestinal Neoplasias

Prompt recognition of cutaneous manifestations is of extreme importance in recognizing individuals with neoplasias or those predisposed to develop cancer. In this section, we will discuss the most common cutaneous manifestations of gastrointestinal neoplasias: Gardner's syndrome, Müir–Torre syndrome, Peutz–Jeghers syndrome, Bazex's syndrome, and necrolytic migratory erythema.

Gardner's Syndrome

Gardner's syndrome, a variant of familial adenomatous polyposis (FAP), is an autosomal dominant disorder caused by the mutation of the adenomatous polyposis coli (APC) gene on chromosome [5]. Cutaneous features appear in approximately 50% of affected individuals and are often present

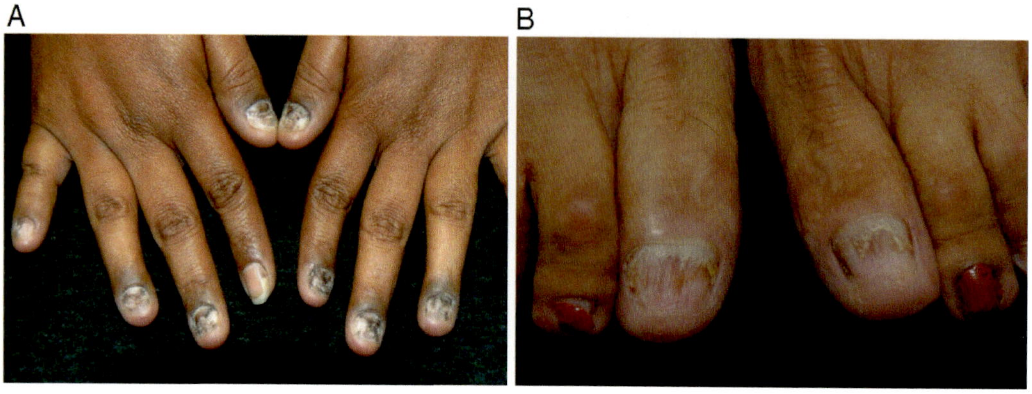

Fig. 12 (**a**, **b**) Lichen planus: nail dystrophy and a violaceous periungual discoloration

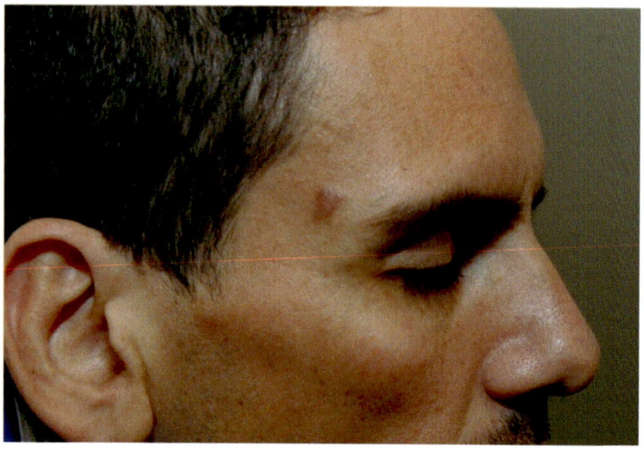

Fig. 13 Kaposi's sarcoma on the face

before the polyps become symptomatic. It is characterized by multiple epidermoid cysts of the face, scalp, and extremities, as well as multiple osteomas and desmoid tumors [51, 52]. The earliest marker of disease is the presence of multiple osteomas at the angles of the mandible. Although most osteomas are asymptomatic, the patient can present with headaches, facial pain, rhinorrhea, and sinusitis [53]. An oral manifestation of supernumerary teeth can also occur. Desmoid tumors occur in approximately 10% of patients [52]. Although surgery is widely accepted as the first-line of treatment, the high recurrence rate has led some authors to suggest that surgery should be avoided, except for bypass of bowel obstructions or relief of ureteric obstructions caused by intraabdominal desmoids tumors. Pharmacological pain control with nonsteroidal anti-inflammatory drugs and an anti-estrogen agent are the most widely documented management. Chemotherapy and radiotherapy are also alternatives considered in symptomatic patients who do not respond to conventional medical therapy [54].

The importance of recognizing this syndrome is that the colonic polyps have a 100% chance of developing into colonic carcinomas before the age of 40, so referral to a gastroenterologist for colonoscopy is urgent and mandatory [2].

Surgical management with prophylactic colectomy is recommended to prevent the evolution of the adenomatous polyps to adenocarcinoma [55]. Other neoplasms that may be seen are duodenal carcinomas, endocrine tumors, thyroid carcinomas, or hepatoblastomas [2].

Müir–Torre Syndrome

Müir–Torre syndrome (MTS) is a rare, autosomal dominant disorder that presents with multiple sebaceous neoplasms (with or without keratoacanthomas) and a visceral malignancy, usually of the proximal colon [56]. Familial aggregation has been reported, suggesting an association with hereditary nonpolyposis colorectal cancer (HNPCC) or Lynch syndrome. This syndrome is caused by a germline mutation in at least one of the DNA mismatch repair genes, most commonly MLH-1 and MSH-2, the same genes known to cause Lynch syndrome. This insight has led MTS to be considered a phenotypic variant of Lynch syndrome [57, 58]. The criteria for the clinical diagnosis of Lynch syndrome (Amsterdam II criteria) are (1) three or more relatives with an Lynch syndrome-associated cancers (colon, rectum, endometrium, small bowel, ureter, or renal pelvis), (2) one is a first-degree relative of the other two, (3) at least two successive generations are affected, (4) at least one is diagnosed before age 50, and (5) FAP has been excluded [59]. Tumors of the genitourinary tract (especially ureter and endometrium) are the most common visceral neoplasms seen in MTS after colorectal cancer [58].

The most common cutaneous manifestions are sebaceous neoplasms of the head and neck region (Fig. 14). Clinically, MTS diagnosis requires the presence of a cutaneous sebaceous adenoma, a sebaceous epithelioma, a basal cell epithelioma with sebaceous differentiation, a keratoacanthoma with sebaceous differentiation, or a sebaceous carcinoma in addition to at least one visceral malignancy. Alternatively, the diagnosis of MTS can be made with the presence of multiple keratoacanthomas and visceral malignancies in the context of a family history of MTS [56, 60].

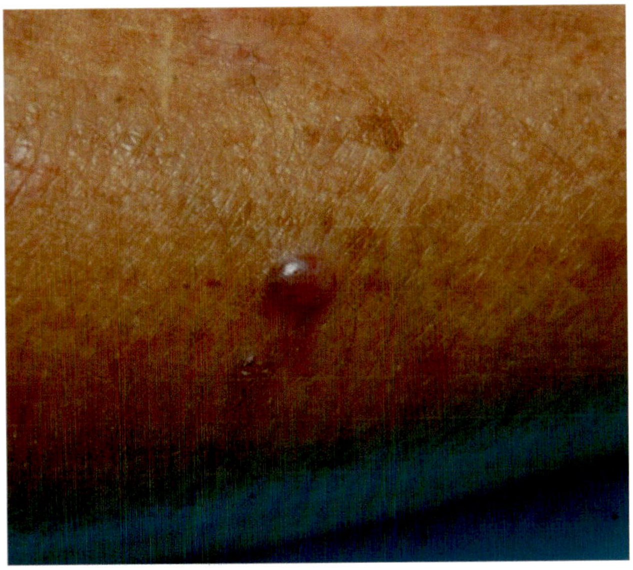

Fig. 14 Müir–Torre syndrome. Sebaceous carcinoma in a colon cancer patient

Evaluation includes a meticulous family history and timely referral to a gastroenterologist for colonoscopy and appropriate search for gastrointestinal malignancy in the patient. If Lynch syndrome is suspected, the patient and relatives must undergo gastroenterological, gynecological, and genetic counseling evaluation for malignancy screening or diagnosis. The benign sebaceous tumors can be treated with curettage, excision, cryosurgery, or radiotherapy. Sebaceous carcinoma lesions should be excised using Mohs micrographic surgery. Oral retinoids with or without interferon-alpha may be useful in the prevention of new skin tumor development [61, 62].

Peutz–Jeghers Syndrome

Peutz–Jeghers syndrome is an autosomal dominant disorder composed of mucocutaneous hyperpigmentation and hamartomatous polyps in the gastrointestinal tract. Hamartomas are lesions that resemble neoplasms but actually results from faulty development in an organ. This syndrome was first described in 1921 by Johannes L. Peutz and in 1949 by Harold J. Jeghers [63, 64]. It is now known that Peutz Jeghers syndrome is caused by germline mutations in the *STK11/LKB1* gene [65, 66]. The lesions appear in early childhood and consist of dark brown 0.1–1 cm macules on the lips, oral mucosa, acral and periorbital areas, and anus. The malignancy most commonly associated with this syndrome is colorectal, gastric and duodenal cancer which arises from the hamartomatous polyps. Female patients also have an increased incidence of developing tumors of the ovary and breast [67]. Large hamartomatous polyps can lead to bleeding, intussusception, or obstruction [1]. For these reasons, once mucocutaneous lesions are seen, a referral to a gastroenterologist is desirable to evaluate for gastrointestinal hamartomatous polyp presence and removal. Genetic testing for the mutation is also available [1]. Cancer surveillance guidelines have been published, but the efficacy is unproven [68].

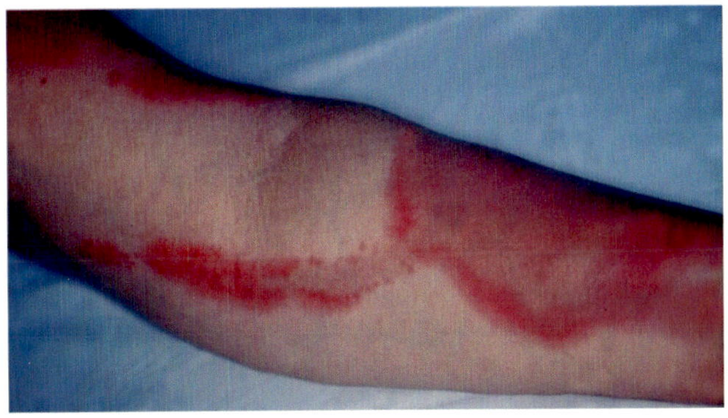

Fig. 15 Necrolytic migratory erythema: annular, migratory erythematous plaques affecting the extremities

Bazex's Syndrome

Paraneoplastic acrokeratosis of Bazex, or Bazex's syndrome, is a rare acquired syndrome associated primarily with squamous cell esophageal carcinoma that mostly affects mostly men over 40 years old [69]. It is also associated with carcinoma of the larynx and tongue [2]. The characteristic cutaneous finding is a psoriasiform eruption that favors acral areas, eventually progressing to the nose, ears, scalp, and face [70]. Other findings are thickening of the periungual skin with marked nail dystrophy and thickening of the palms and soles. The skin findings precede diagnosis of the tumor by approximately 1 year in 63% of patients [70].

The finding of such characteristic lesions allows for opportune referral to a gastroenterologist for esophagogastroduodenoscopy, searching for upper gastrointestinal malignancy. Bazex's syndrome usually responds to successful treatment of the underlying tumor.

Necrolytic Migratory Erythema

The presence of a glucagonoma, a tumor of the pancreatic islet cells, may lead to the development of necrolytic migratory erythema of the skin, although this skin condition has been reported with other malignancies as well [71, 72]. This rash consists of periods of painful erythema with blisters and erosions around flexural regions, fingers, and orifices (Fig. 15). Angular cheilitis and painful glossitis can also occur. On histological evaluation, there is necrosis of the upper portions of the epidermis. The pathogenesis is related to the metabolic disarrangements of amino acids as a result of excess glucagon production [71]. Acrodermatitis enteropathica is on the differential diagnosis.

The finding of the distinctive lesions requires referral to a gastroenterologist for evaluation of a pancreatic tumor. The cutaneous symptoms usually resolve with successful surgical removal of the tumor.

Conclusions

As previously discussed, some gastrointestinal diseases have a variety of cutaneous manifestations: IBD (Crohn's disease and ulcerative colitis), nutritional and metabolic disorders (dermatitis herpetiformis), gastrointestinal hemorrhage (Kaposi's sarcoma), and gastrointestinal neoplasias (Gardner's syndrome, MTS, Peutz–Jeghers syndrome, Bazex's syndrome, and necrolytic migratory erythema), among others. Early recognition by dermatologists of cutaneous manifestations associated with gastrointestinal diseases or neoplasia will lead to prompt referral of the patient (and relatives if indicated) for gastroenterological evaluation and successful prevention, diagnosis, or therapy of these illnesses. This, in turn, may guide the patient to early intervention, management, and decreased risk of progression to advanced disease.

References

1. McQuaid KR. Alimentary tract. In: Tierney LM, McPhee SJ, Papadakis MA, editors. Lange current medical diagnosis & treatment. 43rd ed. New York: McGraw-Hill; 2004. p. 515–622.
2. Boh EE, al-Smadi RM. Cutaneous manifestations of gastrointestinal diseases. Dermatol Clin. 2002;20:533–46.
3. Cribier B, Caille A, Heid E, Grosshans E. Erythema nodosum and associated diseases. A study of 129 cases. Int J Dermatol. 1998;37:667–72.
4. Garcia-Porrua C, Gonzalez-Gay MA, Vazquez-Caruncho M, et al. Erythema nodosum: etiologic and predictive factors in a defined population. Arthritis Rheum. 2000;43:584–92.
5. Mert A, Ozaras R, Tabak F, et al. Erythema nodosum: an experience of 10 years. Scand J Infect Dis. 2004;36:424–7.
6. Berger TG. Skin, hair, & nails. In: Tierney LM, McPhee SJ, Papadakis MA, editors. Lange current medical diagnosis & treatment. 43rd ed. New York: McGraw-Hill; 2004. p. 81–144.
7. Yotsu R, Mii S, Hayashi R, Harada H, Furukawa K, Eto H. Erythema nodosum associated with *Yersinia enterocolitica* infection. J Dermatol. 2010;37(9):819–22.
8. Senturk T, Aydintug O, Kuzu I, et al. Adhesion molecule expression in erythema nodosum-like lesions in Behcet's disease. A histopathological and immunohistochemical study. Rheumatol Int. 1998;18:51–7.
9. Hanauer SB. How do I treat erythema nodosum, aphthous ulcerations, and pyoderma gangrenosum? Inflamm Bowel Dis. 1998;4:70. discussion 73.
10. Horio T, Imamura S, Danno K, Ofuji S. Potassium iodide in the treatment of erythema nodosum and nodular vasculitis. Arch Dermatol. 1981;117:29–31.
11. Marshall JK, Irvine EJ. Successful therapy of refractory erythema nodosum associated with Crohn's disease using potassium iodide. Can J Gastroenterol. 1997;11:501–2.
12. Vavricka SR et al. Frequency and risk factors for extraintestinal manifestations in the Swiss inflammatory bowel disease cohort. Am J Gastroenterol. 2011;106(1):110–9.
13. Jorizzo JL, Solomon AR, Zanolli MD, Leshin B. Neutrophilic vascular reactions. J Am Acad Dermatol. 1988;19:983–1005.
14. Huang W, McNeely MC. Neutrophilic tissue reactions. Adv Dermatol. 1997;13:33–64.
15. Fox LP, Geyer AS, Husain S, Grossman ME. Bullous pyoderma gangrenosum as the presenting sign of fatal acute myelogenous leukemia. Leuk Lymphoma. 2006;47:147–50.
16. Wiseman DH, Hunter HJ, Dennis M. Bullous pyoderma gangrenosum in acute myeloid leukaemia. Eur J Haematol. 2007;79:91–2.
17. Shankar S, Sterling JC, Rytina E. Pustular pyoderma gangrenosum. Clin Exp Dermatol. 2003;28:600–3.
18. Langan SM, Powell FC. Vegetative pyoderma gangrenosum: a report of two new cases and a review of the literature. Int J Dermatol. 2005;44:623–9.
19. Hurwitz RM, Haseman JH. The evolution of pyoderma gangrenosum. A clinicopathologic correlation. Am J Dermatopathol. 1993;15:28–33.
20. Powell FC, O'Kane M. Management of pyoderma gangrenosum. Dermatol Clin. 2002;20:347–55, viii.
21. Powell FC, Collins S. Pyoderma gangrenosum. Clin Dermatol. 2000;18:283–93.
22. Powell FC, Su WP, Perry HO. Pyoderma gangrenosum: classification and management. J Am Acad Dermatol. 1996;34:395–409. quiz 410–2.
23. Reguiai Z, Grange F. The role of anti-tumor necrosis factor-alpha therapy in Pyoderma gangrenosum associated with inflammatory bowel disease. Am J Clin Dermatol. 2007;8:67–77.
24. Regueiro M, Valentine J, Plevy S, et al. Infliximab for treatment of pyoderma gangrenosum associated with inflammatory bowel disease. Am J Gastroenterol. 2003;98:1821–6.
25. Kirsner RS. Biological agents for chronic wounds. Am J Clin Dermatol. 2010;11 Suppl 1:23–5.
26. Chiba T, Isomura I, Suzuki A, Morita A. Topical tacrolimus therapy for pyoderma gangrenosum. J Dermatol. 2005;32:199–203.
27. Sweet RD. An acute febrile neutrophilic dermatosis. Br J Dermatol. 1964;76:349–56.
28. Whittle CH, Beck GA, Champion RH. Recurrent neutrophilic dermatosis of the face – a variant of Sweet's syndrome. Br J Dermatol. 1968;80:806–10.
29. Fett DL, Gibson LE, Su WP. Sweet's syndrome: systemic signs and symptoms and associated disorders. Mayo Clin Proc. 1995;70: 234–40.
30. Kurkcuoglu N, Aksoy F. Sweet's syndrome associated with Helicobacter pylori infection. J Am Acad Dermatol. 1997;37: 123–4.
31. Cohen PR, Kurzrock R. Sweet's syndrome and malignancy. Am J Med. 1987;82:1220–6.
32. Cohen PR, Talpaz M, Kurzrock R. Malignancy-associated Sweet's syndrome: review of the world literature. J Clin Oncol. 1988;6:1887–97.
33. Cohen PR, Kurzrock R. Sweet's syndrome and cancer. Clin Dermatol. 1993;11:149–57.
34. Cohen PR, Kurzrock R. Sweet's syndrome: a neutrophilic dermatosis classically associated with acute onset and fever. Clin Dermatol. 2000;18:265–82.
35. Cohen PR, Kurzrock R. Sweet's syndrome revisited: a review of disease concepts. Int J Dermatol. 2003;42:761–78.
36. Thompson DF, Montarella KE. Drug-induced Sweet's syndrome. Ann Pharmacother. 2007;41:802–11.
37. Giasuddin AS, El-Orfi AH, Ziu MM, El-Barnawi NY. Sweet's syndrome: is the pathogenesis mediated by helper T cell type 1 cytokines? J Am Acad Dermatol. 1998;39:940–3.
38. Going JJ. Is the pathogenesis of Sweet's syndrome mediated by interleukin-1? Br J Dermatol. 1987;116:282–3.

39. Rugo HS. Cancer. In: Tierney LM, McPhee SJ, Papadakis MA, editors. Lange current medical diagnosis & treatment. 43rd ed. New York: McGraw-Hill; 2004. p. 1577–635.
40. Tabanlioglu D, Boztepe G, Erkin G, Gokoz O, Karaduman A. Sweet's syndrome and erythema nodosum: a companionship or a spectrum? – A case report with review of literature. Int J Dermatol. 2010;49(1):62–6.
41. Cohen PR, Kurzrock R. Sweet's syndrome: a review of current treatment options. Am J Clin Dermatol. 2002;3:117–31.
42. Bianchi L, Masi M, Hagman JH, et al. Systemic interferon-alpha treatment for idiopathic Sweet's syndrome. Clin Exp Dermatol. 1999;24:443–5.
43. Duhring LA. Landmark article, Aug 30, 1884: dermatitis herpetiformis. By Louis A. Duhring. JAMA. 1983;250:212–6.
44. Hall RP, Sanders ME, Duquesnoy RJ, et al. Alterations in HLA-DP and HLA-DQ antigen frequency in patients with dermatitis herpetiformis. J Invest Dermatol. 1989;93:501–5.
45. Olbricht SM, Flotte TJ, Collins AB, et al. TJ. Dermatitis herpetiformis. Cutaneous deposition of polyclonal IgA1. Arch Dermatol. 1986;122:418–21.
46. Rose C, Brocker EB, Zillikens D. Clinical, histological and immunopathological findings in 32 patients with dermatitis herpetiformis. J Dtsch Dermatol Ges. 2010;8(4):265–71.
47. van der Meer JB. Gluten-free diet and elemental diet in dermatitis herpetiformis. Int J Dermatol. 1990;29:679–92.
48. Irla N, Schneiter T, Haneke E, Yawalkar N. Nail Lichen Planus: successful treatment with Etanercept. Case Rep Dermatol. 2010; 2(3):173–6.
49. NCI. Kaposi sarcoma treatment (PDQ®): patient version: U.S. National Institutes of Health; 2007.
50. Potthoff A, Brockmeyer NH, Stucker M, Wieland U, Krenter A. Kaposi Sarcoma in a HIV uninfected man who has sex with men. Eur J Med Res. 2010;15(2):79–80.
51. Wijn MA, Keller JJ, Giardiello FM, Brand HS. Oral and maxillofacial manifestations of familial adenomatous polyposis. Oral Dis. 2007;13:360–5.
52. Finan MC, Ray MK. Gastrointestinal polyposis syndromes. Dermatol Clin. 1989;7:419–34.
53. Alexander AA, Patel AA, Odland R. Paranasal sinus osteomas and Gardner's syndrome. Ann Otol Rhinol Laryngol. 2007;116: 658–62.
54. Chung J, Namkoong S, Jung KE, Park JW, Park BC, Cinn YW, et al. A case of Gardner's syndrome associated with desmoid tumor. Ann Dermatol. 2010;22(4):418–21.
55. Nunez Nunez R, Galan Gomez E, Moreno Hurtado C, et al. [Familial adenomatous polyposis: Gardner's syndrome]. Cir Pediatr. 2006;19:111–4.
56. Schwartz RA, Torre DP. The Muir-Torre syndrome: a 25-year retrospect. J Am Acad Dermatol. 1995;33:90–104.
57. Lachiewicz AM, Wilkinson TM, Groben P, et al. Muir-Torre syndrome. Am J Clin Dermatol. 2007;8:315–9.
58. Lynch MC, Anderson BE. Ileocecal Adenocarcinoma and unilateral transitional cell carcinoma with multiple sebaceous tumors and keratoacanthomas in a case of Muir-Torre syndrome. Dermatol Res Pract. 2010;2010. pii:173160.
59. Vasen HF, Watson P, Mecklin JP, Lynch HT. New clinical criteria for hereditary nonpolyposis colorectal cancer (HNPCC, Lynch syndrome) proposed by the International Collaborative group on HNPCC. Gastroenterology. 1999;116:1453–6.
60. Morales A, Figueroa LD. Muir-Torre syndrome. Caribb J Dermatol Ther. 2006;3:33–5.
61. Spielvogel RL, DeVillez RL, Roberts LC. Oral isotretinoin therapy for familial Muir-Torre syndrome. J Am Acad Dermatol. 1985;12:475–80.
62. Graefe T, Wollina U, Schulz H, Burgdorf W. Muir-Torre syndrome – treatment with isotretinoin and interferon alpha-2a can prevent tumour development. Dermatology. 2000;200:331–3.
63. Peutz JL. Very remarkable case of familial polyposis of mucous membrane of intestinal tract and nasopharynx accompanied by peculiar pigmentations of skin and mucous membrane (Dutch). Nederl Maandschrift voor Geneeskunde. 1921;10:134–46.
64. Jeghers H, Mc KV, Katz KH. Generalized intestinal polyposis and melanin spots of the oral mucosa, lips and digits; a syndrome of diagnostic significance. N Engl J Med. 1949;241:1031–6.
65. Jenne DE, Reimann H, Nezu J, et al. Peutz-Jeghers syndrome is caused by mutations in a novel serine threonine kinase. Nat Genet. 1998;18:38–43.
66. Hemminki A, Markie D, Tomlinson I, et al. A serine/threonine kinase gene defective in Peutz-Jeghers syndrome. Nature. 1998;391:184–7.
67. Mangili G, Taccagni G, Garavaglia E, et al. An unusual admixture of neoplastic and metaplastic lesions of the female genital tract in the Peutz-Jeghers Syndrome. Gynecol Oncol. 2004;92:337–42.
68. Bond JH. Polyp guideline: diagnosis, treatment, and surveillance for patients with colorectal polyps. Practice Parameters Committee of the American College of Gastroenterology. Am J Gastroenterol. 2000;95:3053–63.
69. Karabulut AA, Sahin S, Sahin M, et al. Paraneoplastic acrokeratosis of Bazex (Bazex's syndrome): report of a female case associated with cholangiocarcinoma and review of the published work. J Dermatol. 2006;33:850–4.
70. Bolognia JL, Brewer YP, Cooper DL. Bazex syndrome (acrokeratosis paraneoplastica). An analytic review. Medicine (Baltimore). 1991;70:269–80.
71. Vandersteen PR, Scheithauer BW. Glucagonoma syndrome. A clinicopathologic, immunocytochemical, and ultrastructural study. J Am Acad Dermatol. 1985;12:1032–9.
72. Gregory B, Ho VC. Cutaneous manifestations of gastrointestinal disorders. Part I. J Am Acad Dermatol. 1992;26:153–66.

Cutaneous Manifestations of Common Endocrine Disease

Inés M. Hernández and Yanira Marrero

In all specialties of medicine, physicians are approached by patients with skin complaints which may be associated with a systemic illness. It is challenging for physicians to attempt to relieve these symptoms, meanwhile identifying the underlying causative conditions which give rise to these lesions. Endocrine diseases, through hormonal excess or deficiency, may cause general skin changes in texture, temperature, color, morphology or may manifest specific lesions. These lesions are often the most visible signs of the hormonal disease for which the patient seeks medical care. In this chapter, we describe the most common skin changes encountered in patients with diabetes mellitus, thyroid, and adrenal disorders. Identification of these lesions and knowledge of their causative endocrine imbalance is vital to achieve cure or relief.

Thyroid Disease

Thyroid hormone disorders include hyperthyroidism, hypothyroidism, and autoimmune thyroid disease; the most common of the latter being Graves' disease and Hashimoto's thyroiditis. Thyroid hormones stimulate epidermal oxygen consumption, protein synthesis, mitosis, and aid in the determination of layer thickness. Hair growth and formation may be affected by triiodothyroxine (T3) and thyroxine (T4). However, the dermal effects of thyroid hormones are poorly understood [1].

I.M. Hernández (✉)
Department of Medicine, University of Puerto Rico School of Medicine, Medical Sciences Campus, San Juan, Puerto Rico
e-mail: ineshndez@hotmail.com

Y. Marrero
Department of Endocrinology, University of Puerto Rico School of Medicine, Medical Sciences Campus, San Juan, Puerto Rico

Hyperthyroidism

Hyperthyroidism, or thyrotoxicosis, affects almost 1% of all Americans, and the disease occurs in women five to ten times more often than in men [2]. Causes of hyperthyroidism are Graves' disease, toxic multinodular goiter, toxic adenoma, subacute thyroiditis, postpartum thyroiditis, silent thyroiditis, excessive iodine ingestion, and exogenous thyroid ingestion or overmedication. Generally, patients who are suffering from hyperthyroidism have signs and symptoms which are systemic in nature, and the skin is no exception. In the hyperthyroid state, patient's skin is often warm, moist, and erythematous; scalp hair is fine and soft and up to 40% of patients may experience some degree of hair loss [3]. Hyperhidrosis of the palms and feet may also be present. Nails become shiny, soft, and friable. They may have a distal separation of the nail plate from its underlying bed with an upward curvature, forming the shape of a spoon, often called Plummer's nails [4]. Onycholysis, which is characterized by the distal separation of the nail from the nail bed, may only be present in 5% of patients with hyperthyroidism. It may be seen in other thyroid and dermatologic conditions, including psoriasis and allergic contact dermatitis. The most common clinical form of hyperthyroidism is Graves' disease, which affects 60–90% of all patients [4]. These patients may develop other autoimmune conditions such as vitiligo, and specific skin lesions such as pretibial myxedema and thyroid achropachy.

Pretibial myxedema is a diffuse or circumscribed mucinous dermopathy [5]. It is a misnomer because it can arise in the hands, arms, shoulders, ankles, feet, ears, face, surgical scars, skin grafts, and animal bites, as such, it is often referred to as thyroid dermopathy [1]. These lesions are typically bilateral, asymmetric, firm, nonpitting, and painless nodules and plaques present on the extensor aspects of the lower legs and feet. A waxy swelling and induration of the skin ensues, often with variable colors (Fig. 1). Infiltrative thyroid dermopathy is an uncommon systemic autoimmune feature of GD, occurring in approximately 5% of patients with GD.

N.P. Sánchez (ed.), *Atlas of Dermatology in Internal Medicine*,
DOI 10.1007/978-1-4614-0688-4_5,

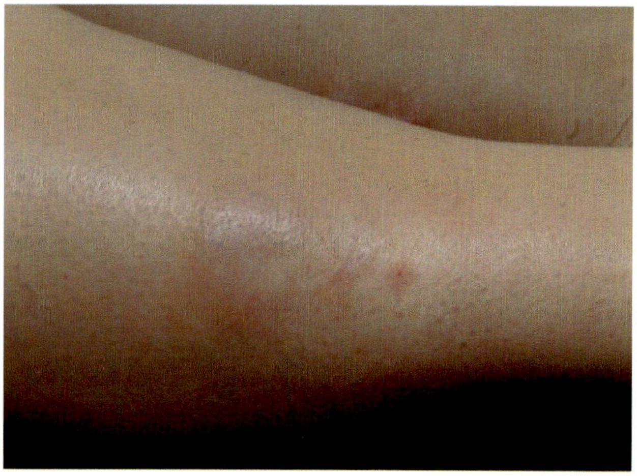

Fig. 1 Pretibial myxedema can present as firm, nonpitting edematous erythematous plaques on the lower legs of a patient

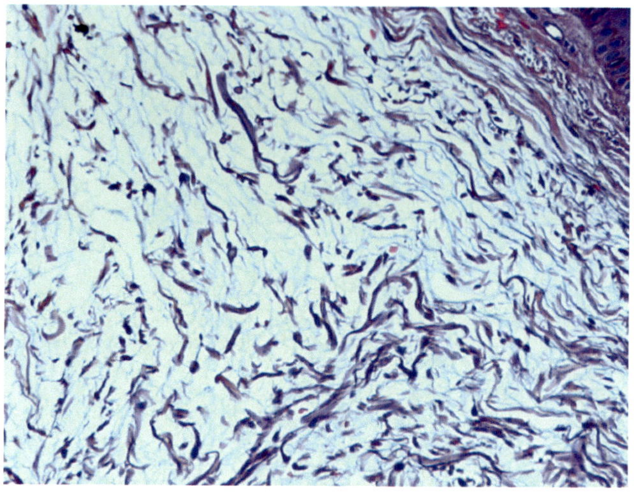

Fig. 2 Pretibial myxedema histopathology: increased spaces between the collagen bundles which represent an accumulation of mucin

One study using ultrasonography found that pretibial skin thickness was increased in 33% of patients with autoimmune thyroid disease, implying that infiltrative dermopathy is likely to have a higher subclinical prevalence [6]. It may be present in up to 15% of patients with Graves' ophthalmopathy, but it has also been described in Hashimoto's thyroiditis and in euthyroid states [7]. As such, lesions do not necessarily correlate with thyroid hormone levels [1]. There are five clinical variants of thyroid dermopathy: nonpitting, nodular, plaque-like, polypoid, and elephantiasic [7]. The nonpitting variant of pretibial myxedema is the most common presentation of the disorder, accounting for 58% of patients, whereas the nodular and plaque-like variants occur in 20% of patients. The polypoid and elephantiasic variants rarely occur, affecting only 1% of patients with Graves disease and thyroid dermopathy [8].

The mechanism that causes the accumulation of glycosoaminoglycans is unknown. However, it has been shown that circulating levels of immunoglobin G auto-antibodies in patients with Graves' disease and pretibial myxedema seem to stimulate glycosoaminoglycan production in fibroblasts and in keratinocytes [1]. Histologic characteristics of this disorder include the accumulation of glycosoaminoglycans (such as hyaluronic acid and chondroitin sulfate) within the papillary dermis of both affected and normal skin (Fig. 2).

After identification of the lesion and the underlying thyroid state, it is very challenging to manage thyroid dermopathy because it does not necessarily remit after thyroid hormone levels normalize [1]. The lesions may persist or resolve slowly over a number of years. Data available is limited in regards to treatment due to the small number of patients treated and the variable response rate. In a 20-year study by Fatourechi of 150 patients treated with topical triamcinolone response was described as "valuable" [7]. In another study seven of nine patients with Graves' ophthalmopathy responded to octreotide. Treatment with intravenous immunoglobin and pulse steroids followed by oral steroids has a reported effective response rate [1]. Another particular study recommended adjunctive therapy with compression therapy regardless of the therapeutic regimen. Monitoring the lesion with ultrasonography for the evaluation of skin thickness response to therapy has proven promising [9, 10].

Thyroid achropachy (clubbing of the fingers and toes) is a rare manifestation of autoimmune thyroid disease and appears in only 0.1–1% of patients with Graves' disease in association with ophthalmopathy and pretibial myxedema. Thyroid achropachy is a triad consisting of digital clubbing, soft tissue swelling of the hands and feet, and periosteal new bone formation on the shafts of the phalanges, and distal long bones [4, 11]. It is asymptomatic and requires no therapy. The first, second, and fifth metacarpals and the proximal phalanges of the hand, and the first metatarsal and proximal phalanges of the feet are most commonly affected. The pathogenomic radiographic osseous changes are lamellar periosteal reactions paralleling the diaphyses of the hands and wrists. Bone spicule formation develops perpendicularly to the long axis of the bone [1]. Even though the cause is unknown [12], it has been proposed that there is stimulation of local fibroblasts by an autoimmune process that increases mucopolysaccharide synthesis and deposition [12].

Hypothyroidism

Hypothyroidism affects approximately 25 million Americans, and it is thought that approximately 50% remain undiagnosed [2]. The most common cause in the USA is autoimmune

Hashimoto's thyroiditis, but worldwide, iodine deficiency remains to be the most common cause. Other causes of this thyroid hormone deficiency state include radioactive iodine treatment, thyroidectomy, medications, postpartum, and subacute thyroiditis [4].

General skin changes include cold, pale, thin, and dry skin. Cutaneous vasoconstriction and reduced core temperature account for the changes in skin temperature [13]. The paleness of the skin is attributed to an altered light refraction due to increased water content and mucopolysaccharides in the dermis of the skin. There is a yellowish tinge of the palms, soles, and nasolabial folds due to the defective conversion by the liver of β-carotene to vitamin A leading to the accumulation of carotene in the stratum corneum [14]. A study designed to determine whether there is a significant association between alopecia areata and other autoimmune diseases found that thyroid disorders showed the highest frequency. Among the thyroid disorders, hypothyroidism was the most frequent association (14.1%) [15]. Hair loss is a common complaint in hypothyroid patients and its texture dull, coarse and brittle, leading to partial alopecia. Loss of the outer third of the eyebrow is a classic finding [16]. Perhaps the most characteristic feature of hypothyroidism is generalized myxedema. There are no distinct lesions as in thyroid dermopathy, but histologically there is deposition of hyaluronic acid and chondroitin sulfate in the skin causing it to appear swollen, dry, pale, and firm to the touch. Facial features look puffy with involvement of eyelids, lips, tongue, and nose. Dryness of the skin (xerosis) may be severe enough to develop into ichthyosis vulgaris, a hyperkeratotic condition characterized by rough, dry, and scaly skin [8]. Scales are small, fine, irregular, and polygonal in shape, varying in size from 1 to 1 cm, occurring mostly on the extensor surfaces of the lower extremities. Myxedematous changes resolve with thyroid hormone replacement, but recur if treatment is abandoned or if therapeutic levels of thyroid hormones are not met.

Diabetes Mellitus

Approximately 7% of the US population suffers from diabetes mellitus (20.8 million), and approximately 30% of these patients experience some cutaneous involvement during the course of their illness [17]. About 6.2 million of these patients are undiagnosed [18]. This means that a large amount of patients may present with skin manifestations of diabetes mellitus without knowing that they suffer from the disease. The clinician must become familiarized with the most common skin manifestations of diabetes mellitus to establish a prompt diagnosis and initiate treatment. This metabolic disease, characterized by hyperglycemia, may be due to defects in insulin production (type I), insulin action, or both [18]. Among the various skin disorders associated with diabetes mellitus are acanthosis nigricans, necrobiosis lipoidica diabeticorum (NLD), Scleredema adultorum of Buschke, and diabetic dermopathy [4]. Skin infections are also common in diabetic patients [13].

Acanthosis Nigricans

Acanthosis nigricans is defined by diffuse velvety thickening and hyperpigmentation of the skin, mostly involving the axillae, neck, skin folds, groin, and perineum [4] (Fig. 3). It is a common manifestation of endocrine and malignant diseases [8]. Histological features include hyperkeratosis, epidermal papillomatosis, and increased numbers of melanocytes [19].

Necrobiosis Lipoidica Diabeticorum

Necrobiosis lipoidica diabeticorum (NLD) is a rare skin manifestation of diabetic mellitus. It occurs in 0.3% of diabetic patients per year and 80% of patients affected are women [20]. Although uncommon, due to large population

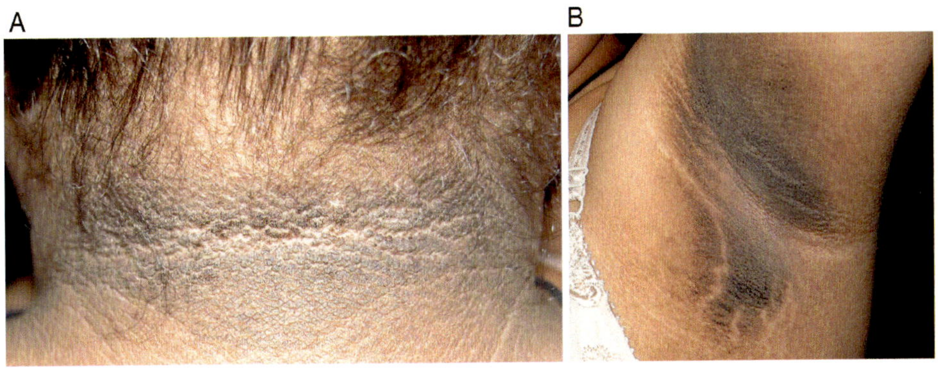

Fig. 3 (**a**, **b**) Acanthosis nigricans often presents with thick, velvety, and hyperpigmented areas of the neck and axillae

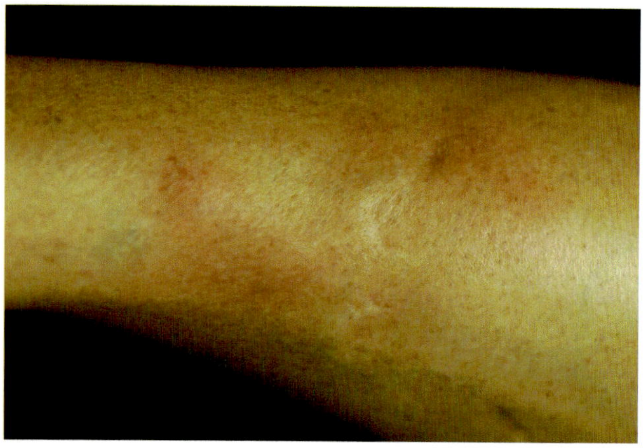

Fig. 4 Necrobiosis lipoidica diabeticorum: on the pretibial area of the lower extremity, one can see erythematous, non-scaly plaques with a *yellowish* atrophic center and prominent superficial telangiectasias

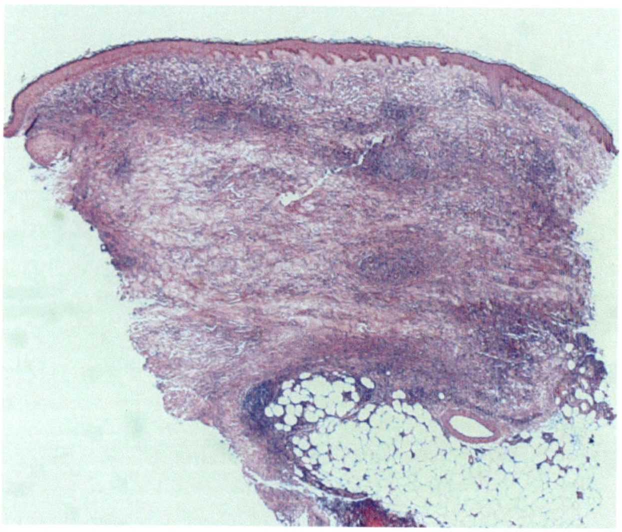

Fig. 5 Necrobiosis lipoidica diabeticorum histopathology demonstrates a granulomatous infiltrate arranged in a characteristic palisading pattern with degeneration of collagen

of undiagnosed diabetics, this number is significant. Typically, lesions develop on the pretibial area of lower extremities. These are erythematous, nonscaly plaques with a yellowish atrophic center, and prominent superficial telangiectasias [20] (Fig. 4). Biopsy may be necessary in early lesions or in patients without a diagnosis of diabetes mellitus, to rule out other conditions such as sarcoidosis, stasis dermatitis, lichen sclerosus et atrophicus, and granuloma annulare [20]. On histologic examination, the presence of fibrin and palisading histiocytes suggests that the process is due to a delayed hypersensitivity reaction [21] (Fig. 5). Treatment consists of local application of potent steroids or intralesional triamcinolone injections. Despite the chronicity of the lesions, 10–20% may remit spontaneously.

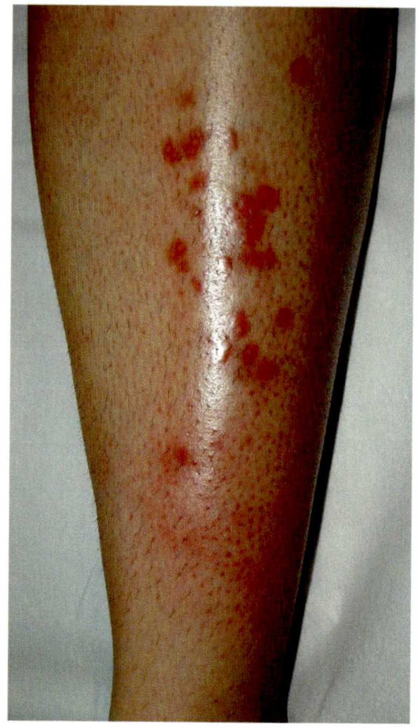

Fig. 6 Diabetic dermopathy. Atrophic *reddish-brown* macules on the pretibial areas of the lower extremities

Miscellaneous Conditions

Other common skin lesions seen in patients afflicted by this metabolic disorder include diabetic scleredema, diabetic dermopathy and thickening of the skin on the fingers.

Scleredema is more common in males and associated with obesity. There is taught thickening of the skin over the upper back, neck, and shoulders, sometimes with extension to the face, arms, and chest [4]. A biopsy must be performed to distinguish scleroderma from dermatomysitis [20].

Diabetic dermopathy consists of pigmented papules and is seen in over 70% of men over 60 years with diabetes mellitus. The lesions, consisting of pigmented papules, are localized to the shins of the lower extremities (Fig. 6). They initially present as pink patches that evolve into depressed brown papules with fine scaling and surface atrophy [4, 20].

Type I diabetics are susceptible to develop waxy thickening of collagen on the fingers, the so-called diabetic thick skin of the fingers [20]. It can limit joint mobility and result in contractures of the interphalangeal joints. It can also be present in adult diabetics who suffer from retinopathy and/or nephropathy.

Adrenal Disorders

Cushing's syndrome and Addison's disease are the most common diseases associated with adrenal cortisol excess and deficiency, respectively. Cortisol excess may be due to pituitary hypersecretion of ACTH (adrenocorticotropic hormone) due to a pituitary adenoma (Cushing's disease); adrenal hypersecretion of glucocorticoids due to an adrenal adenoma or carcinoma; ectopic ACTH secretion by other tumors or exogenous administration of cortisol. The cutaneous manifestations of Cushing's syndrome are centripetal obesity, wasting of the extremities, purple striae and thin, fragile skin. The skin may peel after being covered with adhesive tape (Liddle's sign) [4]. In addition, the loss of subcutaneous tissues leads to easy bruising after minimal trauma.

In regards to skin cell physiology, the dermal effects of corticosteroids include the inhibition of epidermal cell division, decreased collagen synthesis, thinning of the stratum corneum, and a loss of subcutaneous fat [22]. The accumulation of adipose tissue in Cushing's syndrome leads to what has been characterized as moon facies (cheeks), buffalo hump (dorsocervical), supraclavicular fat pads (supraclavicular fossae), and exophthalmos (retro-orbital fat). Fat also accumulates internally in the mediastinum and mesentery [23, 24].

Purple striae are wide (>1 cm) and are most commonly located on the abdomen and lower flanks, but may be also present on the breasts, axillae, and upper thighs [4]. These are due to the reduced tensile strength of dermal structures and the loss of underlying connective tissue caused by excess cortisol.

If hypercortisolism is secondary to ectopic ACTH secretion, hyperpigmentation may also be present with a generalized pattern similar to that found in Addison's disease. If the patient has Cushing's secondary to an adrenal carcinoma, the concomitant androgen excess leads to hirsutism, acne, temporal balding, and signs of virilization [4].

Hirsutism is defined as the presence of terminal coarse hairs in females in a male-like distribution. It is a common clinical condition seen in female patients of all ages. It affects around 5–10% of women and is a common presenting complaint in the dermatological outpatient department for cosmetic reasons. The cause is mainly hyperandrogenism, which may be ovarian or adrenal. It may be part of a rare metabolic syndrome, drug induced, or just idiopathic. Hirsutism requires indepth clinical evaluation and investigation for treatment [25].

A study comparing ovarian morphology and prevalence of polycystic ovary syndrome (PCOS) in reproductive aged women with or without mild acne and hirsutism showed that the prevalence of PCOS was 17.1% (19/111) in all women included in this study. In the acne group, the prevalence of PCOS was 26.9% (14/52), and significantly more prevalent than in control group 8.4% (5/59). Total ovarian volume was significantly larger and stromal thickness of the ovary was thicker in women with acne than women without acne [26].

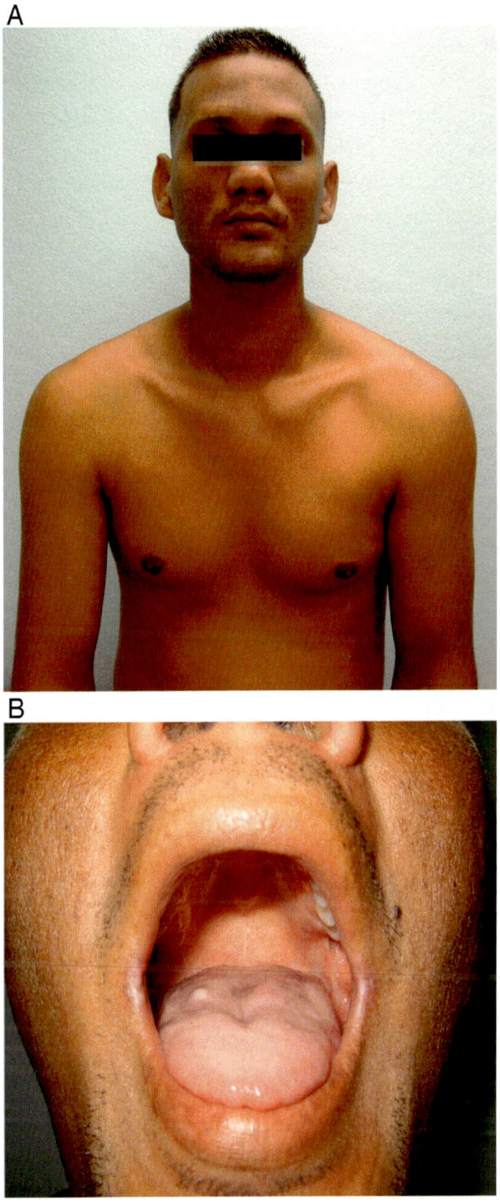

Fig. 7 (**a**, **b**) Addison's disease: (**a**) hyperpigmented skin is most noticeable in areas exposed to the sun; (**b**) hyperpigmented macules on the oral mucosa

Addison's disease, or cortisol deficiency, is most commonly caused by autoimmune destruction of the adrenal glands by cytotoxic lymphocytes [27]. Other causes of adrenal destruction are hemorrhage, infection, or metastases from solid tumors. Hyperpigmentation is the most common skin manifestation of Addison's disease, caused by increased melanin content in the skin. The hyperpigmentation is generalized, but most noticeable in areas exposed to sunlight (face, neck, and hands), friction or pressure (elbows, knees, knuckles), and palmar creases (Fig. 7a). In dark skin individuals or those living in tropical countries, it is best to identify the hyperpigmentation on the buccal mucosa, under the tongue, on the hard palate, and in the anal and vaginal mucosa (Fig. 7b). Scars acquired during the untreated disease will be permanently pigmented until the disease is treated. Those scars acquired before the disease or during treatment, remain unpigmented [28].

The skin cell physiology of the hyperpigmentation is due to increased melanin content in the skin. Melanin is synthesized in epidermal melanocytes located in the basal layer of the epidermis and is stored in secretory structures, called melanosomes [28]. ACTH production within the pituitary is preceded by POMC (propiomelanocortin), a large precursor protein which is later cut in several fragments, producing ACTH, MSH (melanocyte stimulating hormone), and β-lipoprotein. Due to low levels of cortisol, POMC production augments, resulting in higher levels of ACTH and MSH, resulting in melanocyte stimulation and the hyperpigmentation typical of Addison's disease. Patients may also have androgen deficiency leading to loss of secondary sex characteristics, such as axillary and pubic hair.

Conclusion

There are multiple cutaneous manifestations of endocrine disorders which both the dermatologist and the primary care physician must have a thorough understanding of in order to diagnose, treat or refer the patient to an endocrinologist for the appropriate management of the underlying condition.

References

1. Ai J, Leonhardt JM, Heymann WR. Autoimmune thyroid diseases: etiology, pathogenesis, and dermatologic manifestations. J Am Acad Dermatol. 2003;48:641–59.
2. American Association of Clinical Endocrinologists. http://www.thyroidawareness.com.
3. Rook A. Endocrine influences on hair growth. Br Med J. 1965; 1:609–14.
4. Jabbor SA. Cutaneous manifestations of endocrine disorders. A guide for dermatologists. Am J Clin Dermatolol. 2003;4:315–31.
5. Stadlmayr W, Spitzweg C, Bichlmair AM, Heufelder AE. TSH receptor transcripts and TSH receptor-like immunoreactivity in orbital and pretibial fibroblasts of patients with Graves' ophthalmopathy and pretibial myxedema. Thyroid. 1997;7:3–12.
6. Rice SA, Peden NR, Mc Glynn S, Morton C. Atypical presentation of infiltrative thyroid dermopathy. Clin Exp Dermatol. 2010;35(1):56–8.
7. Fatourechi V, Pajouhi M, Fransway AF. Dermopathy of Graves disease (pretibial myxedema). Medicine (Baltimore). 1994; 73:1–7.
8. Leonhardt JM, Heymann WR. Thyroid disease and the skin. Dermatol Clin. 2002;20:473–81.
9. Appetecchia M, Castelli M, Delpino A. Anti-heat shock protein autoantibodies in autoimmune thyroiditis: preliminary study. J Exp Clin Cancer Res. 1997;16:395–400.
10. Salvi M, De Chiara F, Gardini E, et al. Echographic diagnosis of pretibial myxedema in patients with autoimmune thyroid disease. Eur J Endocrinol. 1994;131(2):113–9.
11. Abu HN. Exophthalmos, digital clubbing and pretibial myxedema in thyroiditis. J Clin Endocrinol. 1963;23:215–7.
12. Vanhoenacker FM, Pelckmans MC, De Beuckeleer LH, et al. Thyroid acropachy: correlation of imaging and pathology. Eur Radiol. 2001;11:1058–62.
13. Freinkel RK. Cutaneous manifestations of endocrine diseases. In: Fitzpatrick TB, Eisen AZ, Wolff K, et al., editors. Dermatology in general medicine. 4th ed. New York: McGraw-Hill; 1993. p. 2113–31.
14. Lang Jr PG. Cutaneous manifestations of thyroid disease. Cutis. 1978;21:862–6.
15. Thomas EA, Kadyan RS. Alopecia areata and autoimmunity: a clinical study. Indian J Dermatol. 2008;53(2):70–4.
16. Donnelly A. Skin signs of systemic disease. Aust Fam Physician. 1999;28:1217–22.
17. Ahmed I, Goldstein B. Diabetes mellitus. Clin Dermatol. 2006;24: 237–46.
18. National Diabetes Statistics, 2007. http://diabetes.niddk.nih.gov/dm/pubs/statistics/index.htm#7. Accessed 5 Dec 2007.
19. Goldstein, Beth G, Goldstein, Adam O. Metabolic and inherited diseases affecting the Skin. http://www.utod.com.
20. Sibbald RG, Landol SJ, Toth D. Skin and diabetes. Endocrinol Metab Clin North Am. 1996;25:463–72.
21. Nieboer C, Kalsbeek GL. Direct immunofluorescence studies in granuloma annulare, necrobiosis lipoidica and granulomatosis disciformis Miescher. Dermatologia. 1979;158:427–32.
22. Ferguson JK, Donald RA, Wetson TS, et al. Skin thickness in patients with acromegaly and Cushing's syndrome and response to treatment. Clin Endocrinol (Oxf). 1983;18:347–53.
23. Findling JW, Raff H. Diagnosis and differential diagnosis of Cushing's syndrome. Endocrinol Metab Clin North Am. 2001;30: 729–47.
24. Panzer SW, Patrinely JR, Wilson HK. Exophthalmos and iatrogenic Cushing's syndrome. Ophthal Plast Reconstr Surg. 1994;10: 278–82.
25. Sachdeva S. Hirsutism: evaluation and treatment. Indian J Dermatol. 2010;55(1):3–7.
26. Kelekci KH, Kelekci S, Incki K, Ozdemir O, Yilmaz B. Ovarian morphology and prevalence of polycystic ovary syndrome in reproductive aged women with or without mild acne. Int J Dermatol. 2010;49(7):775–9.
27. Oelkers W. Adrenal insufficiency: current concepts. N Engl J Med. 1996;335:1206–12.
28. Nieman L. Clinical manifestations of adrenal insufficiency. http://www.utod.com. Accessed 7 Dec 2007.

Cutaneous Manifestations of Internal Malignancy and Paraneoplastic Syndromes

Zelma C. Chiesa-Fuxench, Liliana Ramírez, and Néstor P. Sánchez

In this chapter, an attempt is made to examine the wide spectrum of cutaneous manifestations related to internal malignancies and the most important paraneoplastic syndromes. In medicine, cutaneous manifestations are an invaluable marker because they may well be the presenting manifestation of an underlying neoplasm. Primary care specialists, as well as specialty and subspecialty doctors, would greatly benefit from knowing the most common cutaneous manifestations associated with malignancies. Increased clinician awareness could prove beneficial for the patient by promoting earlier screening and diagnosis, as well as increased intervention measures, thereby significantly affecting the chances of survival and/or improving the quality of life of the patient.

Cutaneous manifestations of internal malignancies can be classified into a number of ways. One can look at dermatologic involvement as direct malignant involvement or as symptoms of internal malignancy. Common malignant signs include xerosis, pruritus, pallor, ecchymoses, Sister Mary Joseph nodule, Paget's disease of the breast, or paraneoplastic dermatoses. The following discussion will focus on those cutaneous lesions which involve metastasis to the skin from internal malignancies, cutaneous signs and symptoms of internal malignancies, and some of the most important and well-recognized paraneoplastic syndromes.

Cutaneous Metastasis of Internal Malignancies

Internal malignancies rarely metastasize to the skin. The estimated prevalence has been reported to vary from 0.7 to 10.4% of all patients with cancer [1–4]. In contrast to paraneoplastic syndromes, metastatic lesions are rarely the presenting sign in patients with internal malignancies. These lesions usually develop months to years after the primary diagnosis and their reappearance may be an indicator of disease recurrence. The morphology and behavior of the metastatic lesions tends to be similar, despite place of origin. Although, specific characteristics have been identified corresponding to its organ of origin [4]. The most common metastatic malignancies in men are carcinoma of the lung, colon, and kidney, while in women breast and colon carcinoma are most common [1, 5].

Malignancies may metastasize to the skin through different pathophysiological mechanisms. Direct tumor invasion, extension through the bloodstream or lymphatic vessels, and accidental implantation at surgery. Direct invasion may present with unspecific symptoms of inflammation such as erythema, pain, or edema. Metastatic lesions tend to be multiple and affect skin at location close to primary tumor [6].

The scalp is a primary site of distant tumor metastases, with lesions that appear either nodular or as circumscribed areas of hair loss, also known as alopecia neoplastica [7]. Direct metastases occur in association with neoplasms of the lung or kidney in men and breast in women [8]. These can also present with ulceration of the overlying skin [9].

The cutaneous metastases that present as solitary or multiple nodules tend to have a predilection for areas of old surgical scars [1, 6]. They are usually firm or rubbery, but they may also show ulceration; they vary in color from flesh colored, pink, brown, or black [9]. The location of the metastases can give an idea of what is the possible organ of origin [4]. The majority of tumor cell metastases develop in regions close to the primary malignancy. For example, lesions found on the skin of the chest wall tend to arise from carcinomas of the lung or breast, while lesions found on the abdominal wall usually arise from cancers of the gastrointestinal, genitourinary, or reproductive systems [9, 10].

Cancers of the breast as well as cancers of the oral cavity usually metastasize directly to the skin (Fig. 1). Breast metastases are particularly intriguing because of their mechanism.

Z.C. Chiesa-Fuxench (✉) • N.P. Sánchez
Department of Dermatology, University of Puerto Rico School of Medicine, Medical Sciences Campus, San Juan, Puerto Rico
e-mail: chifu14@hotmail.com

L. Ramírez
Department of Medicine, University of Puerto Rico School of Medicine, Medical Sciences Campus, San Juan, Puerto Rico

N.P. Sánchez (ed.), *Atlas of Dermatology in Internal Medicine*,
DOI 10.1007/978-1-4614-0688-4_6,

The lymphatic obstruction from tumor cells leads to extensive thickening of the skin, and fibrosis of the dermis and subcutaneous tissue (Fig. 2). Other histopathology findings include the presence of neoplastic cells within the dermis between the collagen bundles arranged in a linear pattern ("Indian file") (Fig. 3). The term carcinoma en cuirasse is applied when these changes are seen, because the lymph stasis and fibrosis results in a hard and infiltrated plaque with a characteristic leathery or woody appearance [6, 11]. Carcinoma en cuirasse is usually a sign of recurrence in breast cancer after mastectomy with tumor spreading well beyond the limits of standard surgical or radio therapeutic boundaries [12, 13].

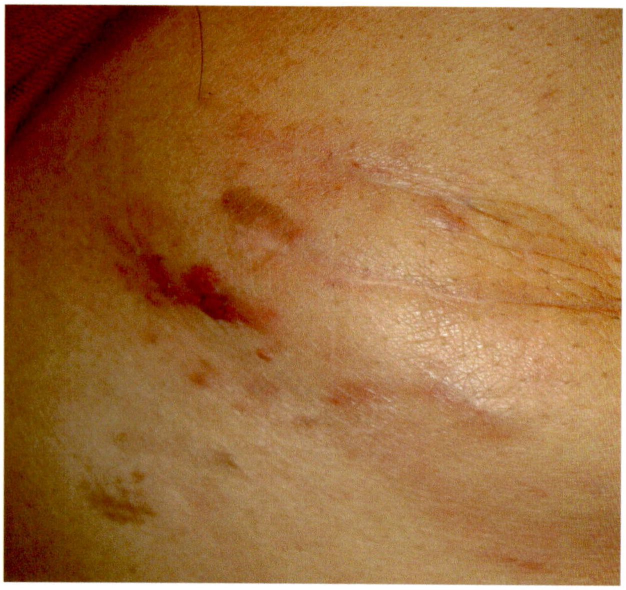

Fig. 1 Breast cancer metastases presenting clinically with nodules on the anterior wall of the chest

Inflammatory carcinoma, also known as carcinoma erysipelatoides, is described as a tender, erythematous, and edematous area which may be the presenting sign of an underlying breast malignancy [6] (Fig. 4). Aside from breast cancer, inflammatory carcinoma has also been seen with metastases from the uterus and lung [9]. The suspicion of inflammatory carcinoma of the breast should arise in any patient with a primary diagnosis of cellulitis of the breast or erysipelas, which does not show an adequate response to antibiotic therapy [9, 13]. In the absence of systemic therapy, nearly all patients with a diagnosis of inflammatory carcinoma die within 5 years of the initial diagnosis [13]. Preoperative chemotherapy in patients with inflammatory breast carcinoma produces a response rate of almost 80%, with the majority of patients achieving subsequent surgical resection with clear margins [13].

Although the appearance of cutaneous metastases is a poor prognostic factor, the period that extends from initial detection and treatment of the primary tumor to the onset of

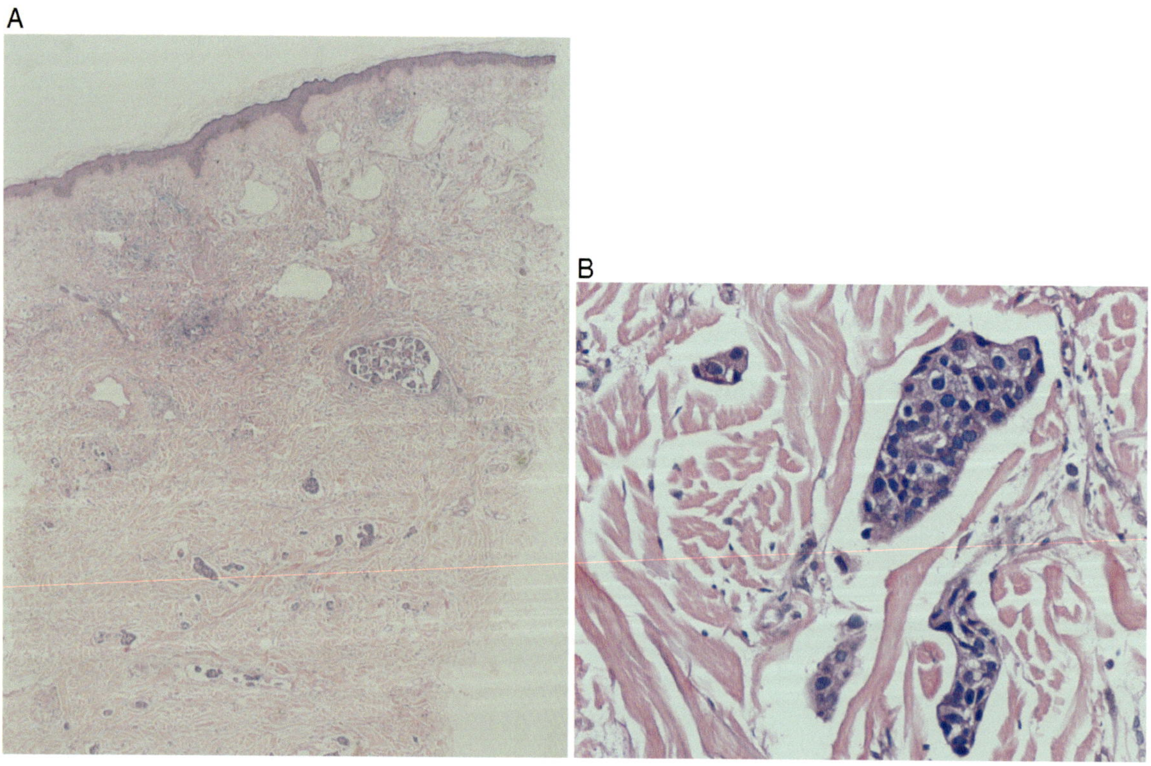

Fig. 2 (**a**, **b**) Breast metastases. Lymphatic obstruction by tumor cells, resulting in extensive thickening of the skin with fibrosis of the dermis and subcutaneous tissue

A

B

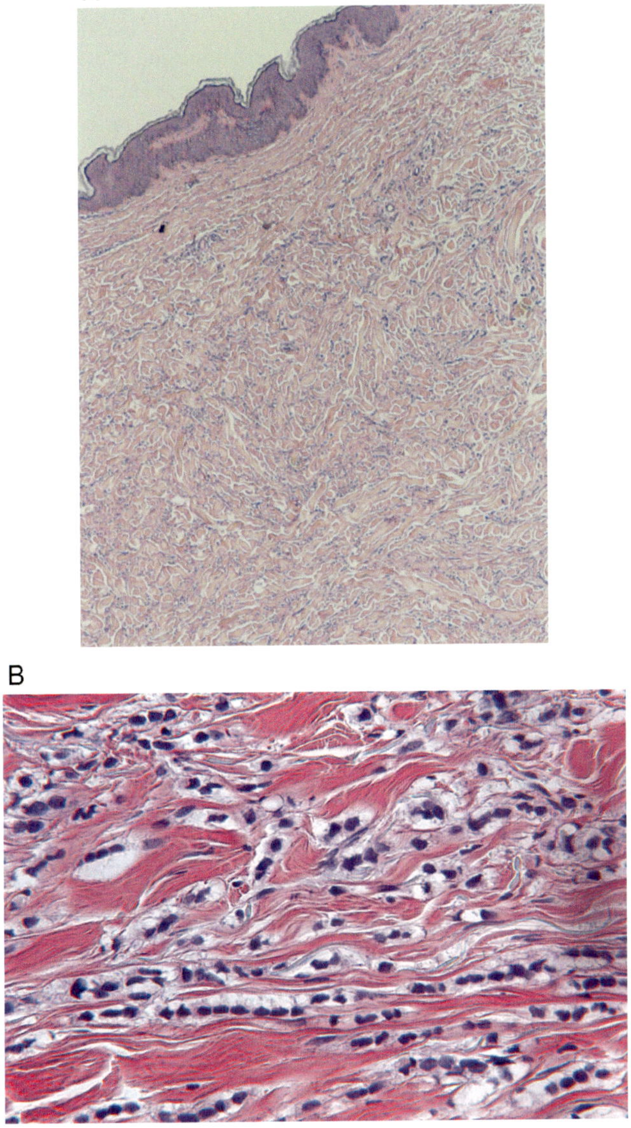

Fig. 3 (a, b) Breast metastases. Histological examination of breast metastases showing the characteristic *Indian file* pattern of tumor cells

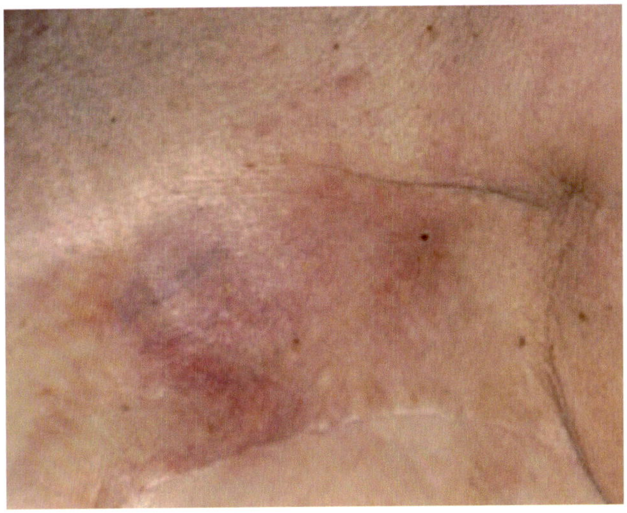

Fig. 4 A tender and erythematous plaque simulating an infectious process (cellulitis)

metastases can be particularly long [1, 6, 14]. Previously published studies have reported a delay from the recognition of primary malignancy to the development of metastases from 5 to 10 years in cancers of the ovaries, bladder, larynx, and colon [9, 15].

Ocular melanoma has also been shown to metastasize as late as 32 years after the removal of the primary tumor [9].

Treatment of the primary tumor takes precedence over the management of skin lesions [1, 16]. If cutaneous metastases are present, surgical treatment is necessary and the lesions need to be excised. In contrast to skin lesions observed with paraneoplastic syndromes, it is important to know that the management of the internal malignancy does not entail a resolution of skin metastasis since these two entities do not necessarily follow a parallel course.

Sister (Mary) Joseph's Nodule

Sister Mary Joseph's nodule is a broad term that refers to any malignant metastatic nodule near the umbilical area, with the primary sites of origin most commonly being malignancies of the stomach, colon, ovaries, pancreas, gallbladder, and lymphomas [17]. Although extremely rare, Sister Mary Joseph's nodule has also been found in association with carcinomas of the lung and endometrium [18, 19]. The term was coined by Sir William Bailey in honor of Sister Mary Joseph, a scrub nurse of the well-known physician William Mayo, because she was the first to notice the association between palpable umbilical lymph node enlargement and advanced stage cancer [20]. The clinical presentation of a Sister Mary Joseph's nodule is variable. In a study of 85 patients with tumors metastatic to the umbilicus, skin lesions were observed as firm, indurated nodules, with fissuring or ulceration [21]. Lesions can also present with hyperpigmentation, erythematous, or non-erythematous changes, without discharge [22]. The histology of the nodule depends on the primary site of the tumor, but is most commonly an adenocarcinoma [21, 22]. The clinician should be aware that the differential diagnosis of Sister Mary Joseph's nodule can include epidermoid cysts, seborrheic keratosis, dermal nevi, polyps, congenital malformations of the omphalomesenteric duct or urachus, foreign bodies, talc granulomas, pyogenic granulomas, angiokeratomas or lymphangiomas, and basal cells epitheliomas or melanomas, although these rarely occur as primary tumors of the umbilicus [22]. Since benign tumors of the umbilicus are uncommon, it is recommended that all lesions near this area be biopsied [17].

A number of mechanisms have been proposed as the pathophysiologic basis of metastasis to this region. The most common route of metastasis is direct tumor extension from the anterior peritoneal surface, since most of the tumors originate in the abdominal area [20]. Other possibilities include arterial, venous, and/or lymphatic spread. Another interesting possible route is through the ligaments of embryonic origin such as the round ligament of the liver or the median umbilical ligament of the urachus [22].

The prognosis of patients with umbilical metastases is generally poor because the appearance of such lesions is usually indicative of advanced metastatic disease [22]. Some studies report that the mean survival period in patients presenting with umbilical metastases is 10 months, with the majority of tumors being inoperable at the time of initial diagnosis [21, 22]. However, other studies have suggested, depending on the site of the primary tumor, a more aggressive approach, such as combining surgical interventions with chemotherapy and radiotherapy, may result in improved survival [17, 21].

Cutaneous Manifestations of Internal Malignancies: Symptoms, Signs, and Other Distinct Disease Entities

Even though there is a great variety of conditions that can cause pruritus, primary physicians and subspecialists should recognize that pruritus could be a sign of an occult malignancy [23]. Generalized pruritus may be the initial symptom present in patients with solid tumors [24]. The origin of pruritus is complex and a lot is unknown about the mechanisms responsible [23]. It can be either peripheral or central in origin. The production of pruritogenic mediators such as histamine, serotonin, eicosanoids, and cytokines stimulate the free nerve endings of specialized C fibers found in the skin, which then transmit information to the central pathways [24]. Pruritus is commonly found in hematologic malignancies. Nearly 50% of patients with a diagnosis of polycythemia vera experience itching, while almost 30% of patients with Hodgkin's lymphoma report itching [25]. Pruritus in non-Hodgkin's lymphoma is rare, with the exception of Sezary's syndrome, in which the incidence is nearly 100%. A localized itch may offer a diagnostic clue to an underlying malignancy, for example: (1) scrotal itch may be associated with prostate cancer; (2) nostril itching associated with brain tumors infiltrating the floor of the fourth ventricle; (3) vulval itch with cervical cancer; and (4) perianal itch with colon or rectal cancer [24]. Although localized pruritus is fairly uncommon, in patients with an already established history of cancer, localized pruritus may portend a worse prognosis [1].

The use of corticosteroids or H2 receptor blockers, such as cimetidine, is not useful in the treatment of pruritus associated with solid tumors [24]. Twycross et al. proposed a treatment ladder for the management of pruritus in these patients, the first step of which consists of using paroxetine 5–20 mg daily [22]. The drug of choice for the treatment of polycythemia vera is low-dose aspirin. Platelet degranulation is increased in polycythemia vera releasing pruritogenic mediators such as serotonin and prostanoids. Therefore, it is theorized that the antipruritic effect of aspirin could be related to its action over platelet function [24, 26].

Hematologic malignancies often show numerous other skin signs that are rather nonspecific; however, their presence should alert the astute physician to search for their cause as they may suggest the presence of cancer. Examples of such nonspecific lesions associated with leukemia and lymphomas include: petechiae, pruritus, pallor, ichthyosis, urticaria, bullous eruptions, erythema nodosum, alopecia, stomatitis, and phlebitis, among others. Pallor and ecchymoses are more frequently observed in patients with leukemia due to the underlying anemia and/or thrombocytopenia. Ichthyosis and pruritus are more commonly found in patients with Hodgkin's lymphoma [6, 27]. The localization and distribution of skin lesions may also give a clue in determining the primary malignancy. Skin lesions localized on the extremities and face are more common in acute and chronic lymphocytic leukemia, whereas truncal lesions are more common in chronic granulocytic leukemia [6, 27]. Gingival hypertrophy and bleeding are common findings in acute monocytic leukemia [6, 27].

Paget's Disease of the Breast and Extramammary Paget's Disease

Paget's disease of the breast and extramammary Paget's disease are both recognized as skin markers of internal malignancies. Paget's disease was first described in 1874 by Sir James Paget, who recognized that this condition usually followed the development of breast cancer within 1 year of diagnosis [13]. Paget's disease of the breast is a rare form of breast cancer that typically affects the nipple and areola and is characterized clinically by the appearance of erythematous, keratotic patches with crusting or weeping [13] (Fig. 5).

The diagnosis of Paget's disease should be considered in patients with a diagnosis of atopic eczema or atopic dermatitis not responsive to topical therapy. When Paget's disease is diagnosed, the clinician should examine both breasts carefully because the occurrence of cancer in one breast is a predisposing factor for the development of cancer in the contralateral breast [6]. Aside from the clinical presentation and results of mammography, the diagnosis of Paget's disease is also made based on histological findings found on biopsy of an eczematous lesion. These include the presence of Paget's cells, which are large cells with large nucleoli and a pale cytoplasm, located within the epidermis [13] (Fig. 6). In a study of 104 patients with Paget's disease of the breast, nearly 93% of patients had an underlying carcinoma. A total

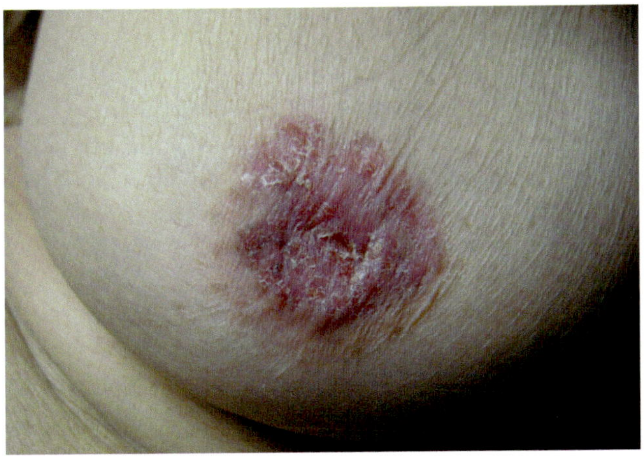

Fig. 5 Paget's disease of the breast. Erythematous scaly plaque affecting the right areola

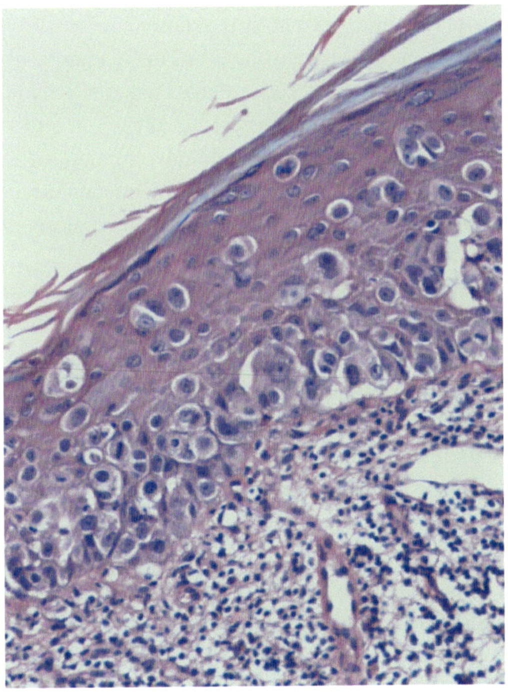

Fig. 6 Histopathological examination of Paget's disease. Clear cells with large nuclei (Paget cells) are seen throughout the epidermis

of 33% were ductal carcinoma in situ (DCIS), while 36% had multifocal disease [26]. Researchers from this study concluded that their findings were similar to those published by previous studies, and thus confirmed the high frequency of underlying carcinoma associated with Paget's disease [28].

Extramammary Paget's disease is most commonly seen in the anogenital region (Fig. 7). Evidence of perianal involvement has been reported to be associated with underlying cancer in 25–35% of patients, whereas only 4–7% of those with genital involvement are associated with cancer [9, 29]. If evidence of perianal involvement is found, the presence of

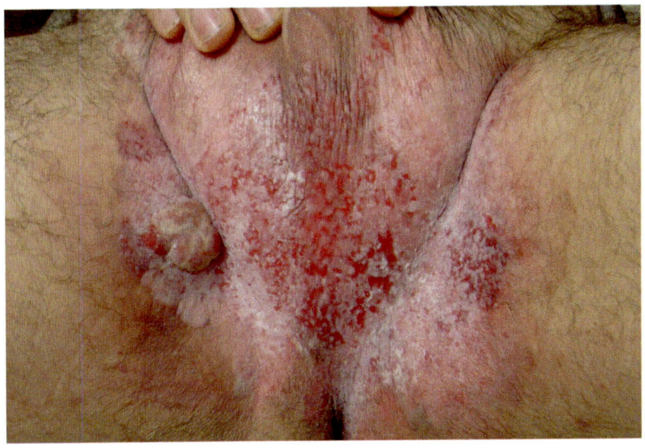

Fig. 7 Extramammary Paget's disease. A pruritic, erythematous, and well-demarcated plaque with erosions and white crusts

rectal cancer should be excluded. In contrast, if the genital area is affected, cancers from the urogenital or reproductive tracts should then be excluded [9, 29].

Clinicians may confuse the diagnosis of extramammary Paget's disease as eczema, candidiasis, leukoplakia, or lichen simplex chronicus [6]. Therefore, a thorough and pertinent patient history and assessment of possible risk factors for the development of cancer should be obtained.

Although the treatment of extramammary Paget's disease is primarily targeted towards the underlying malignancy, the management of Paget's disease of the breast has been more controversial, because it presents either in conjunction with an underlying invasive cancer, DCIS, or without any underlying malignancy. Treatment varies from total mastectomy to breast conserving surgery with adjuvant radiotherapy, depending on the tumor type, size, and level of lymph node involvement [29]. Previous studies have shown that mastectomy was not associated with increased survival outcomes when compared with patients who had undergone breast conserving therapy with central lumpectomy [28–30]. However, the use of radiotherapy is strongly recommended in patients undergoing breast conserving therapy to ensure adequate local control of malignant disease [30, 31]. Furthermore, the use of sentinel lymph node biopsy (SNLB) has also been recommended for all cases of Paget's disease in which the evidence of invasive cancer is confirmed to evaluate for the involvement of the axillae [32]. The use of SLNB in patients with DCIS or Paget's disease alone continues to be questionable [32].

Ultimately the decision of choosing breast conserving therapy versus mastectomy should be made on an individual basis. Some researchers argue that even though breast conserving therapy may seem a feasible alternative for patients with Paget's disease, findings on clinical examination and mammography results may underestimate the true extend of underlying disease [33, 34]. In a study of 40 cases with a benign mammogram and no evidence of a palpable mass, these researchers found evidence of invasive cancer or DCIS of 5 and 68%, respectively [33]. Most recently, the use of MRI has been considered as an appropriate imaging modality to help in the selection of patients with Paget's disease and no evidence of a palpable mass or other abnormal mammography findings [34]. The prognosis in Paget's disease of the breast is related to the staging of breast disease and is similar to those seen in other types of breast cancer [13]. Although Paget's disease of the breast remains a rare form of breast cancer, it is a neoplasm nonetheless and should be treated accordingly [30]. In the event that invasive breast cancer is found, the use of adjuvant systemic chemotherapy should be used following the same guidelines, similar to those of other types of breast cancer [13].

Paraneoplastic Syndromes: A Brief Overview

Paraneoplastic syndromes affect a wide variety of systems, including the endocrine, nervous, and dermatologic systems [35]. The primary focus of this discussion will be those syndromes with cutaneous manifestations. Curth et al. was first to establish a group of characteristics needed to be met before one could suggest that a particular skin disease is part of a paraneoplastic syndrome. These included: (1) both conditions start at approximately the same time; (2) both conditions follow a parallel course; (3) in syndromes, neither the onset, nor the course of either condition is dependent on the other; (4) a specific tumor occurs with a specific skin manifestation; (5) the dermatosis is not common in the general population; and (6) a high percentage of association is noted between the two conditions [36]. Although the criteria for diagnosing a cutaneous manifestation as a paraneoplastic syndrome per se has varied throughout the years, a current review of the literature demonstrates that only two criteria are essential for the diagnosis of a paraneoplastic syndrome: (1) both entities follow a parallel course and (2) the development of the dermatosis occurred after the formation of the malignant tumor [1, 37]. Furthermore, an abrupt appearance or rapid changes in skin lesions may suggest a paraneoplastic phenomenon, for example, the sudden worsening of multiple seborrheic keratosis is the sign of Leser–Trélat [35]. It is understood that many of the pathological processes or malignancies causing paraneoplastic phenomena are difficult to recognize because they produce subtle physiologic changes [38]. Studies have shown that almost 15% of patients with cancer present with a paraneoplastic syndrome at the moment of their initial diagnosis and almost 50% of all patients with cancer will develop a paraneoplastic syndrome during the course of their disease [39, 40]. Therefore, it is of utmost importance to recognize these cutaneous signs because failure to do so may delay the diagnosis of cancer and thus adversely affect therapeutic interventions [41].

Acanthosis Nigricans

In simple terms, acanthosis nigricans is defined as hyperpigmentation of the skin that primarily affects the flexural areas. It is a clinical diagnosis based on the appearance of small hyperkeratotic papules with a velvety texture [39, 42, 43]. Hyperkeratosis alone, not an increase in melanin production, is what gives rise to the hyperpigmentation of acanthosis nigricans [39]. Transforming growth factor-1 (TGF-1) has been considered a likely culprit of the development of such lesions. A product of tumor secretion, TGF-1, promotes the proliferation of keratinocytes and thus the appearance of the lesions [41, 42, 44].

Acanthosis nigricans can be classified into three different subgroups: the hereditary benign acanthosis nigricans, acanthosis nigricans related to obesity, or malignant acanthosis nigricans [9]. When suspecting the diagnosis of acanthosis nigricans in an obese patient, it is usually benign and related to an increase in insulin resistance. A family history of endocrinopathies, as well as chronic steroid use, may also lead to its development in benign cases [1, 9, 39].

Causes for concern are the rapid development of lesions, a lack of family history of acanthosis nigricans, and extension beyond that of the typical intertriginous regions, such as the neck, axillae, antecubital, and popliteal fossae. When areas such as the palms, soles, anus, periocular areas, lip vermilion, and oral mucosa (including the gingival areas) are affected, the suspicion of malignant acanthosis nigricans should prompt a meticulous investigation for related malignancies [39, 42, 45] (Fig. 8).

As a paraneoplastic syndrome, the occurrence of malignant acanthosis nigricans has been associated with gastrointestinal malignancies, specifically gastric adenocarcinoma in 45–95% of cases. It has also been found to occur in relation to other malignancies, such as hepatocellular carcinoma, cholangiocarcinoma, lung cancer, endometrial carcinoma, ovarian cancer, non-Hodgkin's lymphoma, and mycosis fungoides [39, 41, 46, 47]. Malignant acanthosis nigricans may precede the diagnosis of malignancy by as much as 5 years, although this may vary considerably. Malignant acanthosis nigricans may have a simultaneous onset with cancer in approximately 60% of cases, 20% may occur almost 2 years after the cancer is diagnosed and almost 18% may precede the diagnosis [9, 45]. Cancers associated with acanthosis nigricans, as well as other paraneoplastic phenomena, are generally highly aggressive malignancies. The average survival period varies from 12 to 24 months [9, 45].

Once the diagnosis of malignant acanthosis nigricans is established, the primary focus of treatment is directed at the underlying malignancy. Topical and systemic agents may also be used to control the additional symptoms of pruritus and improve the patient's quality of life [39]. To the best of

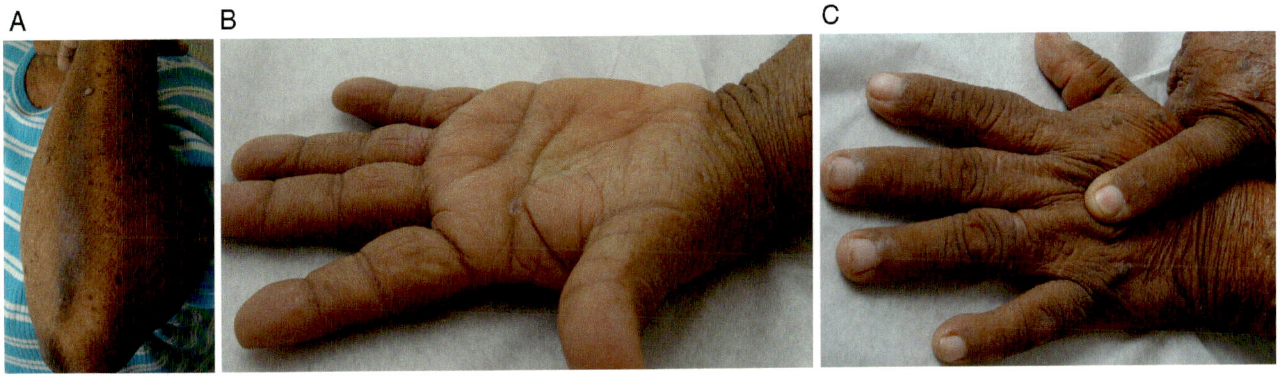

Fig. 8 (**a–c**) Acanthosis nigricans and "tripe palms." Hyperpigmented, velvety skin on the forearms, palms and dorsum of the hands

our knowledge, the use of systemic photochemotherapy for the treatment of malignant acanthosis nigricans was used successfully in one patient. Treatment consisted of therapy with oral 8-methoxypsoralene (8-MOP) and a total UVA dose of 52 J/cm^2, with a final exposure of a maximum dose of 4 J/cm^2. This treatment has been found to alleviate the pruritus and cause significant regression of the pigmented lesions. Although systemic chemotherapy has also been proposed, others contend that no effective treatment exists for malignant AN as the underlying malignancy involves a generally poor prognosis [39, 44, 48–51].

The Sign of Leser–Trélat

The sign of Leser–Trélat is believed to have first been described by two European surgeons. By definition, it is used to refer to the acute onset of multiple seborrheic keratoses with or without pruritus [39, 41, 52, 53]. Seborrheic keratoses are a common finding in the elderly population and are usually described as waxy, dark papules which have a "stuck on appearance." These lesions are generally located on the trunk and especially the back. As a paraneoplastic syndrome, it is most commonly associated with gastric or colon adenocarcinoma, gallbladder carcinoma, bile duct adenocarcinoma, leukemia or lymphoma, breast, lung, ovarian, or uterine cancer [44, 45, 47, 53–58].

The pathogenesis of the sign of Leser–Trélat is similar to that of acanthosis nigricans; transforming growth factor-α (TGF-α) production by tumor cells, similar to epidermal growth factor (EGF), and the subsequent disruption of the regulation of epidermal cell turnover promotes the development of these and other paraneoplastic lesions [41, 45, 59].

As a paraneoplastic syndrome, its validity has been routinely questioned. Some argue that because of their high prevalence in the elderly population as well as in pregnancy, they provide no adequate role in the clinical diagnosis of malignancies [1, 45, 53, 60, 61]. However, it is not the quantity of lesions but the precipitous onset which should alert the physician to the possibility of an internal malignancy.

There is no specific therapy for the sign of Leser–Trélat, however when found in association with a malignancy, treatment of the underlying disease may result in the regression of seborrheic keratoses in almost 50% of cases [41, 60]. They may also serve as a marker for relapse after tumor treatment. Interestingly, one study describes the case of a patient with an adenocarcinoma of the colon whose lesions almost completely resolved with chemotherapy for the primary tumor, and then reappeared when the tumor began to expand 6 months later [9, 61].

The majority of patients who present with multiple seborrheic keratoses are not at an increased risk for internal malignancies. However, if these lesions begin to develop or expand rapidly, and if other paraneoplastic phenomena such as malignant acanthosis nigricans and tripe palms are noted, a thorough search for internal malignancies should be undertaken [40, 44, 45].

Tripe Palms (Pachydermatoglyphy)

The term tripe palms are derived from its resemblance to the rugose surface of tripe found in the bovine foregut. It is defined as hyperkeratotic palms with accentuation of normal skin dermographics creating a wrinkled, velvety appearance (Fig. 8b). It is a distinct paraneoplastic sign, and over 90% of cases of tripe palms are found to be associated with malignancies [42, 62, 63]. The dermatopathology of tripe palms is characterized by hyperkeratosis, acanthosis, dermal mucin deposition, and an increase in the number of dermal mast cells [42, 62].

Tripe palms is occasionally grouped within the spectrum of papulosquamous disorders, which may also include the sign of Leser–Trélat, malignant acanthosis nigricans and other florid cutaneous dermatoses because it often occurs in conjunction with other paraneoplastic manifestations.

Some consider tripe palms to be a subset of malignant acanthosis nigricans due to their histological resemblance, but unlike malignant acanthosis nigricans, it is not common for tripe palms to affect the soles [45]. Malignant acanthosis nigricans is present in about 72% of cases of tripe palms and almost 10% are associated with Leser–Trélat [45, 62]. Tripe palms are most commonly associated with lung cancer when no other paraneoplastic phenomena are present [41, 63, 64]. The appearance of malignant acanthosis nigricans in conjunction with tripe palms is most suggestive of gastric adenocarcinoma [41]. Interestingly, a case of early stage ovarian cancer in a 52-year-old female was recently described as presenting with all three entities: tripe palms, malignant acanthosis nigricans, and the sign of Leser–Trélat [47].

Although the pathological mechanisms involved in the development of tripe palms are still unknown, the role of cytokines in the development of lesions is highly probable, and TGF-α, again, appears to be the most likely candidate. In a previously published case report of a patient with systemic mastocytosis and associated tripe palms, the level of TGF-α produced by the abnormal mast cells was found to correlate with the severity of skin lesions. The systemic mastocytosis was successfully treated with interferon-α (IFN-α), and the tripe palms completely regressed [65].

Acrokeratosis Paraneoplastica (Bazex's Syndrome)

Bazex's syndrome was first described by Gougerot and Rupp in 1922 [66]. It is a rare paraneoplastic syndrome characterized by the development of papulosquamous plaques, resembling psoriasiform dermatitis, primarily localized on the nose, hands, feet, and acral surfaces of the ears, such as the helix [41]. Nail changes are also a common finding, characterized by subungual hyperkeratosis with onycholysis, nail thickening and discoloration, and longitudinal or horizontal ridges. Because the diagnosis of Bazex's syndrome is mainly clinical, physicians should familiarize themselves with the classic distribution of skin lesions to make the correct diagnosis [67]. It is also of great importance to talk about risk factors such as smoking, alcohol use, and family history, because of their high association with internal malignacies [38]. The differential diagnosis of Bazex's syndrome includes acral psoriasis, pityriasis rubra pilaris, systemic lupus erythematous, treatment-resistant eczema, and superficial skin infections [39, 41, 68, 69]. Patients diagnosed with Bazex's syndrome are usually white, middle-aged men [23, 122, 123, 125, 126]. The histological examination of Bazex's syndrome is characterized by vacuolar degeneration of keratinocytes, acanthosis, parakeratosis, and a lymphocytic perivascular infiltration of the superficial dermis [68].

The malignancies most likely to be associated with Bazex's syndrome are those related to the oropharynx, larynx, lung, or esophagus. Although rare, it has also been associated with cancers of the stomach, colon, bladder, and prostate [70–74]. Most recently, a case of infiltrating ductal carcinoma of the breast was found in association with Bazex's syndrome [70]. The most common tumor histology encountered in these patients was squamous cell carcinoma, but poorly differentiated carcinomas as well as adenocarcinomas were also observed [66]. In a significant number of reported cases, however, the primary site of malignancy was unknown [75]. Almost 60% of patients with Bazex's syndrome demonstrate symptoms of this disorder prior to the diagnosis of a malignancy [1, 41, 69, 70, 76, 77].

Similar to other paraneoplastic syndromes, there is much speculation about the pathogenesis of Bazex's syndrome. Most studies agree with the theory of a tumor-derived growth factor which stimulates abnormal proliferation of keratinocytes [41, 78]. Other proposed mechanisms include antigen cross-reactivity with the basal membrane as well as a T cell-mediated response to antigens present in the epidermis [66, 69, 75]. An autoimmune mechanism has also been proposed because Bazex's syndrome has been found in association with other autoimmune diseases such as alopecia areata and vitiligo [68, 79].

Definitive treatment of Bazex's syndrome is dependent on the removal of the primary tumor. However, studies also report the use of adjuvant therapy, such as systemic or topical steroids, vitamin D, psoralen, and ultraviolet A light (UVA) [68, 70, 76, 80]. If one suspects the diagnosis of Bazex's syndrome, the physician should have a high clinical suspicion for malignancy and work up the patient as indicated. A study published by Valdivielso et al. proposed a diagnostic algorithm for further evaluation in which the most important aspects were the complete history and physical exam, including an otolaryngological examination, plus pertinent studies, such as a chest X-ray [68]. If no abnormalities are found but clinical suspicion persists, patients should continue to be monitored at least every 3 months for the occurrence of possible malignancies.

Necrolytic Migratory Erythema

Necrolytic migratory erythema (NME) is a paraneoplastic sign which has generally been regarded as part of a paraneoplastic syndrome known as the glucagonoma syndrome [1, 81]. The first reported case of NME was seen in a patient with a pancreatic islet cell tumor and was reported by Becker et al. in the year 1942. In 1966, more than 20 years later, the association between NME and hyperglucagonemia was established; but it was not until 1973 that Wilkinson first used the term NME to describe these typical skin lesions [82, 83].

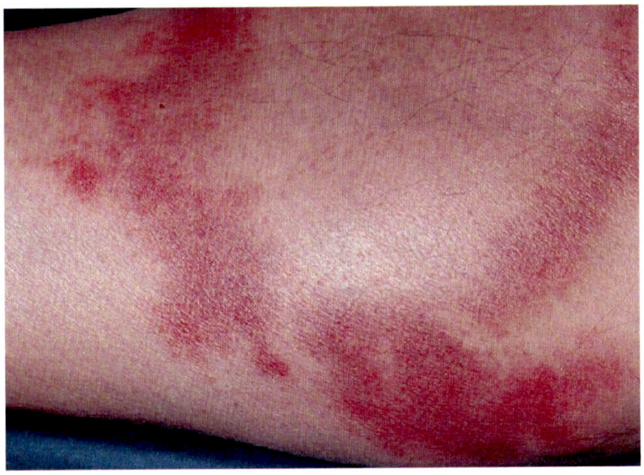

Fig. 9 Necrolytic migratory erythema. Annular erythematous plaques with central clearing affecting the extremities

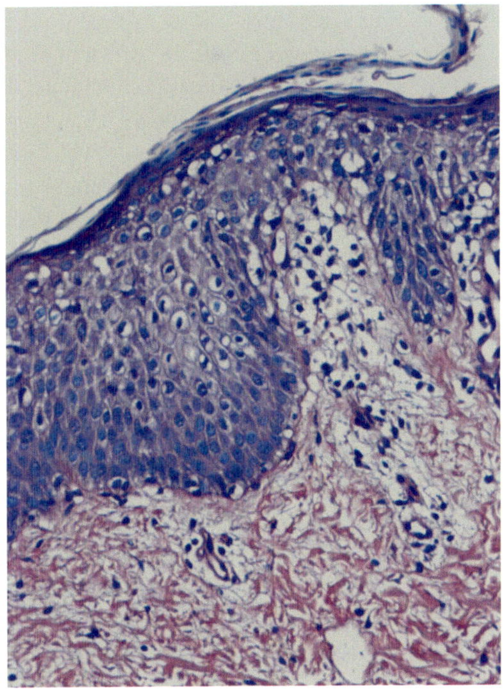

Fig. 10 A lesion in the early stages of the glucagonoma syndrome reveals pale-vacuolated keratinocytes in the upper epidermis

Glucagonoma syndrome is extremely rare, with an estimated incidence of 1 in 20 million; for which it also carries a very poor prognosis (5-year survival rate is usually less than 50%). Because of its rarity, the time elapsed until a correct diagnosis is made is usually prolonged, even up to 12 years [82]. NME is the presenting problem in nearly 70% of patients with a glucagonoma, even so, NME often goes undiagnosed for prolonged periods of time [41, 84–86]. Because almost 75% of glucagonomas are already metastatic at the time of diagnosis, the physician should be highly aggressive when clinical suspicion of NME arises [41, 87–89]. Glucagonoma syndrome is often described as the constellation of NME, diabetes mellitus, stomatitis, cheilitis, weight loss, and diarrhea. Glucagonoma syndrome is also commonly referred to as the 4D syndrome because of the common findings of dermatosis, diarrhea, deep vein thromboses, and depression [86]. The term pseudoglucagonoma syndrome is used when skin lesions suggestive of NME are found in patients with other types of pancreatic cancers, malabsorption syndromes, chronic pancreatitis, jejunal adenocarcinoma, or liver cirrhosis [82, 90]. Furthermore, thromboembolic events, such as deep vein thrombosis or pulmonary embolism, have been found in nearly 30% of patients with a glucagonoma [39].

Skin lesions in NME are characterized by widespread areas of erythema over the face, abdomen, buttocks, thighs, perineum, and other intertriginous areas (Fig. 9). They typically begin as erythematous macules which then progress into flaccid, central bulla that rupture, leaving an area of denudation and crusting. New lesions form simultaneously, with progressive spreading of bullae, vesicles, and skin desquamation [9]. Once healing has occurred, post-inflammatory hyperpigmentation is usually evident. The disease waxes and wanes, with most lesions running a 1–2-week course. The clinician must be able to recognize the natural course of lesions in NME because the correct diagnosis is often missed due to its resemblance to other dermatoses such as pemphigus, psoriasis, pellagra, contact or seborrheic eczema, and acrodermatitis enteropathica [82].

The hallmark histological findings of NME are necrolysis of the upper epidermis and vacuolated keratinocytes which leads to the formation of areas of confluent necrosis [85, 91] (Fig. 10). A perivascular lymphocytic infiltrate is also present in the papillary or upper dermis. Another histological pattern, which is not commonly observed, is psoriasiform hyperplasia of the epidermis with areas of parakeratosis [1, 92].

The pathophysiology of NME is not well understood. Multiple theories have been proposed, but none have proven to be mutually exclusive of the others. Most recently, NME has come to be recognized as a true deficiency dermatosis [85]. The metabolic effects of glucagon are variable. In simple terms, hypoglycemia stimulates glucagon secretion, which results in increased fat and muscle protein catabolism, inhibition of glycogen synthesis and glycolysis, and an increase in hepatic gluconeogenesis and glycogenolysis; finally resulting in increased blood glucose levels. Skin manifestations in hyperglucagonemia are thought to result from depletion of the Vitamin B complex, due to increased carbohydrate metabolism, and a decrease in the essential fatty acids, due to increased lipolysis [85, 93–95]. NME has also been suggested to occur by the direct action of glucagon because when glucagon secreting tumors are surgically removed or treated with a glucagon antagonist, such as somatostatin or octreotide, skin lesions resolve [95, 100, 101].

Deficiency of amino acids is also considered a possible theory for the development of NME. In previous studies of patients with glucagonoma and/or pseudoglucagonoma, researchers have observed that patients have low total protein levels or selective amino acid deficiencies in which replacement of said amino acids results in the resolution of NME [97]. Furthermore, specific amino acid deficiencies such as histidine and tryptophan deficiency are also known to cause a scaly, erythematous rash [96]. Zinc deficiency has also been considered as a possible cause of NME because the clinical and histologic findings of inherited zinc deficiency (acrodermatitis enterohepathica), and acquired zinc deficiency are very similar to those changes seen in NME [96, 98, 99]. Patients with NME and low zinc levels show improvement of skin rashes once therapy with 200 mg oral zinc three times daily for 3–6 weeks is given [96, 98]. The release of inflammatory mediators also appears to play a role in the pathogenesis of NME. When glucagon levels are elevated, there is also an increase in the levels of inflammatory mediators in the epidermis such as arachadonic acid, prostaglandins, and leukotrienes. With additional trauma to the skin, these inflammatory mediators are released causing inflammatory lesions such as those observed in NME [96, 103]. The direct injection of these mediators to the skin produces local induration, erythema, increased vascular permeability, and infiltration of the skin with neutrophils [96, 102].

As with the majority of paraneoplastic syndromes, an early diagnosis is essential for successful treatment. Surgery is considered the gold standard for the treatment of solitary glucagonomas. Most cases of NME have rapid resolution of lesions once the primary tumor is excised [41, 82, 85, 110]. In addition, palliative therapy with somatostatin analogs, IFN-α, and the supplementation of essential fatty acids, zinc, and amino acids can improve the patient's skin lesions [85, 96, 104–109].

Erythema Gyratum Repens

Erythema gyratum repens is a rare paraneoplastic syndrome which is sometimes grouped in conjunction with NME as part of a much broader category of annular erythemas. Skin lesions in erythema gyratum repens are characterized by the acute development of intensely pruritic annular rings of erythema, primarily localized on the trunk and proximal extremities [41, 111, 112]. These lesions may migrate up to 1 cm/day and such extension has been described as giving the skin a "wood-grained" appearance [1]. The estimated prevalence of an internal malignancy in patients with erythema gyratum repens has been found to vary between 77 and 82% [1, 113, 114]. Erythema gyratum repens is commonly associated with malignancies of the breast, lung, pharynx, esophagus, stomach, colon, bladder, anus, and cervix [41, 112].

In a report of 21 cases associated with cancer, the most common malignancy was bronchial carcinoma (41%) [1, 114]. Erythema gyratum repens has been shown to precede the diagnosis of malignancy in 60–80% of cases, with men affected twice as commonly as women [1, 41, 112, 115, 116].

The histological findings in erythema gyratum repens include hyperkeratosis, parakeratosis, spongiosis, acanthosis, and a perivascular infiltrate primarily localized within the papillary dermis. Because direct immunofluorescence studies have demonstrated the presence of IgG and/or C3 deposits in the basement membrane, an immune mechanism of action has been theorized. Patients with bronchial carcinoma often have tumor invasion of the pulmonary basement membrane, which exposes previously protected antigens to the immune system. This may, in turn, induce the production of antibodies that cross-react with those antigens present in the basement membrane of the skin, resulting in these characteristic lesions [1, 117, 118].

Although no specific therapies for erythema gyratum repens exist, as with other paraneoplastic syndromes, improvement and resolution of symptoms is observed with the management of the underlying malignancy. No specific complication has been found associated to cutaneous manifestations of erythema gyratum repens. The morbidity and mortality are directly related to the malignancy causing the syndrome [38].

Acute Febrile Neutrophilic Dermatosis (Sweet's Syndrome)

Sweet's syndrome, or acute febrile neutrophilic dermatosis, was first described by Dr. Robert Sweet in 1964 and was also known as Gomm-Button's disease in honor of the first two patients identified with the disease [119, 120]. Sweet's syndrome, is an entity characterized by the development of painful, erythematous papules, nodules, and/or plaques, with an associated fever (>38°C) and increased neutrophil count. A polymorphonuclear or neutrophilic infiltrate localized within the upper dermis can be seen histologically. It can be divided into classical or idiopathic Sweet's syndrome, malignancy-associated Sweet's syndrome, and drug-induced Sweet's syndrome. All three categories are briefly described, but for the purposes of our discussion, we will be mainly focused on malignancy-associated Sweet's syndrome.

The skin manifestations in malignancy-associated Sweet's syndrome are frequently localized to the face, neck, and upper extremities [119–121] (Fig. 11). These lesions begin as extremely tender, erythematous plaques, or nodules which may develop into bullae and become ulcerated, similar to pyoderma gangrenosum [119, 122, 123]. Multiple lesions can coalesce to form larger plaques in a period of days to weeks. These lesions usually heal without marked evidence of scarring.

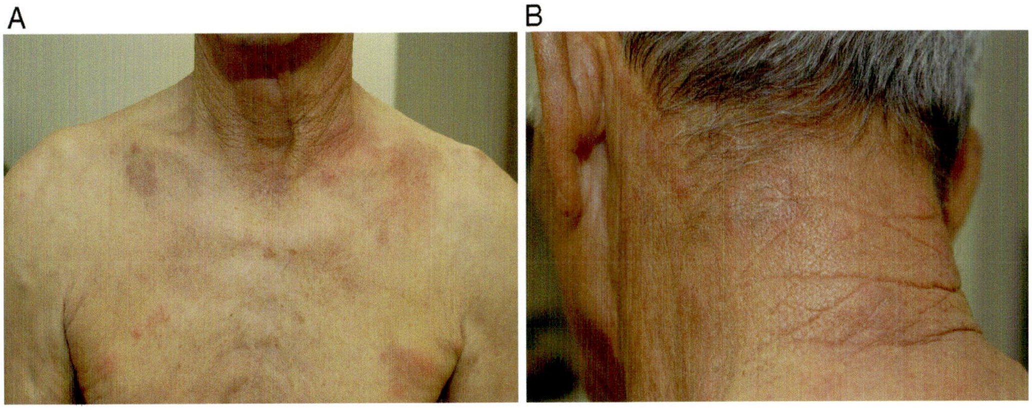

Fig. 11 (**a**, **b**) Sweet's syndrome. A patient with a history of laryngeal cancer presents with well-demarcated erythematous plaques

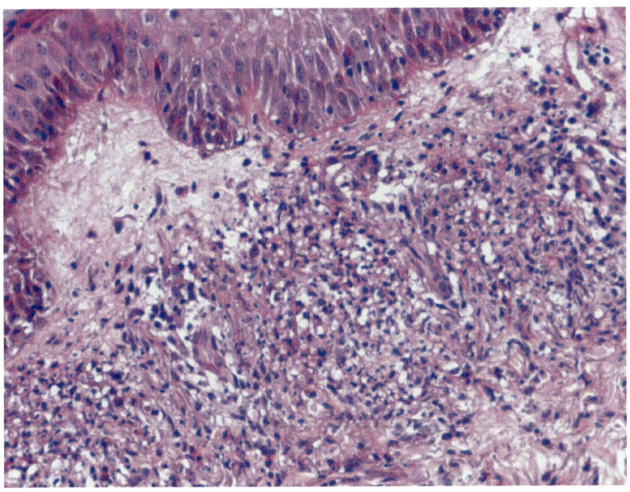

Fig. 12 Sweet's syndrome. Histopathological examination in Sweet's syndrome demonstrates numerous neutrophils infiltrating the superficial dermis, and significant edema of the papillary dermis

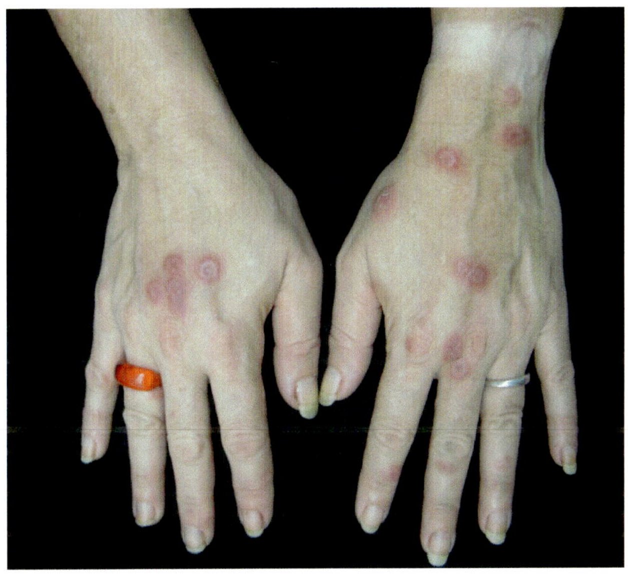

Fig. 13 Sweet's syndrome. Well-demarcated erythematous plaques affecting the dorsum of the hands

As with other cases of Sweet's syndrome, the histopathological findings in malignancy-associated Sweet's syndrome are characterized by edema of the dermis and an infiltrate of mature neutrophils primary localized within the papillary dermis (Fig. 12). Fragmentation of neutrophil nuclei, also known as karyorrhexis or leukocytoclasia, swelling of the endothelial cells, and dilation of blood vessels are all common findings [119, 120]. Other characteristics once considered exclusionary for Sweet's syndrome, such as fibrinoid degeneration of vessels and vascular inflammation, have also been seen in a number of cases [124–130, 134]. Most recently, a new variant of Sweet's syndrome has been proposed, named "histiocytoid Sweet syndrome" [129, 134]. This entity is characterized by clinical signs and symptoms similar to those of Sweet's syndrome, but the histology is marked by a predominantly mononuclear dermal infiltrate. The main differential diagnosis of "histiocytoid Sweet syndrome" is granulocytic sarcoma, also known as leukemia cutis and extramedullary myeloid tumor [129, 134]. Granulocytic sarcomas have been found to be associated with a number of hematologic malignancies, including acute myeloid leukemia, myelodysplastic syndromes, and myeloproliferative disorders [134]. Sweet's syndrome colonized by circulating leukemic cells can be difficult to distinguish from leukemia cutis or differentiated granulocytic sarcoma [124, 130, 134]. Therefore, cases in which "histiocytoid Sweet syndrome" is suspected, long-term follow-up is recommended to exclude the possibility of granulocytic sarcoma [134].

Classical Sweet's syndrome is more commonly found in women ages 30–50 [119, 131] (Fig. 13). The diagnosis of classical Sweet's syndrome requires that both major criteria and at least two of four minor criteria are met [14, 119, 132].

The major criteria are (1) acute development of painful erythematous papules or nodules and (2) neutrophilic infiltration of the dermis without leukocytoclastic vasculitis. The minor criteria are (1) a recent history of an upper respiratory tract infection, gastrointestinal infection, or vaccination or an association with underlying malignancy, inflammatory disease, or pregnancy; (2) fever (>38°C); (3) excellent response to treatment with systemic corticosteroids or potassium iodine; and (4) at least three of four laboratory values significant for an increase in erythrocyte sedimentation rate more than 20 mm/h; a positive C-reactive protein; and an increase in leukocytes more than 8,000 consisting of more than 70% neutrophils [119]. Drug-induced Sweet's syndrome has been found to occur in patients exposed to antibiotics, antiepileptic drugs, anti-thyroid hormones, contraceptives, nonsteroidal anti-inflammatory drugs, and colony-stimulating factors [119]. In drug-induced Sweet's syndrome, there is a concurrent relationship between drug ingestion and the clinical presentation, with the resolution of lesions once the offending agent is removed or the patient is treated with systemic corticosteroids [119, 131].

Malignancy-associated Sweet's syndrome follows the same diagnostic criteria as classical Sweet's syndrome. However, the suspicion of malignancy-associated Sweet's syndrome should arise in those patients with the characteristic skin lesions who are older in age, have hematologic disorders and develop ulcerations of the oral mucosa, and whose complete blood counts demonstrate anemia, a normal to low neutrophil count, and/or an abnormal platelet count [1, 119, 120, 131, 133].

Cases associated with malignancy are not usually preceded by upper respiratory tract infections and it equally affects men and women [119]. The most common cancers found in patients with malignancy-associated Sweet's syndrome are hematological malignancies, such as acute myelogenous leukemia (AML) [119, 134, 135]. In a series of 41 patients with malignancy-associated Sweet's syndrome, the most common non-hematological cancers were genitourinary (37%), breast (23%), and gastrointestinal carcinoma (17%); with the most common histological type being an adenocarcinoma (57%) [119, 136].

Malignancy-associated Sweet's syndrome has also been diagnosed in patients with adenocarcinoma of the lung [137]. Malignancy-associated Sweet's syndrome preceded the diagnosis of hematologic, recurrent or asymptomatic metastases in 61% of cases of those patients with solid tumors [136].

The evaluation of patients with new onset Sweet's syndrome, in which malignancy is suspected, should include a complete history and physical examination with emphasis on the thyroid, lymph nodes, oral cavity and skin; digital rectal examination; breast, ovary, and pelvic examination in women; and prostate and testicular examination in men [41]. Further evaluation should be based on previously established guidelines for early cancer detection, including age-appropriate screening procedures. Since a number of cases of Sweet's syndrome associated with hematologic malignancies were diagnosed within 11 years of the appearance of skin lesions, it has been proposed as reasonable to order a complete blood count with differential every 6–12 months until a more precise diagnosis can be made [136]. However, because most non-hematological malignancies were diagnosed within 12 months of the appearance of skin lesions in previously cancer-free patients, keep in mind that it is highly unlikely that a subsequent detection of Sweet's syndrome associated with a solid tumor will be made following 1 year of continued evaluation [136].

Although numerous theories regarding the etiology of malignancy-associated Sweet's syndromes, as well as other acute febrile neutrophilic dermatoses have been proposed, the exact pathological mechanisms are still unknown. Circulating antigens, immune complexes, human leukocyte antigens, dermal dendrocytes, and cytokines (granulocyte colony-stimulating factor, granulocyte–macrophage colony-stimulating factor, interferon-γ, interleukin (IL)-1, IL-3, IL-6, and IL-8) have all been considered as plausible causes. The production of granulocyte colony-stimulating factor may be responsible for the dermatological lesions in patients with malignancy-associated Sweet's syndrome [119, 138–140].

Spontaneous resolution often occurs in patients whose malignancy is treated successfully [141]. Treatment with systemic corticosteroids is one of the primary modalities of therapy [120]. A review of 79 patients with malignancy-associated Sweet's syndrome, in which the most common malignancy was AML, showed marked improvement in the skin lesions of all patients treated with corticosteroids, regardless of the efficiency of tumor-directed therapy [142]. Intralesional and high-potency topical steroids have also been used successfully in the treatment of individual lesions, but the response varies depending on the underlying malignancy [141]. Potassium iodide and colchicine are also effective treatment options when the use of corticosteroids is contraindicated. The use of cyclosporine in a patient with myelodysplastic syndrome showed marked resolution of skin lesions and lack of progression of the hematologic disease [141, 143]. Cyclosporine has also been used as a second-line agent or in patients where corticosteroid use is also not indicated [141, 143–145]. Treatment with cytotoxic chemotherapy and antimetabolic drugs, including methotrexate, are not routinely used for the management of Sweet's syndrome, except when combined with systemic corticosteroids. The successful use of etretinate and IFN-α in patients with malignancy-associated Sweet's syndrome has also been reported. Etretinate was used in a patient with idiopathic myelofibrosis or agnogenic myeloid metaplasia that did not improve after therapy with 100 mg/day of methylprednisolone, potassium iodine, or clofazimine. After 5 days of therapy, there was marked improvement not only of plaque lesions but also of his general medical condition. IFN-α was used as adjunct therapy with corticosteroids in a patient with chronic myelogenous leukemia. The patient experienced resolution of skin lesions, but the effect was only transient [141, 146]. To the best of our knowledge, these represent isolated cases and further studies are indicated to determine the true efficacy of the treatment options.

Acquired Ichthyosis

Acquired ichthyosis is a rare paraneoplastic syndrome whose diagnosis should alert the clinician to the possibility of internal malignancies. It is characterized by the presence of rhomboidal scales, localized to the extensor surfaces of the extremities, often sparing the flexural areas, palms, and soles. Histological changes include hyperkeratosis with a decreased or absent granular layer. The most common malignancies associated with acquired ichthyosis are lymphoreticular malignancies such as Hodgkin's or non-Hodgkin's lymphoma [38]. Kaposi's sarcoma, multiple myeloma, breast cancer, lung cancer, and female reproductive tract cancers have also been found in association with acquired ichthyosis [1, 41, 147–149]. Acquired ichthyosis can be caused by systemic illnesses such as lepra, hypothyroidism, and acquired immunodeficiency syndrome. It has also been associated with the use of nicotinic acid, triparanol, and butirofenones [38].

The clinical and histological presentation is very similar to that of ichthyosis vulgaris. Unlike ichthyosis vulgaris, an autosomal-dominant disease, acquired ichthyosis, is not hereditary and usually manifests after the detection of cancer [1]. The pathological mechanism is unknown, but the secretion of TGF-α by tumor cells is considered the primary suspect in the development of this condition [1, 150].

Improvement of the skin lesions in acquired ichthyosis occurs with adequate treatment of the underlying malignancy. Keratinolytics and emollients can be used palliatively. Inadequate resolution of this condition should prompt a search for disease persistence or tumor recurrence since acquired ichthyosis follows a parallel course with its underlying malignancy.

Paraneoplastic Pemphigus

Paraneoplastic pemphigus was first proposed as a distinct paraneoplastic syndrome by Anhalt and colleagues in 1990. In their land mark study of five patients with a previous diagnosis of cancer, Anhalt et al. proposed a definition of paraneoplastic pemphigus based on the following five criteria: (1) painful mucosal ulcerations and polymorphous skin lesions with the progression to blister formation and erosion most commonly of the trunk, extremities, palms, and soles in the context of a confirmed or occult neoplasm, (2) intraepidermal acantholysis, necrosis of keratinocytes, and vacuolar interface changes, (3) IgG and complement deposition in the epidermal intercellular spaces, (4) autoantibodies that bind the cell surface of the skin and mucosa similar to other types of pemphigus, but in addition they also bind to simple, columnar, and transitional epithelia, and (5) a four protein complex immunoprecipitated from keratinocytes consisting of 250, 230, 210, and 190 kDa, respectively [151].

Throughout the years, researchers have come to propose a reorganization of the criteria used in the diagnosis of paraneoplastic pemphigus [151, 153]. Camisa et al. proposed a stratification of these criteria into major and minor subdivisions. The three major criteria include: (1) polymorphous mucocutaneous eruption, (2) concurrent internal neoplasia, and (3) characteristic serum precipitation findings. The three minor criteria include: (1) positive cytoplasmic staining of rat bladder epithelium by indirect immunofluorescence, (2) intercellular and basement membrane zone immunoreactants on direct immunofluorescence of perilesional tissue, and (3) acantholysis on biopsy specimen from at least one anatomic site of involvement [152]. Patients who fulfilled all three major criteria or two major and two or more of the minor criteria were considered likely candidates for a diagnosis of paraneoplastic pemphigus. Most recently revised criteria have expanded to include: (1) identification of newer autoantigens such as envoplakin (210 kDa), periplakin (190 kDa), plectin, and desmoglein 3 and 1; (2) lack of correlation of mucocutaneous disease with anti-desmoglein 3 and 1; (3) respiratory involvement; and (4) a lichenoid variant of disease [153]. Most importantly, other key features such as intractable stomatitis, antiplakin antibodies, associated B cell-specific lymphoproliferative neoplasms and progressively worsening disease are refractory to treatment with a fatal outcome in the majority of cases [153]. Intractable stomatitis is most frequently the first sign of disease and is the least likely to respond to treatment [41]. Furthermore, a retrospective study of 22 patients with paraneoplastic pemphigus also found that lympho-proliferative disorders, indirect immunofluorescence of rat bladder, and the immunoblotting recognition of envoplakin and/or periplakin were both sensitive and specific features in the diagnosis of paraneoplastic pemphigus [154]. In a review of 163 cases of paraneoplastic pemphigus diagnosed between 1993 and 2006, 84% of cases were associated with hematologic neoplasms. Non-Hodgkin's lymphoma was found in 38.6% of cases, chronic lymphocytic leukemia in 18.4% of cases and Castleman's disease in 18.4% of cases. Of the 16% of cases that was associated with non-hematologic malignancies, 8.6% were carcinomas of epithelial origin, 6.2% were sarcomas of mesenchymal origin, and 0.6% of cases were associated with malignant melanoma [155].

The basic pathophysiologic mechanism responsible for the development of skin lesions in paraneoplastic pemphigus is still under debate. Some studies suggest that circulating autoantibodies are pathogenic, while others propose that cytotoxic T-lymphocytes are also partially responsible [156–159].

In the majority of cases, treatment of paraneoplastic pemphigus is usually disappointing because treatment of the underlying malignancy is not always associated with the improvement of skin changes [1, 41]. Treatment with high-dose corticosteroid therapy, usually 1–2 mg/kg/day helps improve cutaneous lesions, but stomatitis rarely shows improvement. The use of cyclophosphamide, azathioprine, gold, dapsone, plasmapheresis, or photopheresis is generally ineffective when used alone [156, 157]. Long-standing clinical remission has been achieved with combination therapies using high-dose corticosteroids, cyclophosphamide, and intravenous immunoglobulins [156, 159]. Most recently, the use of rituximab has also been considered as a possible therapeutic option. A review of five patients could not establish whether rituximab was effective in treating paraneoplastic pemphigus due to the small number of cases and differences in protocol used, although 2/5 patients showed recovery and marked improvement of mouth lesions [156, 160, 161]. In an additional study by Schmidt et al., two patients treated with rituximab showed clinical remission with no further therapy necessary, whereas one additional patient showed partial remission [162]. Rituximab has been proven successful in the treatment of other autoimmune diseases mediated by autoantibodies [156]. The precise mechanism of action of rituximab is still unknown, but it is believed to deplete normal and abnormal B lymphocytes, thereby decreasing the abnormal immune response which is presumed to be the basis of paraneoplastic pemphigus [156].

Clinicians should be aware that the presence of progressive diffuse and persistent oral ulcerations or mucocutaneous lesions that are resistant to treatment may suggest that the presence of internal malignancy. Therefore, an extensive malignancy workup should be performed to search for occult neoplasm including a complete blood count, chemistry profile, serum protein electrophoresis, and a CT scan of the chest, abdomen, and pelvis in addition to physical examination of the spleen, liver, and lymph nodes [41, 155]. Furthermore, because the full spectrum of signs or symptoms of paraneoplastic pemphigus may not be present initially, multiple biopsies, direct and indirect immunofluorescence studies, and indirect immunofluorescence on murine bladder are also required for diagnosis [155]. Previous cases published such as lichen planus pemphigoides with associated underlying malignancy, lupus erythematosus with thymoma, erythema multiforme with unusual antibodies, and lichen planus associated with Castleman's tumor may all represent examples of neoplasia-induced pemphigus [152, 163–166]. The importance of early recognition is paramount because paraneoplastic pemphigus is associated with a poor prognosis. The mortality rate is almost 90%, with most patient deaths occurring during 1 month to 2 years after diagnosis [156, 157]. Death is usually secondary to sepsis, bleeding, and respiratory failure [41, 167].

Conclusion

Physician awareness regarding the most common cutaneous manifestations associated with internal malignancies ultimately results in a greater benefit for the patient. Adequate screening, leads to earlier intervention, which in the end helps to determine a more appropriate course of action. Paraneoplastic syndromes may well be the first sign of an occult neoplasm and their persistence may signal disease progression or recurrence. Most importantly, adequate management of these situations may not always result in the prolongation of survival, but an honest attempt can be made towards improving a patient's quality of life.

References

1. Kleyn E, Lai-Cheong JE, Bell HK. Cutaneous manifestations of internal malignancy. Am J Clin Dermatol. 2006;7:71–84.
2. Lookingbill DP, Spangler N, Sexton FMJ. Skin involvement as the presenting sign of internal carcinoma. A retrospective study of 7316 cancer patients. J Am Acad Dermatol. 1990;22:19–26.
3. Spencer PS, Helm TN. Skin metastases in cancer patients. Cutis. 1987;39:119–21.
4. Nashan D, Meiss F, Braun-Falco M, Reichenberg S. Cutaneous metastases from internal malignancies. Dermatol Ther. 2010;23: 567–80.
5. Brownstein MH, Helwig EB. Patterns of cutaneous metastasis. Arch Dermatol. 1972;105:862–8.
6. Poole S, Fenske N. Cutaneous markers of internal malignancy. I. Malignant involvement of the skin and the genodermatoses. J Am Acad Dermatol. 1993;28:1–11.
7. Cohen I, Levy E, Schreiber H. Alopecia neoplastica due to breast carcinoma. Arch Dermatol. 1961;84:490–2.
8. Baum EM, Omura EF, Payne RR, et al. Alopecia neoplastica-a rare form of cutaneous metastasis. J Am Acad Dermatol. 1981;4:688–94.
9. Braverman IM. Skin manifestations of internal malignancy. Clin Geriatr Med. 2002;18:1–19.
10. Reingold IM. Cutaneous metastases from internal carcinoma. Cancer. 1966;19:162–8.
11. Mehregan AH. Metastatic carcinoma to the skin. Dermatologica. 1961;123:311–25.
12. Mullinax K, Cohen J. Carcinoma en cuirasse presenting as keloids of the chest. Dermatol Surg. 2004;30:226–8.
13. DeVita VT, Hellman S, Rosenberg SA. Cancer: principles and practice of oncology, vol. 5. New York: Lippincott-Raven; 1997. p. 1582–3, 1585–6, 2408–10.
14. Freedman DG, Brescia G, Horne M, et al. Cutaneous manifestations of malignancy: metastases to skin are most specific sign of internal cancer. Postgrad Med. 2004;115(1) (online article).
15. Brownstein MH, Helwig EB. Spread of tumors to the skin. Arch Dermatol. 1973;107:80.

16. Gmitter TI, Dhawan SS, Phillips MG, et al. Cutaneous metastases of colonic adenocarcinoma. Cutis. 1990;46:66–8.
17. Lee MY, Li CP, Lee RC, Wang LW, Chao Y. Gastric adenocarcinoma with Sister Mary Joseph's nodule successfully treated with combined chemoradiation. J Gastroenterol Hepatol. 2003;18: 114–5.
18. Dodiuk-Gad R, Ziv M, Loven D, et al. Sister Mary Joseph's nodule as a presenting sign of internal malignancy. Skinmed. 2006;5:256–8.
19. Ikeda S, Yajima M, Hida K, et al. Sister Joseph umbilical nodule coexisting with endometriosis from endometrial carcinoma. Arch Gynecol Obstet. 2006;273:250–2.
20. Hill M, O'Leary JP. Vignettes in medical history. Sister Mary Joseph and her node. Am Surg. 1996;62:328–9.
21. Powell FC, Cooper AJ, Massa MC, et al. Sister Mary Joseph's nodule: a clinical and Histologic study. J Am Acad Dermatol. 1984;10:610–5.
22. Khan AJ, Cook B. Metastatic carcinoma of umbilicus: Sister Mary Joseph's Nodule. Cutis. 1997;60:297–8.
23. Yosipovitch G. Chronic pruritus: a paraneoplastic sign. Dermatol Ther. 2010;23:590–6.
24. Twycross R, Greaves MW, Handwerker H, Jones EA, et al. Itch: scratching more than the surface. Q J Med. 2003;96:7–26.
25. Botero F. Pruritus as a manifestation of systemic disorders. Cutis. 1978;21:873–80.
26. Fjellner B, Hagermark O. Pruritus in polycythemia vera: treatment with aspirin and possibility of platelet involvement. Acta Dermatol Venerol. 1979;59:505–12.
27. Bluefarb EM, editor. Leukemia cutis. Springfield, IL: Charles C. Thomas; 1960.
28. Kawase K, Dimaio DJ, Tucker SL, et al. Paget's disease of the breast: there is a role for breast-conserving therapy. Ann Surg Oncol. 2005;12:391–7.
29. Powell FC, Bjornsson J, Doyle JA, Cooper AJ. Genital Paget's disease and urinary tract malignancy. J Am Acad Dermatol. 1985;13:84.
30. Marshall JK, Griffith KA, Haffty BG, et al. Conservative management of Paget disease of the breast with radiotherapy: 10- and 15-year results. Cancer. 2003;97:2142–9.
31. Polgár C, Orosz Z, Kovács T, Fodor J. Breast-conserving therapy for Paget disease of the nipple: a prospective European Organization for Research and Treatment of Cancer study of 61 patients. Cancer. 2002;94:1904–5.
32. Laronga C, Hasson D, Hoover S, et al. Paget's disease in the era of sentinel lymph node biopsy. Am J Surg. 2006;192:481–3.
33. Zakaria S, Pantvaidya G, Ghosh K, Degnim AC. Paget's disease of the breast: accuracy of preoperative assessment. Breast Cancer Res Treat. 2007;102:137–42.
34. Amano G, Yajima M, Moroboshi Y, et al. MRI accurately depicts underlying DCIS in a patient with Paget's disease of the breast without palpable mass and mammography findings. Jpn J Clin Oncol. 2005;35:149–53.
35. Argawala SS. Paraneoplastic Syndromes. Med Clin North Am. 1996;80:173–84.
36. Curth HO. Skin lesions and internal carcinoma. Cancer of the skin: biology, diagnosis, management. Philadelphia, PA: Saunders; 1976. p. 1308–41.
37. Mclean D, Haynes H. Cutaneous manifestations of internal malignant disease. In: Fitzpatrick TB, Freedberg IM, Eisen AZ, Wolff K, Austen KF, editors. Dermatology in general medicine. New York: McGraw Hill; 1999. p. 2106–20.
38. Abreu-Velez AM, Howard MS. Diagnosis and treatment of cutaneous paraneoplastic disorders. Dermatol Ther. 2010;23:662–75.
39. Weiss P, O'Rourke ME. Cutaneous paraneoplastic syndromes. Clin J Oncol Nurs. 2000;4:257–62.
40. Heaphy Jr MR, Millns JL, Schroeter AL. The sign of Leser-Trélat in a case of adenocarcinoma of the lung. J Am Acad Dermatol. 2000;43:386–90.
41. Boyce S, Harper J. Paraneoplastic dermatoses. Dermatol Clin. 2002;20:523–32.
42. Cohen PR, Kurzrock R. Mucocutaneous paraneoplastic syndromes. Semin Oncol. 1997;24:334–59.
43. Schwartz RA. Acanthosis nigricans. J Am Acad Dermatol. 1994;31:1–19.
44. Scully C, Barrett WA, Gilkes J, et al. Oral acanthosis nigricans, the sign of Leser-Trélat and cholangiocarcinoma. Br J Dermatol. 2001;145:505–26.
45. Pentero M, Carrozzzo M, Pagano M, Gandolfo S. Oral acanthosis nigricans, tripe palms and sign of leser-trélat in a patient with gastric adenocarcinoma. Int J Dermatol. 2004;43:530–2.
46. Mekhail TM, Markman M. Acanthosis nigricans with endometrial carcinoma: case report and review of the literature. Gynecol Oncol. 2002;84:332–4.
47. Kebria MM, Beinso J, Kim R, Mekhail TM. Malignant acanthosis nigricans, tripe palms and the sign of leser-trélat, a hint to the diagnosis of early stage ovarian cancer: a case report and review of the literature. Gynecol Oncol. 2006;101:353–5.
48. Anderson SH, Hudson-Peacock M, Muller AF. Malignant acanthosis nigricans: potential role of chemotherapy. Br J Dermatol. 1999;141:714–6.
49. Bonnekoh B, Thiele B, Merk H, Mahrle G. Systemic photochemotherapy (PUVA) in acanthosis nigricans maligna: regression of keratosis, hyperpigmentation and pruritus. Z Hautkr. 1989;64: 1059–62.
50. Greenwood R, Tring FC. Treatment of malignant acanthosis nigricans with cyproheptadine. Br J Dermatol. 1982;106:697–8.
51. Möller H, Eriksson S, Holen O, Waldenström JG. Complete reversibility of paraneoplastic acanthosis nigricans after operation. Acta Med Scand. 1978;203:245–6.
52. Dantzig PI. Sign of Leser-Trélat. Arch Dermatol. 1973;108: 700–1.
53. Schwartz RA. Sign of Lesser-Trelát. J Am Acad Dermatol. 1996; 35:88–95.
54. Holdiness MR. The sign of Leser-Trélat. Int J Dermatol. 1986;25:564–72.
55. Jacobs MI, Rigel DS. Acanthosis nigricans and the sign of Leser-Trélat associated with adenocarcinoma of the gallbladder. Cancer. 1981;48:325–8.
56. Lee CH, Clark AR, Thorpe ME, et al. Bile duct adenocarcinoma with Leser-Trelat sign and pure red blood cell aplasia. Cancer. 1980;46:1657–60.
57. Holdiness MR. On the classification of the sign of Leser-Trélat. J Am Acad Dermatol. 1988;19:754–7.
58. Koyama S, Ikeda K, Sato M, et al. Transforming growth factor-alpha (TGF-alpha)-producing gastric carcinoma with acanthosis nigricans: an endocrine effect of TGF alpha in the pathogenesis of cutaneous paraneoplastic syndrome and epithelial hyperplasia of the esophagus. J Gastroenterol. 1997;32:71–7.
59. Safai B, Grant JM, Good RA. Cutaneous manifestation of internal malignancies (II): the sign of Leser-Trélat. Intl J Dermatol. 1978;17:494–5.
60. Ellis DL, Yates RA. Sign of Leser-Trélat. Clin Dermatol. 1993;11:141–8.
61. Liddell K, White JE, Caldwell IW. Seborrheic keratoses and carcinoma of the large bowel. Three cases exhibiting the sign of Lester-Trelát. Br J Dermatol. 1975;92:449–52.
62. Cohen PR, Grossman ME, Kurzrock R. Tripe palms and cancer. Clin Dermatol. 1993;11:165–73.
63. Cohen PR, Grossman ME, Almeida L, Kurzrock R. Tripe palms and malignancy. J Clin Oncol. 1989;7:669–78.

64. Stavrianeas AC, Katoulis AC, Neofotistou O, et al. Tripe palms preceding squamous cell carcinoma of the lung by 11 month. Dermatology. 1999;198:173–4.
65. Chosidow O, Bécherel PA, Piette JC, et al. Tripe palms associated with systemic mastocytosis: the role of transforming growth factor-alpha and efficacy of interferon-alpha. Br J Dermatol. 1998;38:698–703.
66. Strobel ES, Bouveret C, Kohl PK. Acrokeratosis paraneoplastica of Bazex as an indicator for underlying squamous cell carcinoma of the lung. J Cancer Res Clin Oncol. 2006;132:376–8.
67. Río-Ramírez MT, Casado-López ME, Peirón Puyal MJ, Penas Herrero JM. Pulmonary Adenocarcinoma and Bazex Syndrome (Paraneoplastic Acrokeratosis). Arch Bronconeumol. 2007;43: 46–8.
68. Valdivielso M, Longo I, Suárez R, Lázaro P. Acrokeratosis paraneoplastica (Bazex Syndrome). J Eur Acta Dermatol Venerol. 2005;19:340–4.
69. Bolognia JL. Bazex syndrome: acrokeratosis paraneoplastica. Semin Dermatol. 1995;14:84–9.
70. Akhyani M, Mansoori P, Taheri A, Asadi Kani A. Acrokeratosis Paraneoplastica (Bazex syndrome) associated with breast cancer. Clin Exp Dermatol. 2004;29:423–36.
71. Douwes KE, Burgdorff T, Szeimies RM, et al. Paraneoplastic Bazex acrokeratosis in adenocarcinoma of the stomach. Dtsch Med Wochenschr. 2001;126:203–6.
72. Obasi OE, Garg SK. Bazex paraneoplastic acrokeratosis in prostate carcinoma. Br J Dermatol. 1987;117:647–51.
73. Hsu YS, Lien GS, Lai HH, et al. Acrokeratosis paraneoplastica (Bazex syndrome) with adenocarcinoma of the colon: report of a case and review of the literature. J Gastroenterol. 2000;35: 460–4.
74. Arregui MA, Ratón JA, Landa N, et al. Bazex's syndrome (acrokeratosis paraneoplastica) – first case report of association with a bladder carcinoma. Clin Exp Dermatol. 1993;18:445–8.
75. Voelter-Mahlknecht S, Bauer J, Metzler G, et al. Bullous variant of Sweet's syndrome. Int J Dermatol. 2005;44:946–7.
76. Neoh CY, Tan AWH, Hg SK. Sweet's syndrome: a spectrum of unusual clinical presentations and associations. Br J Dermatol. 2007;156:480–5.
77. Gross G, Pfister H, Hellenthal B, Hagedorn M. Acanthosis nigricans maligna. Clinical and virological investigations. Dermatologica. 1984;168:265–72.
78. Bolognia JL, Brewer YP, Cooper DL. Bazex syndrome (acrokeratosis paraneoplastica). An analytic review. Medicine (Baltimore). 1991;70:269–80.
79. Hara M, Hunayama M, Aiba S, et al. Acrokeratosis paraneoplastica (Bazex syndrome) associated with primary cutaneous squamous cell carcinoma of the lower leg, vitiligo and alopecia areata. Br J Dermatol. 1995;133:121–4.
80. Halpern SM, O'Donell LJD, Makunura CN. Acrokeratosis paraneoplastica of Bazex in association with a metastatic endocrine tumor. J R Soc Med. 1995;88:353–4.
81. Chastain MA. The glucagonoma syndrome: a review of its features and discussion of new perspectives. Am J Med Sci. 2001;321:306–20.
82. Kovács RK, Krom I, Dobozy A, et al. Necrolytic migratory erythema. J Cutan Pathol. 2006;33:242–5.
83. Becker SW, Kahn D, Rothman S. Cutaneous manifestations of internal malignant tumors. Arch Dermatol Syphilol. 1942;45: 1069.
84. McGavran MH, Unger RH, Recant L, et al. A glucagon-secreting alpha-cell carcinoma of the pancreas. N Engl J Med. 1966;27: 1408–13.
85. Van Beek AP, de Hass ER, Van Vloten WA, et al. The glucagonoma syndrome and necrolytic migratory erythema: a clinical review. Eur J Endocrinol. 2004;151:531–7.
86. Wermers RA, Fatourechi V, Wynne AG, et al. The glucagonoma syndrome. Clinical and pathologic features in 21 patients. Medicine (Baltimore). 1996;75:53–63.
87. Shepherd ME, Raimer SS, Tyring SK, Smith EB. Treatment of necrolytic migratory erythema in glucagonoma syndrome. J Am Acad Dermatol. 1991;25:925–8.
88. Thompson NW, Eckhauser FE. Malignant islet-cell tumors of the pancreas. World J Surg. 1984;8:940–51.
89. Perry R, Vinik A. Diagnosis and management of functioning islet cell tumors. J Clin Endocrinol Metab. 1995;80:2273–8.
90. Schwartz RA. Glucagonoma and pseudoglucagonoma syndromes. Int J Dermatol. 1997;36:81–9.
91. Stacpoole PW. The glucagonoma syndrome: clinical features, diagnosis, and treatment. Endocr Rev. 1981;2:347–61.
92. Weedon D. Metabolic and Storage diseases. In: Weedon D, editor. Skin pathology. Edinburgh: Churchill Livingstone; 1997. p. 109–59.
93. Almdal TP, Heindorff H, Bardram L, Vilstrup H. Increased amino acid clearance and urea synthesis in a patient with glucagonoma. Gut. 1990;31:946–8.
94. Barazzoni R, Zanetti M, Tiengo A, Tessari P. Protein metabolism in glucagonoma. Diabetologia. 1999;42:326–9.
95. Prendiville JS, Manfredi LN. Skin signs of nutritional disorders. Semin Dermatol. 1992;11:88–97.
96. Tierney EP, Bagder J. Etiology and pathogenesis of necrolytic migratory erythema: review of the literature. MedGenMed. 2004;6:1–8.
97. Leitcher SB. Clinical and metabolic aspects of glucagonoma. Medicine. 1980;59:100–13.
98. Sandstrom B, Cekerblad A, Linbland B, Lonnerdal B. Acrodermatitis enterohepathica, zinc metabolism, copper status and immune function. Arch Pediatr Adolesc Med. 1994;148: 908–85.
99. Sinclair SA, Reynolds NJ. NME and zinc deficiency. Br J Dermatol. 1997;136:783–5.
100. Mullans E, Cohen R. Iatrogenic NME: a case report and review of nonglucagonoma-associated NME. J Am Acad Dermatol. 1998;38:866–73.
101. Alexander EK, Robinson M, Staniec M, Dluhy R. Peripheral amino acid and fatty acid infusion for the treatment of NME in the glucagonoma syndrome. Clinl Endocrinol. 2002;57:827–31.
102. Peterson L, Ahae J, Acott K, et al. Glucagonoma syndrome: in vitro evidence that glucagon increases epidermal arachadonic acid. J Am Acad Dermatol. 1984;11:468–73.
103. Jenkins DK, Mitchell JC, Manku MS. Effects of albumin on fatty acid, protein and eicosanoid levels in rat mesenteric arterial bed perfusions. Can J Physiol Pharmacol. 1988;66:679–82.
104. Chastain MA. The glucagonoma syndrome: a review of its features and discussion of new perspectives. Am J Med Sci. 2001;321:306–20.
105. Bhoopalam N, O'Dorsio T, et al. Use of a somatostatin analog (SMS 201-995) in the glucagonoma syndrome. Surgery. 1986;100:989–96.
106. Faiss S, Pape UF, Böhmig M, et al. Prospective, randomized, multicenter trial on the antiproliferative effect of lanreotide, interferon alpha, and their combination for therapy of metastatic neuroendocrine gastroenteropancreatic tumors– the International Lanreotide and Interferon Alfa Study Group. J Clinil Oncol. 2003;21: 2689–96.
107. Alexander EK, Robinson M, Staniec M, Dluhy RG. Peripheral amino acid and fatty acid infusion for the treatment of necrolytic migratory erythema in the glucagonoma syndrome. Clin Endocrinol (Oxf). 2002;57:827–31.
108. Bewley AP, Ross JS, Bunker CB, Staughton RC. Successful treatment of a patient with octreotide-resistant necrolytic migratory erythema. Br J Dermatol. 1996;134:1101–4.

109. Binnick AN, Spencer SK, Dennison WL, Horton ES. Glucagonoma syndrome. Report of two cases and literature review. Arch Dermatol. 1977;113:749–54.
110. Zhang M, Xu X, Shen Y, et al. Clinical experience in diagnosis and treatment of glucagonoma syndrome. Hepatobiliary Pancreat Dis Int. 2004;3:473–5.
111. Mehregan DA, Mehregan DR. Paraneoplastic syndromes. Adv Dermatol. 1994;9:25–43.
112. Tyring SK. Reactive erythemas: erythema annulare centrifugum and erythema gyratum repens. Clin Dermatol. 1993;11:135–9.
113. Eubanks LE, McBurney E, Reed R. Erythema gyratum repens. Am J Med Sci. 2001;321:302–5.
114. Kawakami T, Saito R. Erythema gyratum repens unassociated with underlying malignancy. J Dermatol. 1995;22:587–9.
115. Anhalt GJ. Paraneoplastic pemphigus: the role of tumors and drugs. Br J Dermatol. 2001;144:1102–4.
116. Skolnick M, Mainman ER. Erythema gyratum repens with metastatic adenocarcinoma. Arch Dermatol. 1975;111(2):227–9.
117. Caux F, Lebbe C, Thomine E, et al. Erythema gyratum repens. A case studied with immunofluorescence, immunoelectron microscopy and immunohistochemistry. Br J Dermatol. 1994; 131:102–7.
118. Holt PJ, Davies MG. Erythema gyratum repens – an immunologically mediated dermatosis? Br J Dermatol. 1977;96:343–7.
119. Cohen PR. Sweet's syndrome – a comprehensive review of an acute febrile neutrophilic dermatosis. Orphanet J Rare Dis. 2007;2:34.
120. Cohen PR, Kurzrock R. Sweet's syndrome revisited: a review of disease concepts. Int J Dermatol. 2003;42:761–78.
121. Cohen PR, Almeida L, Kurzrock R. Acute febrile neutrophilic dermatosis. Am Fam Physician. 1989;39:199–204.
122. Voelter-Mahlknecht S, Bauer J, Metzler G, et al. Bullous variant of Sweet's syndrome. Int J Dermatol. 2005;44:946–7.
123. Neoh CY, Tan AWH, Hg SK. Sweet's syndrome: a spectrum of unusual clinical presentations and associations. Br J Dermatol. 2007;156:480–5.
124. Tomasini C, Aloi F, Osella-Abate S, et al. Immature myeloid precursors in chronic neutrophilic dermatosis associated with myelodysplastic syndrome. Am J Dermatopathol. 2002;22:429–33.
125. Sweet RD. An acute febrile neutrophilic dermatosis. Br J Dermatol. 1964;76:349–56.
126. Jordan HF. Acute febrile neutrophilic dermatosis: a histopathological study of 37 patients and review of the literature. Am J Dermatopathol. 1989;11:99–111.
127. von den Driesch P. Sweet's syndrome and vasculitis. J Am Acad Dermatol. 1996;34:539.
128. Malone JC, Slone SP, Wills-Frank LA, et al. Vascular inflammation (vasculitis) in Sweet syndrome: a clinicopathological study of 28 biopsy specimens from 21 patients. Arch Dermatol. 2002;138:345–9.
129. Requena L, Kutzner H, Palmedo G, et al. Histiocytoid Sweet syndrome: a dermal infiltration of immature neutrophilic granulocytes. Arch Dermatol. 2005;141:834–42.
130. Morgan KW, Callen JP. Sweet's syndrome in acute myelogenous leukemia presenting as periorbital cellulitis with an infiltrate of leukemic cells. J Am Acad Dermatol. 2001;45:590–5.
131. Cohen PR, Kurzrock R. Sweet's syndrome and cancer. Clin Dermatol. 1993;1:149–57.
132. von den Driesch P, Gomez RS, Kiesewetter F, et al. Sweet's syndrome: clinical spectrum and associated conditions. Cutis. 1989;44:193–200.
133. Feliu E, Cervantes F, Ferrando J, et al. Neutrophilic pustulosis associated with chronic myeloid leukemia: a special form of Sweet's syndrome. Report of two cases. Acta Hematol. 1992;88:154–7.
134. Haverstock C, Libecco JF, Sadeghi P, Maytin E. Tender erythematous plaques in a woman with acute myelogenous leukemia. Arch Dermatol. 2006;142:235–40.
135. Disel U, Paydas S, Yavuz S, Tuncer I, Alpay R. Bilateral ear Sweet's syndrome in a case with relapse acute myeloblastic leukemia. Leuk Res. 2006;30:364.
136. Cohen PR, Holder WR, Tucker SB, et al. Sweet syndrome in patients with solid tumors. Cancer. 1993;72:2723–30.
137. Nielsen I, Donati D, Strumia R, et al. Sweet's syndrome and malignancy: report of the first case associated with adenocarcinoma of the lung. Lung Cancer. 1993;10:95–9.
138. Reuss Borst MA, Pawelec G, Saal JG, et al. Sweet's syndrome associated with myelodysplasia: possible role of cytokines in the pathogenesis of disease. Br J Haematol. 1993;84:356–8.
139. Kawakami T, Ohashi S, Kawa Y, et al. Elevated serum granulocyte colony-stimulating factor levels in patients with active phase of Sweet syndrome and patients with active Behçet disease: implication in neutrophil apoptosis dysfunction. Arch Dermatol. 2004;140:570–4.
140. Reuss Borst MA, Müller CA, Waller HD. The possible role of G-CSF in the pathogenesis of Sweet's syndrome. Leuk Lymphoma. 1994;15:261–4.
141. Cohen PR, Kurzrock R. Sweet's syndrome; a review of current treatment options. Am J Clin Dermatol. 2002;3:117–31.
142. Cohen PR, Talpaz M, Kurzrock R. Malignancy-associated Sweet's Syndrome: review of the world literature. J Clin Oncol. 1988;6:1887–97.
143. Sharpe GR, Leggat HM. A case of Sweet's syndrome and myelodysplasia: response to cyclosporine. Br J Dermatol. 1992;127: 538–9.
144. Bourke JF, Keohane S, Long CC, Kemmett D, et al. Sweet's syndrome and malignancy in the U.K. Br J Dermatol. 1997;137: 609–13.
145. Wilson DM, John GR, Callen JP. Peripheral ulcerative keratitis – an extracutaneous neutrophilic disorder: report of a patient with rheumatoid arthritis, pustular vasculitis, pyoderma gangrenosum, and Sweet's syndrome with an excellent response to cyclosporine therapy. J Am Acad Dermatol. 1999;40:331–4.
146. Brodkin RH, Schwartz RA. Sweet's syndrome with myelofibrosis and leukemia: partial response to interferon. Dermatology. 1995;190:160–3.
147. Kato N, Yasukawa K, Kimura K, Yoshida K. Anaplastic large-cell lymphoma associated with acquired ichthyosis. J Am Acad Dermatol. 2000;42:914–20.
148. Roselino AM, Souza CS, Andrade JM, et al. Dermatomyositis and acquired ichthyosis as paraneoplastic manifestations of ovarian tumor. Int J Dermatol. 1997;36:611–4.
149. Griffin LJ, Massa MC. Acquired ichthyosis and pityriasis rotunda. Clin Dermatol. 1993;11:27–32.
150. Ameen M, Chopra S, Darvay A, Acland K, Chu AC. Erythema gyratum repens and acquired ichthyosis associated with transitional cell carcinoma of the kidney. Clin Exp Dermatol. 2000;26:510–2.
151. Anhalt GJ, SooChan K, Stanley JR, et al. Paraneoplastic pemphigus, an autoimmune mucocutaneous disease associated with neoplasia. N Engl J Med. 1990;323:1729–35.
152. Camisa C, Helm TN. Paraneoplastic pemphigus is a distinct neoplasia-induced autoimmune disease. Arch Dermatol. 1993;129:883–6.
153. Mimouni D, Anhalt GJ, Lazarova Z, et al. Paraneoplastic pemphigus in children and adolescents. Br J Dermatol. 2002;147: 725–32.
154. Joly P, Richard C, Gilbert D, et al. Sensitivity and specificity of clinical, histologic and immunologic features in the diagnosis of paraneoplastic pemphigus. J Am Acad Dermatol. 2000;43: 619–26.
155. Kaplan I, Hodak E, Ackerman L, et al. Neoplasms associated with paraneoplastic pemphigus: a review with emphasis on non-hematologic malignancy and oral mucosal manifestations. Oral Oncology. 2004;40:553–62.

156. Barnadas MA, Roe E, Brunet S, et al. Therapy of paraneoplastic pemphigus with Rituximab: a case report and review of the literature. J Eur Acad Dermatol Venerol. 2006;20:69–74.
157. Anhalt GJ. Paraneoplastic pemphigus. Adv Dermatol. 1997;1: 77–97.
158. Amagai M, Nishikawa T, Nousari H, Anhalt GJ. Hashimoto antibodies against desmoglein 3 (pemphigus vulgaris antigen) are present in sera from patients with paraneoplastic pemphigus and cause acantholysis in vivo in neonatal mice. Clin Invest. 1998;102:775–82.
159. Reich K, Brinck U, Letschert M, et al. Graft-verusus-host disease like immunophenotype and apoptotic keratinocyte death in paraneoplastic pemphigus. Br J Dermatol. 1999;141:739–46.
160. Heizmann M, Itin P, Werlin M, et al. Successful treatment of paraneoplastic pemphigus in follicular NHL with Rituximab: report of a case and review of treatment for paraneoplastic pemphigus in NHL and CLL. Am J Hematol. 2001;66:142–4.
161. Borradori L, Lombardi T, Samson J, et al. Anti CD-20 monoclonal antibody (Rituximab) for refractory erosive stomatitis secondary to CD20+ follicular lymphoma associated paraneoplastic pemphigus. Arch Dermatol. 2001;17:269–72.
162. Schmidt E, Hunzelmann N, Zillikens D, et al. Rituximab in refractory autoimmune bullous diseases. Clin Exp Dermatol. 2006;31: 503–8.
163. Feverman E, Sandbanck M. Lichen planus pemphigoides with extensive melanosis. Arch Dermatol. 1971;104:61–7.
164. Cruz Jr PD, Coldiron BM, Southeimer RD. Concurrent features of cutaneous lupus erythematosus and pemphigus erythematosus following myasthenia gravis and thymoma. J Am Acad Dermatol. 1987;16:472–80.
165. Matsuoka LY, Wortsman J, Stanley JR. Epidermal autoantibodies in erythema multiforme. J Am Acad Dermatol. 1989;21:677–80.
166. Plewing G, Jansen T, Jungblunt RM, Roher HD. Castleman tumor, lichen ruber and pemphigus vulgaris: paraneoplastic association of immunological diseases. Hautarzt. 1990;41:662–70.
167. Camisa C, Helm TN, Yao-Chang L, et al. Paraneoplastic pemphigus: a report of three cases including one long term survivor. J Am Acad Dermatol. 1992;27:547–53.

Cutaneous Manifestations of Infectious Diseases

Elena Montalván Miró and Néstor P. Sánchez

Skin infections account for a significant portion of dermatologic diseases. Infections of the skin and subcutaneous tissues are highly diverse in respect to incidence, etiologic organisms, and clinical manifestations. Most cases are potentially treatable, thus, it is vital for the clinician to become familiar with the cutaneous expression of local and systemic processes. This chapter covers the clinical presentation, diagnosis, and treatment of the most common bacterial, viral, and fungal mucocutaneous infections encountered in internal medicine.

Bacteria, Spirochetes, and Mycobacteria (Table 1)

Bacteria

Impetigo

Impetigo is considered the most common superficial bacterial skin infection in children 2–6 years) [2]. It may be classified as bullous or non-bullous and is frequently caused by *Staphylococcus aureus* or *Streptococcus pyogenes* (see Fig. 1) [3]. For more information on impetigo, refer to the Cutaneous Disorders in the Intensive Care Unit chapter.

Folliculitis

Introduction

Inflammation of the hair follicle is referred to as folliculitis. It is categorized by the depth of involvement of the follicle (superficial versus deep) and the etiology of the inflammation.

Incidence and Prevalence

Superficial folliculitis is common. Due to its self-limited nature, patients rarely present to the physician with this complaint. Therefore, the incidence is unknown and can be estimated only with cases of recurrent or persistent superficial folliculitis and deep folliculitis, for which patients more commonly seek medical attention [3].

Etiology

Hair follicles may become inflamed by physical injury, chemical irritation, nutritional deficiencies, or an infectious origin as in syphilitic, fungal, viral, parasitic, and bacterial folliculitis. There are numerous predisposing factors that lead to bacterial folliculitis and they include: follicular occlusion, maceration, hyperhydration, nasal harboring of *S. aureus*, pruritic skin diseases, vigorous application of topical corticosteroids, exposure to oils and certain chemicals, shaving against the direction of hair growth, diabetes mellitus, and exposure to heated or contaminated water [4, 5]. *S. aureus* is the most frequent cause of infectious folliculitis [4, 6, 7] but *Streptococcus*, *Pseudomonas*, *Proteus*, and coliform bacteria have also been implicated [8].

Clinical Features

The most common infectious form is superficial folliculitis. It manifests as a pustule on the follicle orifice over an erythematous base and it heals without scarring (see Fig. 2). Multiple (Impetigo of Bockhart) or single lesions mostly appear in hair bearing areas of the skin, predominantly the head, neck, trunk, buttocks, axillae, and groin [4]. Clinically, lesions may be tender or painless; however, pruritus is the most common complaint. Systemic symptoms or fever rarely coexist [5].

Deep folliculitis results from the involvement of portions of the follicle beyond the isthmus [3]. Clinically, these lesions are tender, erythematous papules or nodules that may scar, unlike superficial folliculitis. Major forms of deep folliculitis are furuncles, sycosis (barbae, lupoid, and mycotic) (see Fig. 3), pseudofolliculitis barbae, acne keloidalis, and hidradenitis suppurativa [5].

Pseudomonal folliculitis, also known as "hot-tub folliculitis," is caused by *Pseudomonas aeruginosa*. It is

E. Montalván Miró (✉) • N.P. Sánchez
Department of Dermatology, University of Puerto Rico School of Medicine, Medical Sciences Campus, San Juan, Puerto Rico
e-mail: elena.montalvan@upr.edu

N.P. Sánchez (ed.), *Atlas of Dermatology in Internal Medicine*,
DOI 10.1007/978-1-4614-0688-4_7, © Springer Science+Business Media, LLC 2012

Table 1 Characteristics of some common skin and subcutaneous bacterial infections

Terminology	Subgroups	Location	Etiology
Pyoderma	Non-bullous impetigo	Superficial skin of the face (perioral and perinasal) or extremities	*Staphylococcus aureus* (*S. aureus*), *Streptococcus pyogenes* (*S. pyogenes*)
	Bullous impetigo	Superficial skin of the face, trunk, perineum or extremities	*S. aureus*
	Folliculitis (pustulosis)	Skin, hair follicles	*S. aureus*
	Folliculitis (sycosis) barbae	Skin, hair follicles of the beard	*S. pyogenes*, *S. aureus*
	Hot-tub folliculitis	Skin	*Pseudomonas aeruginosa*
Abscesses	Furuncle (boil, subcutaneous abscess)	Subcutaneous tissue	*S. aureus*
	Hidradenitis suppurativa	Multiple furuncles in sweat glands: axillae, groins	*S. aureus* and other bacteria, including gram-negative bacilli and anaerobes
	Carbuncle	Dense group of furuncles in areas of thick skin: back of neck, shoulders, buttocks	*S. aureus*
Cellulitis		Skin and subcutaneous tissue	*S. aureus*, *S. pyogenes*, Group C and G streptococci, *P. aeruginosa*, *Haemophilus influenzae*, or gram-negative bacilli
	Erysipelas	Skin	*S. pyogenes*
Ecthyma		Skin and subcutaneous tissue	*S. pyogenes*, *S. aureus* or both; *P. aeruginosa*
	Ecthyma gangrenosum	Skin and subcutaneous tissue in neutropenic patients	*P. aeruginosa*

Table adapted from [1]

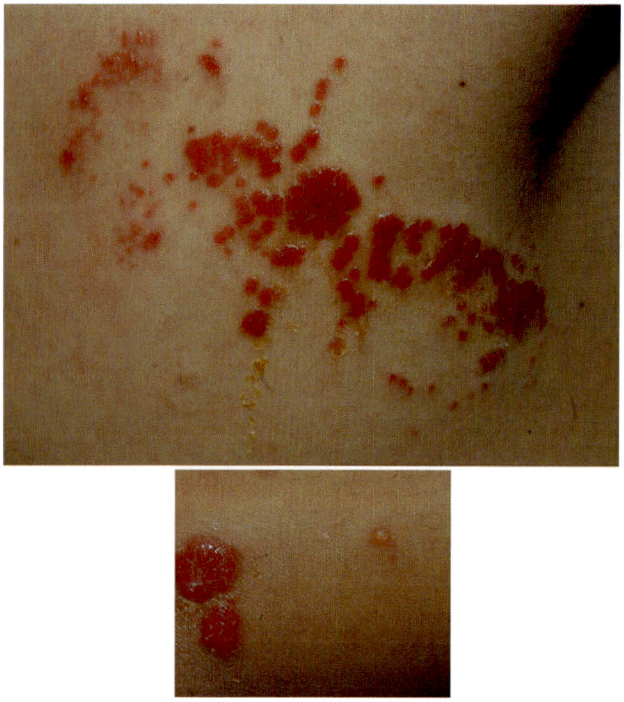

Fig. 1 Non-bullous impetigo. Classic stuck-on, honey-colored crusts overlying confluent erythematous papules. Vesicles and erosions might also be present

characterized by multiple follicular papules or pustules associated with bathing in hot-tubs, whirlpools, or swimming pools. Lesions may appear as early as 6 h after bathing in contaminated or poorly contained waters and are usually self-limiting in immunocompetent individuals lasting up to 14 days [3, 5, 9, 10]. Lesions are pruritic and may be accompanied by symptoms such as earache, painful eyes, sore throat, headache, fever, malaise, and abdominal pain [3, 10].

Diagnosis

The diagnosis of bacterial folliculitis may be established clinically; however, in complicated, recurrent, or treatment-resistant cases, a swab of the pustule contents may be necessary for Gram stain or culture to guide treatment [4].

Pathology

On histology folliculitis presents with inflammatory cells in the wall and ostia of the hair follicle (see Fig. 4). The inflammation may be limited to the superficial aspect of the follicle, involving the infundibulum or it can affect both the superficial and deep aspect of the follicle. The types of inflammatory cells vary depending on the etiology of the folliculitis and/or the stage at which the biopsy specimen was obtained. For example, a neutrophilic infiltrate can be seen in more acute cases, whereas more chronic cases may have histocytic cells [11].

Differential Diagnosis

The differential diagnosis consists of noninfectious folliculitis, acne vulgaris, acne rosacea, milia, acneiform eruptions, dermatologic manifestations of renal diseases, cutaneous candidiasis, coccidioidomycosis, and others.

Complications

Complications, although uncommon, include cellulitis, furunculosis, scarring, and permanent hair loss [4].

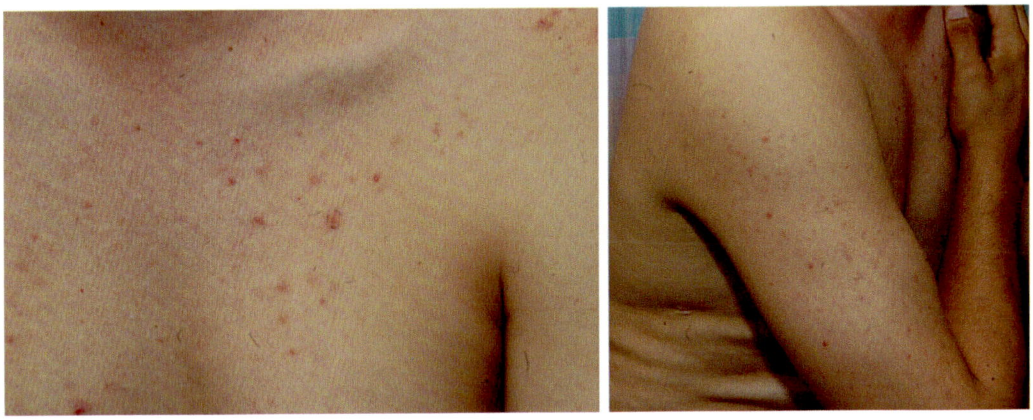

Fig. 2 Folliculitis. Multiple erythematous papules and pustules over trunk and upper extremities

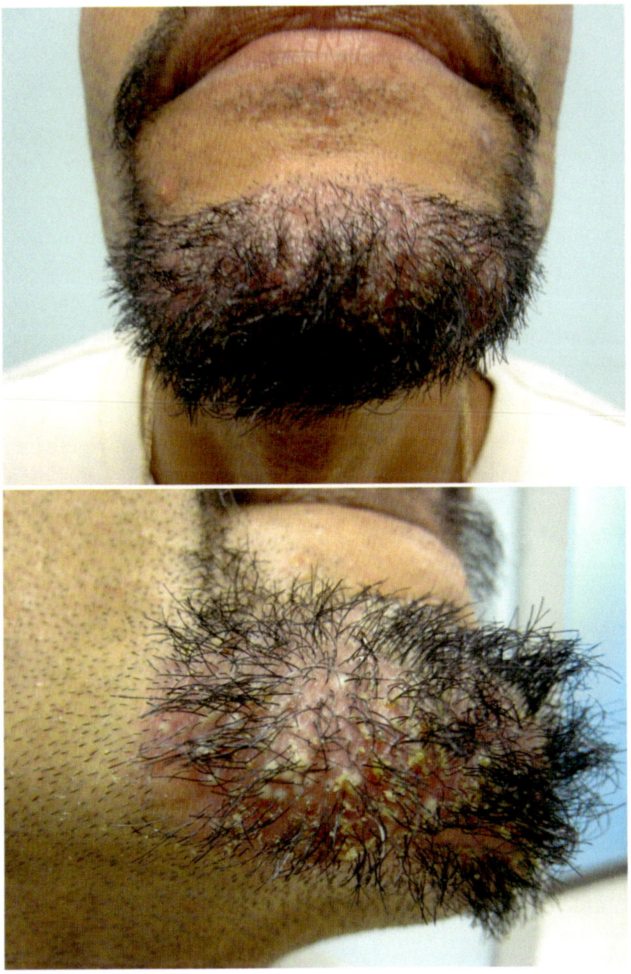

Fig. 3 Folliculitis barbae. Multiple pustules on the orifices of the follicles in the beard area accompanied by crusting in an erythematous base

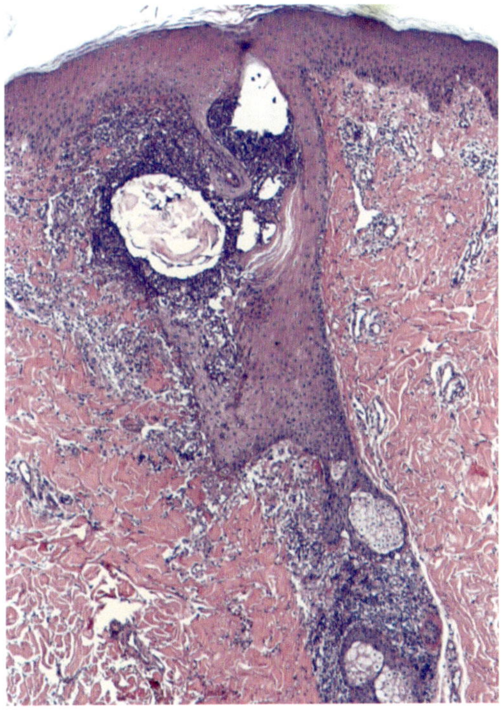

Fig. 4 Histopathologic findings of a folliculitis. Suppurative process involving both the superficial and deep portion of the follicle

Treatment

Treatment of superficial bacterial folliculitis consists cleansing the affected areas thoroughly the affected areas with antibacterial soaps three times daily [12]. Topical antibacterial ointments such as mupirocin are advised for up to 10 days [5, 12]. In recurrent, treatment-resistant, or deep lesions, first generation cephalosporins, penicillinase-resistant penicillin, macrolides and oral clindamycin may be used based on the results of the culture [3, 5, 12]. Some patients may be chronic carriers of *S. aureus* and would consequently benefit from mupirocin ointment application to the nares, axillae, and/or groin twice daily for 5 days and routine washing of towels, linens, and clothing in hot water [4]. If the culture does not reveal any organisms, tetracycline or doxycycline is preferred for their anti-inflammatory properties [5].

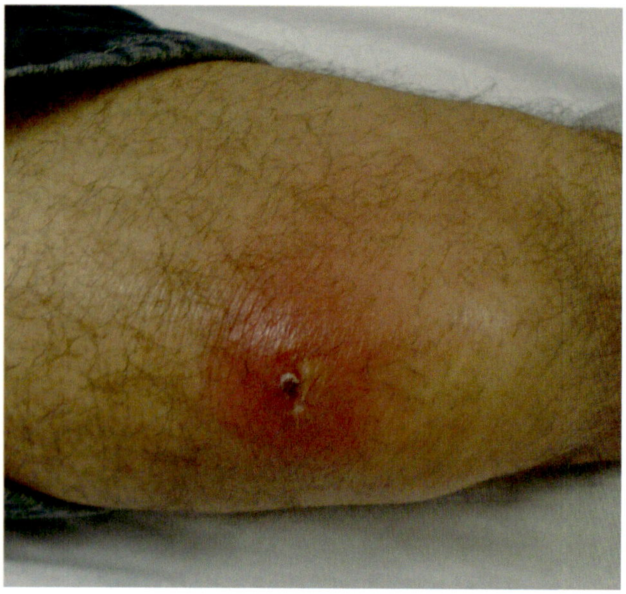

Fig. 5 Furuncle. Erythematous firm nodule in hair bearing skin of areas exposed to friction or minor trauma which may progress into a fluctuant mass that eventually ruptures and suppurates. This particular case was caused by MRSA

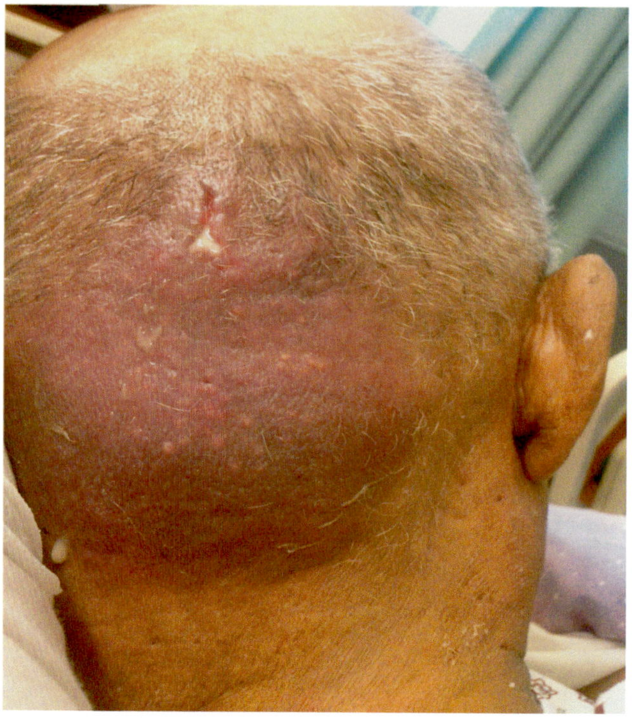

Fig. 6 Carbuncle. Erythematous, edematous, indurated skin with draining sinus, and multiple pustules in a patient that arrived to the hospital for non-resolving fever

"Hot-tub" folliculitis treatment is directed at prevention by maintaining the appropriate chlorine level and the cleaning of the water source [3]. When the course of the disease does not follow its self-limiting nature or manifests with constitutional symptoms, an oral third generation cephalosporin or fluoroquinolone may be beneficial [12].

Furuncles and Carbuncles

Introduction

Folliculitis may progress to form subcutaneous inflammatory abscesses known as furuncles, or boils, which usually drain and resolve spontaneously; however, they may coalesce to form more extensive collections involving multiple hair follicles called carbuncles [1].

Clinical Features

A furuncle presents as an erythematous, painful, and firm nodule in hair bearing skin, especially those areas exposed to friction or minor trauma (see Fig. 5) [1, 3, 5]. The incidence tends to increase after puberty, with *S. aureus* being the most common causative agent [1, 3, 13]. The lesion may progress into a fluctuant mass that will eventually rupture into the skins surface. This drainage of the purulent content diminishes the pain. If multiple or recurrent furuncles (furunculosis) are present, one should suspect chronic *S. aureus* colonization [5]. Constitutional symptoms in furunculosis are rare, in contrast to carbuncles.

Carbuncles present clinically as tender, erythematous, edematous, and multiple draining sinus tracts. They extend deep into the subcutaneous tissue. These lesions occur most often in areas where the dermis is thick such as the nape of the neck, lateral thighs, and back (see Fig. 6). Malaise, chills, and fevers are usually present. Severe infections can result in extensive scarring and are more likely to develop complications such as cellulitis or septicemia [1, 3, 5].

Etiology

As mentioned above, conditions compromising the integrity of the skin are portals for the entry of *S. aureus* thus predispose to the formation of furuncles and subsequently carbuncles. These are most commonly associated with systemic conditions such as diabetes mellitus, eczema, obesity, alcoholism, malnutrition, and immunodeficiency states (Hyper-IgE syndrome) [5, 12, 13]. Nonetheless, healthy individuals with no risk factors can also develop these infections.

Diagnosis

Cultures of pus isolates, gram stains, and antibiotic sensitivities all support the clinical diagnosis and aid in management. They are generally obtained in cases of recurrent abscesses, therapy response failure, systemic toxicity, immunocompromised patients, gas-containing abscesses, and involvement of the face, muscle, or fascia [5].

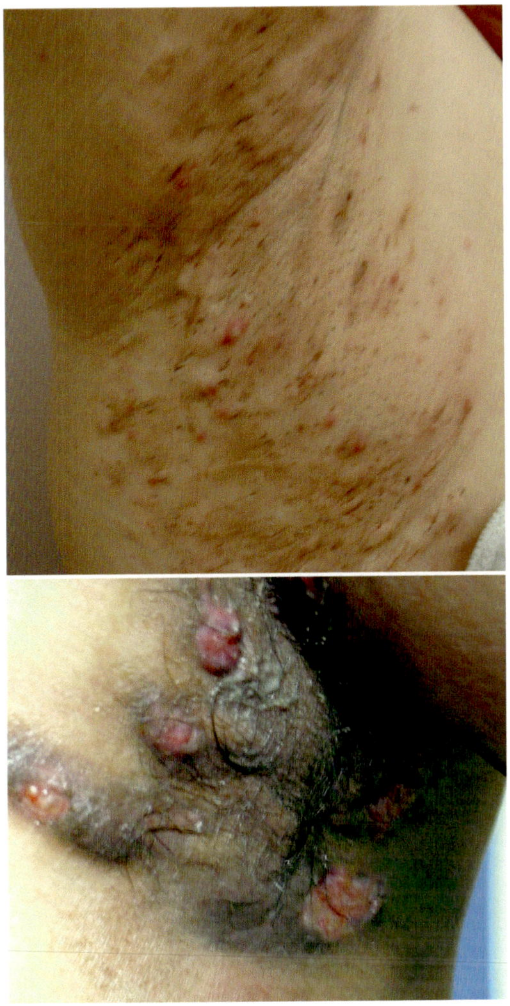

Fig. 7 Hidradenitis suppurativa. Cysts, inflammatory nodules, scarring and draining sinus tracts of the chronic, and suppurative inflammatory disease. It most commonly affects axilla and groin because it affects apocrine gland bearing areas

Pathology

The furuncle is a pyogenic infection with its origin at a hair follicle extending into the deep dermis and possibly to subcutaneous tissue. The carbuncle is visualized as a furuncle with additional loculated abscesses [13].

Differential Diagnosis

Among the differential diagnosis of furuncles and carbuncles the most common are hidradenitis suppurativa (see Fig. 7), ruptured epidermoid or pilar cysts and soft tissue infections [13].

Complications

Most cases resolve after treatment, but some cases are complicated by seeding to the bones, heart valves, or other organs as a result of bacteremia [1].

Treatment

The treatment of furuncles and carbuncles ranges from warm compresses that accelerate the resolution of simple furuncles to surgical and/or medical management for the more complicated cases. Incision and drainage are often adequate therapy in immunocompetent patients. Fluctuant furuncles and carbuncles should be opened and drained with caution so as to avoid rupturing the pseudo-capsule [3]. In addition, the loculations should be broken with a curette or hemostat and the wound packed to encourage complete drainage [1, 3].

Early in the course of furunculosis, antistaphylococcal antibiotics alone may have been useful; however, they have little effect once the lesion is fluctuant. Antibiotics can speed the resolution in healthy individuals and are essential in treating immunosuppressed patients. Oral penicillinase-resistant penicillin or first generation cephalosporins are the mainstay in the outpatient setting. Severe cases should be treated with a parenteral antibiotic that provides empiric coverage for Gram-positive pathogens including *MRSA*, Gram-negative, and anaerobic organisms. Culture and susceptibility results will aid in targeting the antibiotic therapy [12, 13].

Despite treatment, patients with recurrent furunculosis may be experiencing autoinoculation of a pathogenic strain of *S. aureus*. Eradication should be attempted as described previously. If treatment fails, rifampin daily for 10 days combined with cloxacillin four times a day may eradicate the carrier state [12, 13].

Cellulitis

Introduction

Cellulitis is defined as an infection of the deep dermis and subcutaneous tissue.

Incidence and Prevalence

The incidence of lower-extremity cellulitis reaches 199 per 100,000 people/year. The incidence of cellulites increases significantly with age, but there is no statistically significant difference between the sexes [15].

Etiology

Gram-positive pathogens are implicated in the majority of cases of cellulitis with β-hemolytic streptococci being the most common causative agent, followed by *S. aureus*, *MRSA*, and Gram-negative aerobic bacilli [16, 17]. These pathogens gain access through abrasions on the skin, burns, bites, surgical incisions, and intravenous catheters [1, 18]. Toe web *tinea pedis* is the most common portal of entry. There are multiple variants of cellulitis that are caused by specific pathogens of which some are briefly discussed in Table 2.

Table 2 Characteristics of cellulitis variants

Variant	Most common organisms	Etiology	Clinical description	Treatment
Preseptal cellulitis	*S. aureus*, GAS, *S. pneumonia* *H. influenza* was common prior to vaccination	More common in children; following URTI, eye lesions (i.e., Hordeolum) insect bites, trauma	Acute eyelid erythema and edema may suppurate. Pain with EOM movement, affected pupillary reflex and proptosis occurs in orbital cellulitis	Amoxicillin/clavulanate or a first-generation cephalosporin. If no response in 48–72 h consider IV antibiotics
Buccal cellulitis	*H. influenza*	More common in children	Hot, erythematous, edematous cheek area that develops a violaceous hue often accompanied by bacteremia	Ceftriaxone IV
Human bites	Aerobic–anaerobic polymicrobial oral flora	Most occur on the hands (Clenched-fist injury) or occlusional bites	Variable, edema erythema, may suppurate; complication such as OM, tenosynovitis, and septic arthritis if in proximity	Amoxicillin/clavulanate, surgical intervention may be necessary
Dog and cat bites	*P. multocida*	Most commonly in extremities	As in human bites but less severe	Amoxicillin/clavulanate
Marine Trauma	*V. vulnificus*	Exposure of lacerated skin to sea water, systemic illness may ensue in patients with chronic liver disease or DM	Predominantly in extremities bilaterally, hemorrhagic bullae formation, necrotizing vasculitis	Doxycycline and ceftazidime
Fresh water trauma	*Aeromonas* spp.	Exposure of lacerated skin to contaminated fresh water (fisherman) or use of therapeutic leeches	Predominantly in extremities, variable manifestation from indurated erythematous patch to myonecrosis or ecthyma gangrenosum	Ciprofloxacin
Erysipeloid	*E. rhusiopathiae*	Exposure of lacerated skin to raw meat (butchers) and/or fish	Commonly affect the hands, well-demarcated, reddish-violaceous plaques smooth surface, brown with resolution. May manifests as diffuse skin disease or systemic disease	Amoxicillin

GAS Group A streptococci, *EOM* extraocular muscles, *OM* osteomyelitis, *URTI* upper respiratory tract infection, *DM* diabetes mellitus
Adapted from [12, 18–22]

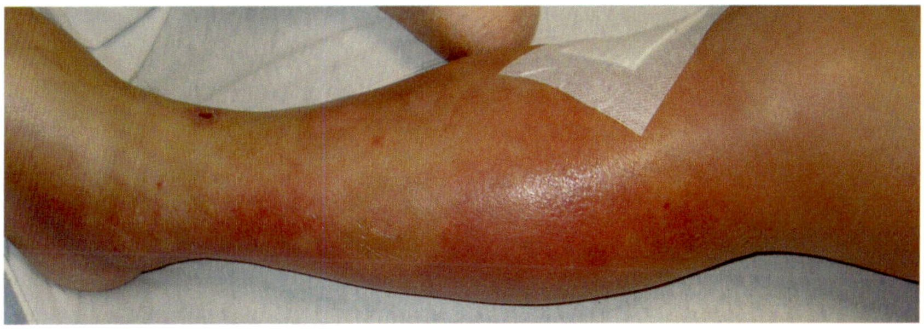

Fig. 8 Cellulitis. Warm localized area of the leg with erythema, edema, induration, and non-palpable, ill-defined borders. In adults the lower extremities are the most affected area of the body

Clinical Features

The clinical features of cellulitis include a localized area of skin of variable size that is painful, erythematous, edematous, and warm with non-palpable and ill-defined borders (see Fig. 8). Patients may present with malaise, fever, and leukocytosis [3]. The area is usually indurated and shows pitting upon pressure. In severe cases, vesicles, bullae, ecchymoses, petechiae, pustules, and necrotic tissue may be observed. Cellulitis may also present with lymphangitis and inflammation of regional lymph nodes that can damage the lymphatic vessels thus leading to recurrent cellulitis. Cellulitis may affect any part of the body, but most commonly involves the lower extremities in adults, followed by the face and hands [3, 23].

Diagnosis

Cellulitis is a clinical diagnosis. In immunocompetent patients, neither blood cultures nor secretion cultures are needed to confirm the diagnosis. Conversely, it may be appropriate to obtain a blood culture, needle aspiration of the leading edge, or a punch biopsy in pediatric cases, immunocompromised patients, lesions with suspected atypical organisms, or states of persistent inflammation. Despite proper needle aspiration or biopsy techniques, these cultures are positive in only 20% of cases thus implying that cellulitis is mainly an inflammatory response of the host elicited by a small number of organisms [1]. Gram-stains and cultures can provide a definitive diagnosis in those lesions that are open, draining or have an obvious portal of entry. Radiographic studies are useful for distinguishing cellulitis from osteomyelitis, necrotizing fasciitis, or gas gangrene but should not be used as routine examination [24].

Pathology

The pathology of these lesions shows mild-to-moderate leukocytic infiltration of the dermis possibly extending into the subcutaneous fat with dilation of the blood vessels and lymphatics. Proliferation of bacteria or other causative organism may be visualized with the appropriate stains [1].

Differential Diagnosis

Rapidly progressive lesions with accompanying signs of systemic toxicity include more severe infections on the differential diagnosis, such as necrotizing fasciitis, gas gangrene, toxic shock syndrome, osteomyelitis, and erythema migrans. Several noninfectious disorders may also resemble cellulitis including thrombophlebitis, Baker's cysts, contact dermatitis, drug reactions, gouty arthritis, and malignancy [25].

Complications

Complications are more common in immunocompromised adults and children. These include abscess formation, involvement of adjacent bones, osteomyelitis, gangrene, and sepsis among others. Recurrence is common if risk factors are neglected [5].

Treatment

Empiric antibiotic therapy for the management of cellulitis should have activity against β-hemolytic streptococci and *S. aureus*. Patients presenting with the first episode of a limited cellulitis and without significant comorbidities can be treated with a 10-day course of oral penicillinase-resistant penicillin, first generation cephalosporin, amoxicillin–clavulanate, or macrolide (i.e., dicloxacillin or cephalexin) [26, 27]. Marking the margins of erythema with ink is a quick and helpful technique for accessing the progression or regression of the cellulitis to a given treatment. If signs and symptoms do not improve after 1–2 days of treatment, cultures and sensitivities should be obtained and antibiotics adjusted accordingly. The antibiotics should be maintained for at least 3 days after the acute inflammation resolves [27].

Limited disease can be treated orally, but initial parenteral therapy is required for cases of extensive cellulitis, signs of systemic toxicity, erythema that has rapidly progressed, or facial cellulitis. A parenteral second- or third-generation cephalosporin (with or without an aminoglycoside) should be considered [27].

Empiric therapy for *MRSA* should be initiated in patients with recurrent infections in the setting of underlying predisposing conditions, risk factors for *MRSA* infections, in communities where the prevalence of *MRSA* is greater than 30%, previous episode of documented *MRSA* infection, and if systemic toxicity is present. Empiric treatment includes linezolid, clindamycin, or penicillin plus TMP-SMX or doxycycline (if outpatient). If parenteral antibiotic therapy is needed, vancomycin (30 mg/kg per 24 h in two divided doses) should be used. For patients who fail to respond to vancomycin or cannot tolerate its side effects, linezolid (600 mg every 12 h) or daptomycin (4 mg/kg once daily) is adequate alternatives [28, 29].

Management of cellulitis should also include immobilization and elevation of the affected area. Maintaining the lesion sufficiently hydrated, especially if bullae are present, helps avoid dryness and cracking. Tetanus immunization should be considered based on patient history. Pain relief medication should be used with caution since they mask the intense pain of a process such as necrotizing fasciitis, which requires emergency surgical attention. As a preventive measure, patients should also be treated for the underlying conditions that predispose them to developing recurrent cellulitis (*tinea pedis*, lymphedema, and chronic venous insufficiency) [18].

These guidelines for empiric antimicrobial therapy should be modified in the setting of known pathogens, underlying conditions such as diabetes, and special circumstances such as animal bites and water exposure. Management of patients in these settings is discussed in Table 2.

Methicillin-Resistant *S. aureus*

Introduction

Methicillin-resistant *S. aureus* (MRSA) was initially described in the1960s in hospitalized populations (HA-MRSA). While patients with community acquired MRSA (CA-MRSA) were first described later in the 1980s. Today, these two are difficult to distinguish from each other because of the introduction of CA-MRSA into the health care setting as well as HA-MRSA being introduced into the community by health care providers. However, given that the strains isolated from CA-MRSA and HA-MRSA are genetically different, it is best to refer to them as "community-type strains" and "health care type strains," regardless of where the infection was actually acquired [30].

Incidence and Prevalence

In the USA surveillance report of nosocomial *S. aureus* infections, isolates with methicillin resistance increased from 22 to 57% from 1995 to 2001, respectively [31]. CA-MRSA was initially reported among intravenous drug users (IVDU) and has since become the most frequent cause of skin and soft tissue infections presenting to the emergency departments and ambulatory clinics in the USA, with an incidence of 15–75% by 2004 [32, 33].

Etiology

MRSA's resistance to methicillin and other beta-lactams antibiotics can be attributed to the production of PBP 2a; an altered penicillin binding protein (PBP) to which these antibiotics have less affinity [34].

The risk factors for HA-MRSA infection include MRSA colonization, proximity to patients with MRSA colonization or infection, prolonged hospitalization (especially if in the intensive care unit), recurrent antibiotic use, and hemodialysis or other invasive procedures.

The risk factors that both HA-MRSA and CA-MRSA infections share are MRSA colonization and proximity to others with MRSA colonization or infection (including domestic animals). The other risk factors for HA-MRSA infection are IVDU, shaving, tattoos, skin trauma, HIV infection, and crowded living conditions (i.e., imprisonment). However, many patients with CA-MRSA have no risk factors [30].

Clinical Features

HA-MRSA is associated with serious invasive disease of the skin, soft tissues, blood, and/or lungs, while at least 85% of CA-MRSA infections present as folliculitis, furunculosis, or abscesses . Less likely, CA-MRSA can manifest as cellulitis, impetigo, scalded skin syndrome, necrotizing fasciitis, osteomyelitis, otitis, urinary tract infections, endocarditis, or bacteremia [30].

Diagnosis

MRSA should be suspected when infectious skin lesions do not respond to the initial antimicrobial treatment directed toward *S. aureus* (methicillin susceptible), mainly in communities with high-MRSA prevalence. For confirmation, bacterial cultures and sensitivities should be performed [34].

Treatment

When treating skin and soft tissue infections, the initial selection of antibiotics should be based upon the severity and the epidemiology in the area.

In all patients with severe, life-threatening infections, empiric antibiotics should be started before sensitivity results are available. However, β-lactam antibiotics are no longer reliable empiric therapy, given the increasing prevalence of MRSA as both a nosocomial and community-associated pathogen. Parenteral therapy with vancomycin is the optimal treatment; new alternative agents, linezolid, daptomycin, tigecycline and quinupristin–dalfopristin have all been FDA approved for the treatment of severe skin and soft tissue infections. Other treatments, such as telavancin, a novel lipoglycopeptide antibiotic with rapid bactericidal activity against a broad spectrum of clinically relevant gram-positive pathogens, may be a promising treatment option in the near future [5].

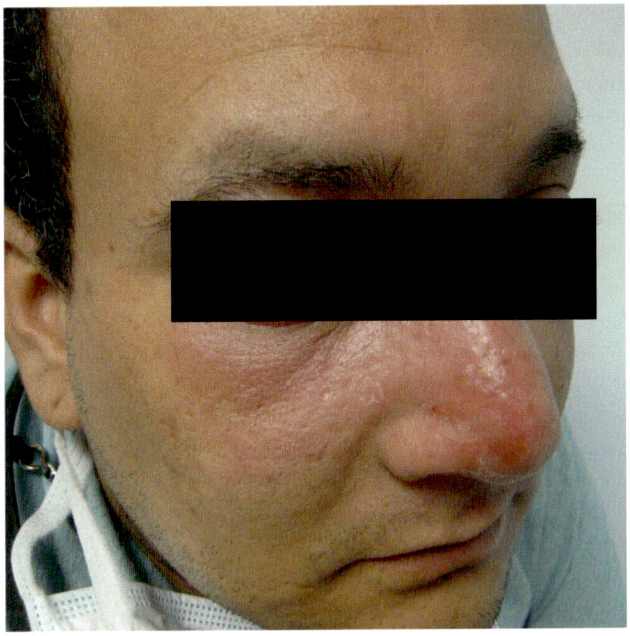

Fig. 9 Erysipelas. *Red*, edematous indurated plaque with sharply demarcated, raised advancing borders

For localized skin and soft tissue MRSA infections, the first-line treatment options include clindamycin, trimethoprim–sulfamethoxazole, tetracycline or linezolid, which are limited by cost, toxicity, and potential for resistance [30, 34].

Abscesses caused by MRSA should undergo surgical treatment because oral antibiotics are an insufficient therapeutic option. For abscesses smaller than 5 cm, therapy with incision and drainage may be sufficient but management of larger abscesses with or without systemic signs of infection should include antimicrobial therapy [35]. Intranasal mupirocin and chlorhexidine washes have proven decolonization in some cases, preventing further episodes of infection. However, colonization may recur [33].

Erysipelas

Introduction

Erysipelas is defined as an acute infection of the upper dermis and superficial lymphatics characterized clinically by the sudden onset of bright red, edematous, and indurated plaque. The plaque has sharply demarcated, raised, and advancing borders which cause intense pain (see Fig. 9). In most patients, constitutional symptoms such as fever are present, generally apparent before skin symptoms, and are more common in erysipelas than in cellulitis or fasciitis [36]. The most common sites of involvement are the legs, arms, and face [37]. The complete blood count may reveal neutrophil leukocytosis.

Etiology

Erysipelas is most commonly caused by β-hemolytic Group A streptococci with occasional cases of Group C and Group G Streptococci [1, 3, 38]. The predisposing factors and diagnosis are similar to those of cellulitis.

Pathology

Pathology reports for erysipelas generally show neutrophilic infiltration of the dermis with accompanying edema. Separation of the dermis from the epidermis can be seen along with dilation of the lymphatic [5].

Differential Diagnosis

In establishing a differential diagnosis, erysipelas can be confused with contact dermatitis, angioedema, scarlet fever, lupus erythematosus, acute tuberculoid leprosy, venous thrombosis, compartment syndrome, and many inflammatory infectious diseases [12, 38].

Complications

Localized abscesses are not rare and should be considered whenever acute erysipelas does not respond to antibiotics. Septicemia and thrombosis are rare complications. Recurrences of erysipelas are relatively high [38].

Treatment

Penicillin continues to be the standard of treatment in uncomplicated erysipelas given the near exclusivity of β-hemolytic Group A streptococci as the causative pathogen. Treatment is administered for 10–20 days [38]. Parenteral antibiotics are reserved for children, immunocompromised patients, and patients with severe constitutional symptoms due to the fact that oral and intravenous efficacy has been found to be equivalent in immunocompetent patients [39]. In patients allergic to penicillin, macrolides may be used. Some clinicians prefer using macrolides, cephalosporins and fluoroquinolones, especially in complicated cases or when the lesion cannot be clearly differentiated from cellulitis. However, due to the increasing resistance of streptococci to macrolides, these antibiotics should be used with care [40].

In patients with recurrent episodes of erysipelas, prophylaxis with penicillin V or erythromycin has resulted in a significant reduction of relapses [41]. Nonetheless, risk factor management is more effective in reducing relapses, morbidity, and costs.

Ecthyma

Introduction

Ecthyma is an ulcerative pyoderma of the skin that extends into the dermis, thus often being referred to as a deeper form of non-bullous impetigo [42].

Incidence and Prevalence

The incidence of ecthyma remains unknown. However, it is known that ecthyma has a predilection for children and the elderly [43].

Etiology

Group A β-hemolytic streptococci initiate the lesion or secondarily infect preexisting ulcerations. The spread of skin streptococci is augmented by crowding, poor hygiene, high temperatures, and humidity. Prior tissue damage, such as excoriations, insect bites, and dermatitis, predispose to ecthyma. It is most commonly seen in children, neglected elderly, and immunocompromised patients such as diabetics. Lesions are often contaminated with staphylococci especially in HIV patients and IVDU [5, 13, 43].

Clinical Features

Ecthyma begins as a vesicle or pustule over an inflamed area of skin which then deepens into a dermal ulceration with an overlying thick hemorrhagic crust. The crust differs from that of impetigo in that it is thicker and harder. A punched-out ulceration is apparent when the crust is removed. Ecthyma commonly manifests as less than 10 lesions that remain fixed in size or progressively enlarge to 0.5–3 cm in diameter. Lesions are painful and may have associated regional lymphadenopathy, even with solitary lesions. Ecthyma usually arises on the lower extremities, most commonly on the ankle and dorsum of the foot. Ecthyma can resolve without treatment, but heals slowly, taking several weeks, and generally producing a scar [42–44].

Diagnosis

The diagnosis of ecthyma is based on clinical features; however, Gram stains and cultures may be performed to confirm Gram-positive cocci infection.

Pathology

The heavy crust covering the surface of the ecthyma ulcer contains superficial and deep granulomatous perivascular infiltrate with endothelial edema. The dermis is affected by necrosis and inflammation [5].

Differential Diagnosis

The differential diagnosis of ecthyma is extensive and includes the following conditions: ecthyma gangrenosum, pyoderma gangrenosum, leishmaniasis, lymphomatoid papulosis, sporotrichosis, tungiasis, *Mycobacterium marinum* infection, papulonecrotic tuberculids, excoriated insect bites, venous or arterial insufficiency ulcers, cutaneous diphtheria, and other bacterial, viral, and deep fungal infections of the skin [12, 13].

Complications

It is unusual for ecthyma to cause systemic involvement or bacteremia. Secondary lymphangitis, cellulitis, gangrene, and osteomyelitis can occur but are very rare. Poststreptococcal glomerulonephritis occurs with an incidence of approximately 1% [42].

Treatment

Treatment of ecthyma begins by maintaining the lesion clean using bactericidal soap and removing crusts by soaking or using wet compresses. For localized ecthyma, consider topical therapy with mupirocin ointment twice daily [45]. However, more extensive lesions may require systemic antibiotics. β-Lactamase resistant penicillin, such as cloxacillin, should be adequate to cover possible secondary *S. aureus* infections or a first generation cephalosporin may also be used [44, 46]. Consider parenteral antibiotics in the event of widespread involvement.

Ecthyma Gangrenosum

Introduction

Ecthyma gangrenosum (EG) is an uncommon cutaneous infection in critically ill and immunocompromised patients, most often associated with bacteremia from *P. aeruginosa* [49].

Incidence and Prevalence

EG develops in 1–13% patients with *P. aeruginosa* sepsis [47].

Etiology

EG is typically caused by *P. aeruginosa*; however, EG-like lesions have been documented in case reports of patients with other bacterial and fungal infections). EG occurs in patients who are immunocompromised by hematologic malignancies, immunodeficiency syndromes, severe burns, malnutrition, immunosuppressive therapy, or other chronic conditions such as diabetes mellitus. Catheterization and instrumentation procedures such as long-term intravenous catheters, indwelling urinary catheters, or surgical procedures can also predispose to pseudomonal sepsis and thus EG [48, 49].

Clinical Features

The primary cutaneous lesion of EG undergoes a rapid transformation. It begins as a painless, round, and erythematous macule that becomes pustular with a surrounding halo of tender inflammation. The initial macule then develops a hemorrhagic vesicle or bulla that ruptures and turns into a gangrenous ulcer with a central gray/black eschar (see Fig. 10) [50].

The patient may have a single lesion or multiple lesions grouped closely. These lesions are usually found on the gluteal area or extremities but may appear on any location of the body [51].

Diagnosis

The lesion of EG described above is unique and distinguishable from most other diseases; therefore, EG should be

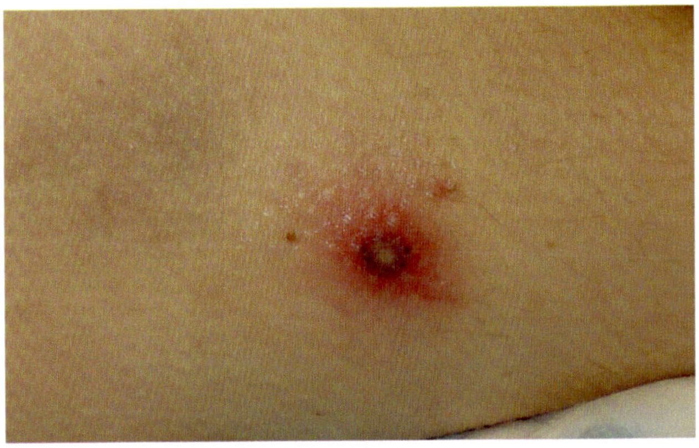

Fig. 10 Ecthyma gangrenosum. The lesion starts as a round erythematous macule that becomes pustular with a surrounding halo of tender inflammation. It then develops a hemorrhagic vesicle or bulla that ruptures and turns into a gangrenous ulcer with a central *gray/black* eschar

suspected if the typical lesion is accompanied by a predisposing clinical picture showing a compromised immune system. For a quick approach to diagnosis, one can analyze the gram stains of the fluid in pustules, vesicles, or the tissue beneath the eschar. Since EG is usually a manifestation of sepsis, blood cultures should be performed, preferably during fever peaks. Cultures of urine and the contents of vesicles or pustules in bacterial, fungal, and mycobacterial media should also be completed to narrow the differential diagnosis and to assure effective antibiotic use by sensitivity studies [51, 52].

Pathology

Histologic examinations of EG lesions show necrotizing hemorrhagic vasculitis. Multiple gram-negative rods are seen within the media and adventitia of the necrotic vessels but not in the intima. Extravasation of blood, edema, and necrosis are typically seen around the involved vessels [52, 53].

Differential Diagnosis

The differential diagnosis includes infectious and noninfectious conditions. EG lesions may be mimicked by septic emboli of other organisms, cryoglobulinemia, polyarteritis nodosa, pyoderma gangrenosum, and necrotizing fasciitis [5].

Complications

EG mortality rates vary significantly, ranging from 15.4% in non-bacteremic patients and up to 96% in bacteremia patients [47]. The factors associated with a dismal prognosis are multiple lesions, delayed diagnosis and treatment, neutropenia, and a high bacterial load [53].

Treatment

Despite pending culture or biopsy results, treatment must be initiated when EG is suspected. It requires parenteral antipseudomonal penicillin, such as piperacillin, in conjunction with an aminoglycoside. The antibiotic selection can be subsequently guided by blood culture and sensitivity results, when feasible [48, 49, 51].

Staphylococcal Scalded Skin Syndrome

Introduction

Staphylococcal scalded skin syndrome (SSSS), also known as Ritter's disease, is a generalized and superficial exfoliative infectious disease.

Incidence and Prevalence

SSSS usually affects neonates, infants, and children under age of 5. Few cases have been reported in adults; since the causative staphylococcal toxin is excreted by the kidneys, these cases have been associated with renal impairment or immune deficiency. When compared with adult patients, children have a greater recovery rate. The mortality rate in children is less than 5% but over 50% in adults [54].

Etiology

SSSS is caused by exfoliative toxins of the phage II *S. aureus* strain. These toxins act as epidermolysins by splitting the epidermis within the granular layer by binding to desmoglein 1, the same desmosomal adhesion molecule targeted in pemphigus foliaceous [55, 56]. The predisposing factors are an impaired immunity and renal insufficiency. Due to the immaturity of both the immune and renal systems, the neonate has an increased risk of SSSS [54].

Clinical Features

Patients with SSSS may first experience prodromal constitutional symptoms (fever and malaise) or symptoms of an upper respiratory tract infection (purulent rhinorrhea or/and conjunctivitis). Erythema ensues cephalad and then generalizes, sparing the palms, soles, and mucous membranes. The skin becomes tender and Nilkosky's sign may become positive. Exfoliation starts 1–2 days later. In the more common and localized form of SSSS, the skin appears wrinkled with superficial erosions on red and moist bases, along with facial edema and/or perioral crusting (see Fig. 11). In less common but more severe forms of the disease, tender, sterile, and flaccid bullae develop in the superficial epidermis. After a couple of days, the bullae rupture exposing moist and denuded skin. Finally, desquamation ensues in flexural areas initially and then generalizes [5, 54, 57].

Diagnosis

SSSS can be diagnosed clinically. Leukocytosis may be present on CBC. Blood cultures are usually negative in children but may be positive in adults. Contrary to bullous impetigo, cultures taken from intact bullae are negative [57]. Children usually rapidly improve thus histology is not necessary.

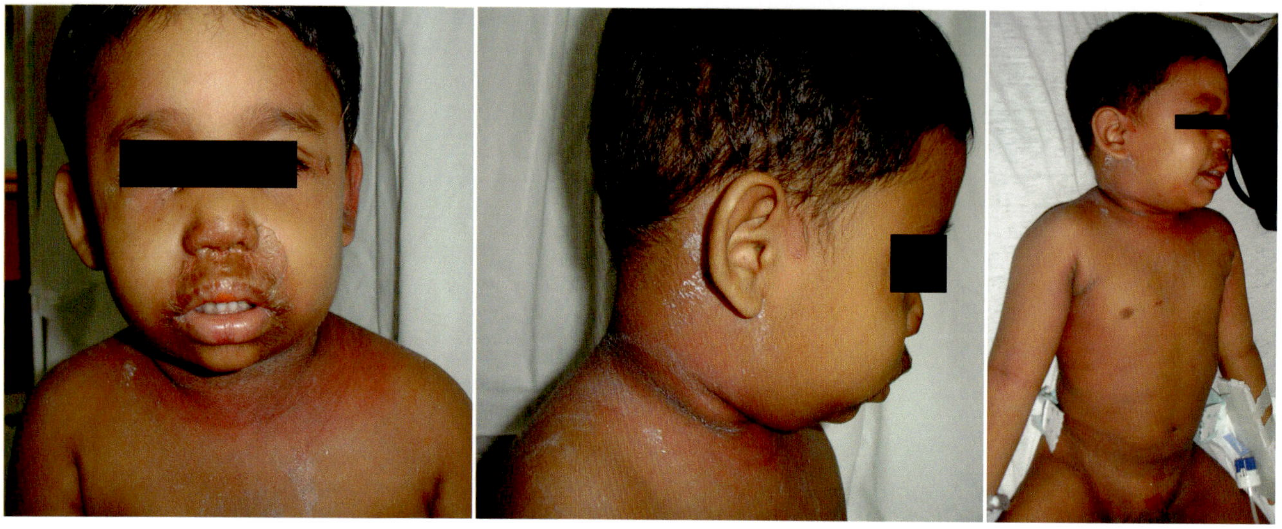

Fig. 11 Staphylococcal scalded skin syndrome (SSSS). In the exfoliation of SSSS skin appears wrinkled with superficial erosions on red and moist bases, along with facial edema and/or perioral crusting

However, in those poorly responding adults, confirmation of the diagnosis may be beneficial. Frozen-section histology of a blister roof is a rapid method for differentiating toxic epidermal necrolysis (TEN), where the roof comprises the whole epidermis, from SSSS, where the cleavage is in the stratum granulosum. Slide latex agglutination and enzyme-linked immunosorbent assay (ELISA) are confirmatory test that identify the exfoliative toxins [54].

Pathology

Pathology of SSSS shows cleavage at the stratum granulosum of the epidermis (see Fig. 12). Due to its toxin-mediated origin, these lesions lack inflammatory infiltrates or organisms in both the dermis and bullae [5].

Differential Diagnosis

The distinction between SSSS and TEN is vital for the management of either disease. SSSS is also confused with other disorders depending on which of the three stages of SSSS the patient presents. These conditions include sunburns, toxic shock syndrome (TSS), viral exanthema, erythema multiforme, drug-induced TEN, extensive bullous impetigo, graft-versus-host (GVH) disease, and pemphigus foliaceous. Child abuse or elderly abuse can also be included in the differential diagnosis when pertinent [12].

Complications

If left untreated or treated poorly, SSSS patients can develop serious and potentially life-threatening complications such as cellulitis, dehydration, electrolyte disturbance, sepsis, shock, and involvement of other body systems [56].

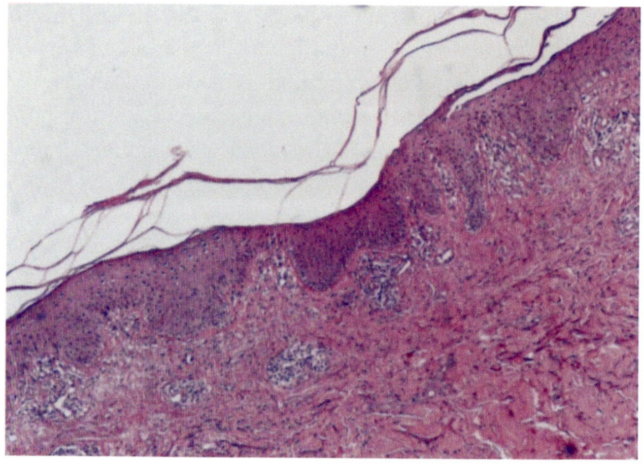

Fig. 12 Histopathological findings of Staphylococcal scalded skin syndrome. Subcorneal blister with some acantholytic cells. Bacteria not present in the blistering toxin-induced lesions

Treatment

Treatment includes systemic anti-staphylococcal antibiotics such as the penicillinase-resistant penicillin, dicloxacillin. Severe cases require hospitalization and parenteral administration of antibiotics. Oral antibiotics should be adequate for mild localized cases. Evidence suggests that parenteral antibiotics are more effective in treating SSSS than oral antibiotics, thus hospital admission is almost always advised due to the rapid progression of this infection. With appropriate treatment, skin lesions resolve within 2 weeks [57].

Pain management is favorable because the lesions are often painful. Oral anti-histamines may be used to control itching. Skin lubrication with emollients is beneficial. Fluid and electrolyte replacement may be necessary. Body temperature should be carefully monitored [58].

Infection control measures include: isolating the patient while they remain infectious during the 48 h after initiating antibiotic treatment, taking culture swabs from the equipment used in the patients room, using gloves and masks at all times, and testing the nursing and medical staff for potential carriers when hospital acquired cases occur [58].

Toxic Shock Syndrome

Introduction

TSS is a capillary leak syndrome caused by the immunological response to a toxin-mediated infection.

Incidence and Prevalence

It was first formally described in 1978; however, major interest did not grow until 1980 when a significant number of staphylococcal TSS cases were reported in healthy young women using high absorbency tampons during menstrual periods [59]. Cases of menstrual TSS have decreased from 9/100,000 women in 1980 to 1/100,000 women since 1986. The menstrual TSS case-fatality rate has also declined from 5.5% in 1979–1980 to 1.8% in 1987–1996 [60].

Currently, more than 50% of reported TSS cases are not related to menstrual tampon use, but rather are seen after surgical procedures, post-partum infections or cutaneous infectious processes, among others [61]. Furthermore, the case-fatality rate for non-menstrual TSS has remained constant at 5% over the past several years, contrary to the decline seen with menstrual TSS cases [60].

TSS has been traditionally associated to *S. aureus*, however, it is known today that group A streptococci causes a similar disease. Group A streptococci (GAS) TSS has been reported with increasing frequency to an estimated 3.5 cases per 100,000 persons and a case-fatality rate of 36% [62, 63].

Etiology

TSS is caused by bacterial superantigens (SAGs) secreted from *S. aureus* and group A streptococci. SAGs bypass normal antigen presentation by binding to class II major histocompatibility complex (MHC) molecules on antigen presenting cells and to specific variable regions on the β-chain of the T-cell antigen receptor. By binding to only one of the five variable elements that conventional antigens need for recognition, SAGs activate T cells at higher orders of magnitude causing massive cytokine release. Cytokines are believed to be responsible for the most severe symptoms of TSS, including hypotension, shock, and multi-organ failure [61].

Staphylococcal TSS may be classified by its etiology: either menstrual or non-menstrual. Menstrual TSS is associated with the prolonged use of high absorbency tampons. Non-menstrual TSS can be seen in several patient populations including post-surgical, post-respiratory tract viral infections, use of contraceptive diaphragms or intrauterine devices, postpartum, concomitant skin infections or lesions, burn patients and after the use of foreign bodies such as nasal packing [61, 64].

Toxic shock syndrome toxin-1 (TSST-1) is the exotoxin believed to be responsible for essentially all cases of menstrual-associated TSS, because of its ability to cross intact mucosa [63]. In most cases of non-menstrual TSS where skin integrity is compromised, TSST-1 and staphylococcal enterotoxin serotype B (SEB) and C (SEC) have been found to be involved [64, 65].

M types 1 and 3 group A streptococci and streptococcal pyrogenic exotoxins (SPE) serotypes A and C have been strongly associated with most cases of streptococcal TSS. However, cases were necrotizing fasciitis and myositis has caused TSS have not been associated with either SPE A or C implying other streptococcal superantigens involvement [66]. For streptococcal TSS to ensue the mucosal or skin barrier must be compromised as in chickenpox, wounds, pharyngitis, postpartum, and after viral infections [61, 67, 68].

Nonetheless, not every patient exposed to a virulent staphylococcal or streptococcal strain develop TSS. This is because the main determining is the lack of antibodies to SAGs [61].

Clinical Features

Staphylococcal TSS is characterized by the sudden onset of high fever, chills, headaches, vomiting, diarrhea, and muscle aches. It generally begins with a severe localized pain out of proportion to the injury and typically found in an extremity. Other initial symptoms may be present: flu-like, fever, chills, muscle aches, sore throat, lymphadenopathy, confusion, vomiting, and diarrhea. Skin manifestations are rarer than in Staphylococcal TSS, but a generalized blanching and macular erythema may be present. A macular erythematous eruption commences on the trunk and spreads centripetally (see Fig. 13). Contrary to SSSS, the palms, soles, and mucous membranes develop erythema. Non-pitting edema of the palms, soles, and occasionally throughout the body occurs. This condition can rapidly progress to severe and intractable hypotension with multisystem dysfunction. When fever is persistent, hypotension and shock may develop and lead to multiorgan failure, myositis, fasciitis, or disseminated intravascular coagulation (DIC). If the patient recovers, desquamation can occur 1–2 weeks after the onset of the illness in 20% of patients, affecting predominantly the palms and soles [61, 67, 68]. Nail and hair shedding may also occur [61, 62, 69].

Diagnosis

The diagnosis criteria for TSS is currently defined by the Center for Disease Control (CDC) and outlined in Table 3. However, patients who do not meet the strict CDC criteria

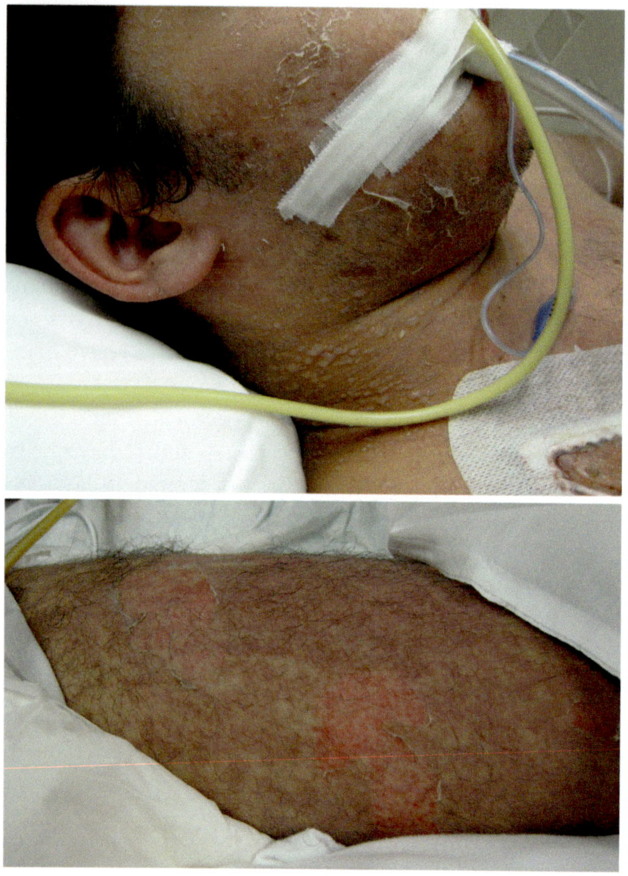

Fig. 13 Toxic shock syndrome (TSS). Denudation of the skin accompanied by hypotension in a critically ill patient

Table 3 Toxic shock syndrome

Fever
Temperature > 38.9°C (102.0°F)
Hypotension
Systolic blood pressure ≤90 mmHg for adults or less than 5th percentile by age for children <16 years; orthostatic drop in diastolic blood pressure ≥15 mmHg
Rash
Diffuse macular erythroderma
Desquamation
1–2 weeks after onset of illness, particularly involving palms and soles
Multisystem involvement (three or more of the following organ systems)
GI: Vomiting or diarrhea at onset of illness
Muscular: Severe myalgia or CPK elevation >2 times the normal upper limit
Mucous membranes: Vaginal, oropharyngeal, or conjunctival hyperemia
Renal: BUN or serum creatinine >2 times the normal upper limit, or pyuria (>5 WBC/hpf)
Hepatic: Bilirubin or transaminases >2 times the normal upper limit
Hematologic: Platelets <100,000/mm^3
Central nervous system: Disorientation or alterations in consciousness without focal neurologic signs in the absence of fever and hypotension
Negative results on the following tests
Blood, throat, or cerebrospinal fluid cultures for a pathogen that is not *S. aureus*
Serologic tests for Rocky Mountain spotted fever, leptospirosis, or measles

Information taken from CDC 1997 case definition

but who clearly have a compatible staphylococcal or streptococcal TSS illness should be managed similarly [70].

Pathology

On histology, one can see a lymphocytic and neutrophilic infiltrate within the upper dermis and edema of the dermal papillae. Other findings may include subepidermal vesiculation, epidermal spongiosis or confluent epidermal necrosis [5].

Differential Diagnosis

A comprehensive differential diagnosis of TSS includes the following conditions: viral exanthema, Kawasaki's disease, scarlet fever, drug eruptions, Rocky Mountain spotted fever, systemic lupus erythematosus, early TEN, SSSS, leptospirosis, meningococcemia, and severe adverse drug reactions [5, 13].

Complications

Multiple complications have been reported in cases of TSS including: renal failure, adult respiratory distress syndrome, vocal cord paralysis, paresthesias, arthralgias, DIC, gangrene, and even death [62].

Treatment

Adequate treatment may result in complete recovery. β-Lactamase resistant systemic antibiotics are required to eradicate organisms and prevent recurrences. Some physicians believe in using antibiotics, such as clindamycin, because it suppresses toxin production by inhibiting protein synthesis, especially in streptococcal TSS [61].

Vigorous fluid therapy should be used to treat hypotension with complementary vasopressors as needed. Removal of the foreign body or causative agent is necessary. If a skin infection is the etiology, drainage of the infected site, debridement, fasciotomy, or even amputation may be required.

The use of corticosteroids in the management of TSS has been in recent debate. Keh in 2004 reported benefit of low-dose corticosteroid use in cases unresponsive to antibiotics. However, many clinicians do not recommend corticosteroid treatment in TSS because of the limited clinical data.

Table 4 Streptococcal toxic shock syndrome

Hypotension
Systolic blood pressure ≤90 mmHg for adults or less than 5th percentile by age for children <16 years
Multi-organ involvement characterized ≥2 of the following
Renal impairment: Creatinine ≥2 mg/dL (≥177 μmol/L) for adults or more than or equal to twice the upper limit of normal for age. In patients with preexisting renal disease, a greater than twofold elevation over the baseline level
Coagulopathy: Platelets ≤ 100,000/mm³ or disseminated intravascular coagulation
Liver involvement: ALT, AST, or total bilirubin levels more than or equal to twice the upper limit of normal for the patient's age. In patients with preexisting liver disease, a greater than twofold increase over the baseline level
Acute respiratory distress syndrome: Acute onset of diffuse pulmonary infiltrates and hypoxemia in the absence of cardiac failure or by the evidence of diffuse capillary leak manifested by acute onset of generalized edema, or pleural or peritoneal effusions with hypoalbuminemia
Rash: A generalized erythematous macular rash that may desquamate
Soft-tissue necrosis: including necrotizing fasciitis or myositis, or gangrene
Isolation of group A streptococcus

Information taken from CDC 1996 case definition [70]

Treatment with intravenous immune globulin (typically, 400 mg/kg in a single dose administered over several hours) has proven to reduce mortality in severe cases of early TSS that has not responded to fluids and vasopressors, particularly in GAS TSS [71]. Because individuals with lack of immunity to SAGs are at greater risk for TSS, a toxoid vaccine that targets the TSS toxin is under investigation [61].

The CDC defines *probable TSS* as any case which meets the laboratory criteria and where four of the five clinical findings described above are present. A *confirmed TSS* is defined by meeting the laboratory criteria and positive findings for all five of the clinical features described previously; including desquamation (unless the patient dies before desquamation occurs) [70] (Table 4).

The CDC defines *probable Streptococcal TSS* as any case that meets the clinical case definition in the absence of another identified etiology and with the isolation of group A streptococcus from a non-sterile site (i.e., throat, vagina, sputum, or superficial skin lesion). CDC defines *confirmed Streptococcal TSS* as any case that meets the clinical case definition with isolation of group A streptococcus from a normally sterile site (i.e., blood or cerebrospinal fluid or, less commonly, joint, pleural, or pericardial fluid) [70].

Blistering Distal Dactylitis

Introduction

Blistering distal dactylitis (BDD) is an uncommon superficial infection of the distal palmar fat pad of the finger described classically in children.

Incidence and Prevalence

Although initially described in children, BDD has also been reported in both immunocompetent and immunocompromised adults.

Etiology

BDD can be caused by the Gram-positive bacteria group A β-hemolytic streptococcus or *S. aureus*. A group of bullae may be a clue of *S. aureus* being the causative agent [72]. BDD can coincide with a gram-positive infection or colonization of the anus, nasopharynx, or conjunctiva due to autoinoculation, prior abrasion, bite, or burn [73].

Clinical Features

BDD manifests as an acral tense blister 10–30 mm in diameter. Most commonly occurs on the volar fat pads of the fingers but can occur on the nail fold, proximal phalangeal, and palmar areas of the hands and rarely on the feet and toes. BDD is usually associated with hyperpigmentation of the surrounding skin. Hyperpigmentation may even occur weeks before the eruption of the blister. The blister may evolve into erosions over the course of several days [74].

Diagnosis

BDD can be diagnosed based on the clinical presentation and confirmatory bacterial cultures or gram stains, although the latter are not necessary.

Differential Diagnosis

The differential diagnosis of BDD includes burns, paronychia, bullous impetigo, and herpetic whitlow [13].

Treatment

The blisters should be incised and drained; wet to dry compresses may be used in the eroded areas. Patient should be started on a 10-day treatment with a β-lactam antibiotic. Nevertheless, β-lactamase-resistant antibiotics are commonly used when *S. aureus* exhibits antibiotic resistance in the area. Systemic therapy is useful in eradicating a focus of inoculation [5, 74].

Necrotizing Soft Tissue Infections

Introduction

Necrotizing soft tissue infections (NSTI) are a dangerous group of rapidly progressive infections that cause necrosis of the skin and underlying subcutaneous tissues. These are

Table 5 Necrotizing soft tissue infections (NSTI)

Type of necrotizing cellulitis	Etiology	Clinical characteristics	Gas content	Risk factors
Clostridial cellulitis	*Clostridium perfringens*	Superficial	Prominent in skin; no involvement of fascia or muscle	Preceded by local trauma or surgery
Non-clostridial anaerobic cellulitis	Mixed anaerobic and aerobic bacteria	Foul odor; often leads to septicemia	Present	Diabetes mellitus
Meleney's synergistic gangrene	Centrally *S. aureus* and peripherally microaerophilic streptococci	Slowly expanding indolent ulcer; confined to superficial fascia	Absent	Preceded by surgery
Synergistic necrotizing cellulitis	Polybacterial: anaerobes and facultative bacteria	Rapid course; systemic toxicity; skin, muscle, fat, and fascia involvement	25% of cases	Diabetes mellitus

Created with information from [78]

divided by depth of involvement, anatomic location, and causative organism or predisposing conditions, but they all share similar pathophysiology, clinical features, and treatment approaches [75]. In this chapter, the most important specific disease entities will be discussed with emphasis on three categories: myonecrosis, necrotizing cellulitis, and necrotizing fasciitis.

Formerly known as gas gangrene, *clostridial myonecrosis* is the most severe form of NSTI. Muscle necrosis and gas formation are prominent as its name implies. Most cases arise after deep wounds or surgery involving muscle tissue, and rarely spontaneously. This condition is caused by the species of the genus *Clostridium*, particularly *C. perfringens*, although other gram-positive rods have been described. The severity of the infection can be explained by the versatility of *C. perfringens*' α (alpha) toxin, which causes tissue necrosis, leukocyte inactivation, red blood cell hemolysis, and direct depression of the cardio-respiratory system. Leukocyte inactivation prevents host response thus predisposes the patient to a fulminant course. This aggressive condition advances in a couple of hours and, unlike other NSTI, there is little inflammation on histologic examination [76].

Of the NSTI's, the category of *necrotizing cellulitis* is characterized by more superficial and insidious involvement, except for *synergistic necrotizing cellulites,* which may also be considered a variant of necrotizing fasciitis [77]. This condition and other types of necrotizing cellulitis are briefly discussed in Table 5 [78].

Necrotizing fasciitis (NF) is a rapidly progressing deep necrotizing infection involving the subcutaneous tissue and fascia. There are approximately 3.5 cases per 100,000 persons, with a case fatality rate of 25% [79].

Etiology

Most NSTI are caused by synergistic aerobic and anaerobic bacteria [75]. Some necrotizing infections are caused by a single organism, as is the case in clostridial myonecrosis and NF type II caused by group A streptococci.

NF is divided, principally, into four groups according to the causative organism and clinical features [80]. NF type I, the most common, is a mixed aerobic–anaerobic bacterial infection that arises generally after trauma or surgical procedures [75]. NF type III is caused by gram-negative bacteria, often marine-related and NF type IV is usually trauma associated with fungal etiology [80]. As in non-clostridial anaerobic cellulitis and synergistic necrotizing cellulitis, patients with NF type I predominantly suffer from a predisposing systemic illness, such as diabetes. NF type II, as mentioned above, is an infection caused by virulent group A streptococci. Factors predisposing to NF type II include varicella lesions, a blunt or lacerating trauma, surgical procedure, exposure to a streptococcal-infected person, and some claim that NSAID use also predispose to NF type II by attenuating the host immune response [75, 77, 81, 82]. In contrast to NF type I, which is generally associated with a systemic illness, NF type II occurs in healthy patients of any age [82]. It evolves more rapidly than NF type I and may progress from group A streptococcal infection to streptococcal TSS.

Clinical Features

Necrotizing fasciitis (NF) is a rapidly progressive, treatment resistant and extremely painful cellulitis. Early recognition of this condition is critical given its rapid progression and extensive tissue destruction. In some patients, the signs and symptoms are not apparent initially and it may spare the overlying skin. In diabetic patients suffering from neuropathy, the exquisite pain typical of necrotizing fasciitis may be absent. Furthermore, if a patient is recovering from trauma or surgery and is receiving pain medications, the symptoms of NF may be disguised [83].

Most NSTI occur in the extremities. Diabetic patients are in greater propensity to develop NF in other less usual areas

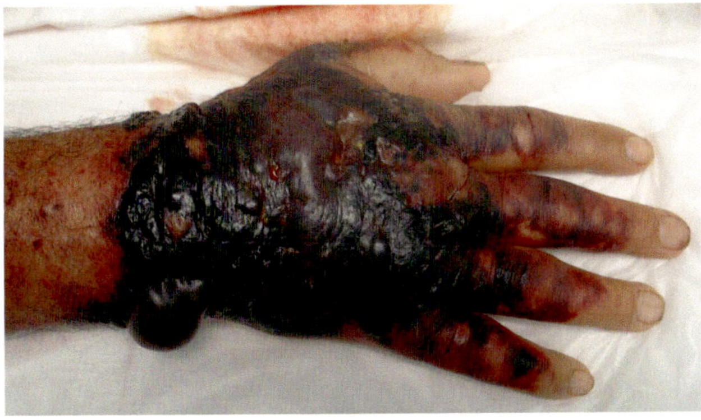

Fig. 14 Gas gangrene. From the beginning, the *red*-violaceous area changes to a *gray-blue* hue with overlying blisters and bullae that contain clear fluid but can progress to hemorrhagic fluid

such as: head and neck region (Ludwig's angina) and perineal area (Fournier's gangrene); these tend to be polymicrobial necrotizing fasciitis [81–83].

In the first 24–48 h, a red-violaceous area changes to a gray-blue hue with overlying blisters and bullae; however, they may also develop over apparently non-affected skin. Initially, the bullae contain clear fluid, but this can progress to hemorrhagic fluid (see Fig. 14). Crepitus can be present in some necrotizing infections as gas enters the soft tissue; however, its absence does not exclude the presence of NSTI. Following the extensive underlying soft tissue destruction, a foul-smelling watery discharge ensues, and the patient usually exhibits signs and symptoms of systemic toxicity. As the infection progresses, anesthesia rather than tenderness is characteristic due to the cutaneous nerve destruction [83].

Diagnosis

A rapidly evolving condition along with the aforementioned clinical features should raise suspicion of an NSTI. Laboratory findings generally are nonspecific. In NF, blood tests typically demonstrate coagulopathy, leukocytosis with a marked left shift, and elevations in serum lactate, creatinine kinase, and creatinine concentrations [81, 85]. Clinical findings with laboratory abnormalities are sufficient to prompt urgent surgical exploration. Surgical exploration should never be delayed for imaging studies. MRI is not sensitive enough to warrant a delayed surgery, nonetheless, it can delineate the depth of infection and it can rule out NSTI when the clinical picture is ambiguous [24, 86, 87].

During surgical exploration, the presence of gas, tissue integrity, and depth of invasion are evaluated. For example, upon entering the muscle compartment in myonecrosis, the muscle is edematous, pale gray, without blood or contraction, and has an obvious release of gas. A tissue biopsy for histologic examination and cultures is more reliable than samples of skin or bullae. Local anesthesia and a small incision may be sufficient for diagnostic purposes; however, since aggressive surgical debridement is the gold standard of therapy, surgical exploration may be performed simultaneously for both [75].

Pathology

Histologic examination of tissue samples generally show neutrophilic infiltrates, thrombosis of blood vessels, abundant bacteria in the upper dermis (polymicrobial in NF type I vs. monomicrobial in NF type II) and widespread necrosis of the subcutaneous fat and fascia while sparing the muscle. Gas may or may not be present in NF type I, but is highly unusual in NF type II [75].

Differential Diagnosis

It is important to distinguish NSTI from cellulitis or other superficial tissue infections that do not present such hazardous prognoses. When approaching a suspected NSTI, also consider conditions such as aspergillosis, pyomyositis, viral myositis, arthritis, bursitis, phlebitis, hematoma, trauma, and bites [75, 77].

Complications

Even with appropriate treatment, the probability of developing shock, multiorgan failure or dying is high. Among the most important prognostic factors are: the time from the onset of infection to treatment, extent of surgical debridement, and location of the lesion. Furthermore, the mortality rate of NF type II is higher than in NF type I because of the possible development of Streptococcal TSS [88].

Treatment

Treatment of NSTI requires early and aggressive surgical debridement with excision of all necrotic tissue. Incision and drainage approach is not sufficient [75]. Parenteral empiric antibiotic coverage should be started immediately with broad spectrum antibiotics and anaerobic coverage until information is gained by surgical exploration and confirmed with Gram stain or culture results. A number of antibiotic combinations may be used; options include: (1) ampicillin and gentamicin or (2) ampicillin–sulbactam plus clindamycin or metronidazole as good first-line choices. In previously hospitalized patients, gram-negative and pseudomonal coverage should be improved by using (3) ticarcillin–clavulanate or piperacillin–tazobactam, instead of the ampicillin or ampicillin–sulbactam. If group A streptococcal infection is suspected, (4) clindamycin and penicillin may be used [75, 77, 84, 89].

Use of hyperbaric oxygen therapy is controversial and should never delay surgical management and antibiotic administration. In specific conditions, such as gas gangrene, hyperbaric oxygen is of greater advantage because of its effects in arresting toxin production [80, 90].

Administration of intravenous immunoglobulin (IVIG) has been reported to be beneficial in cases of severe group A streptococci infections, as discussed previously in TSS. Additional studies, however, are needed before a strong recommendation can be made regarding their use in NSTI.

Rhinoscleroma

Introduction

Rhinoscleroma is a chronic granulomatous, slowly progressing, and disfiguring infection predominantly affecting the upper respiratory tract.

Incidence and Prevalence

Rhinoscleroma is a rare disease without accurate national or international incidence data. More than 16,000 cases have been reported since 1960 [91]. Most cases are from Central Europe, Middle East, Central America, and tropical Africa [92].

Etiology

The causative agent is the encapsulated gram-negative bacilli *Klebsiella rhinoscleromatis*. Due to the fact that it is associated with poor hygiene, malnutrition, and population over crowding it usually affects lower social and economic population classes [92].

Clinical Features

Rhinoscleroma affects most areas of the upper respiratory tract, for which the nose is involved in 95–100% of cases [92]. Clinically the disease progresses in three stages:

1. The catarrhal stage: symptoms of rhinitis that progress to foul-smelling purulent rhinorrhea, crusting, and nasal obstruction which may last for months.
2. The hypertrophic stage: formation of granulation tissue causing deformity and enlargement of the nose, upper lip, and adjacent structures. This lesion appears as a rubbery bluish-purple granuloma that evolves to a pale-indurated mass. Most cases are diagnosed in this because of complaints of epistaxis, anosmia, hoarseness, or anesthesia of the tissues.
3. The sclerotic stage: fibrotic tissue surrounds the granulomatous area with extensive scarring and laryngeal and nasal stenosis [92, 93].

Diagnosis

The distinctive clinical features of the disease along with the patient's living conditions are the two most important assessments needed for diagnosis. Histopathological and bacteriological analyses with PAS, Giemsa, and Warthin–Starry stains confirm the diagnosis [93]. Radiographic studies are of value in assessing the extension.

Pathology

As the clinical stages progress, so do the histologic features of the disease.

1. The catarrhal stage: atrophic mucosa with squamous metaplasia and a subepithelial infiltrate of neutrophils with some granulation tissue.
2. The hypertrophic stage: pseudo-epitheliomatous hyperplasia with hypertrophic collagenous tissue and chronic inflammatory cells including Mikulicz's cells (foamy macrophages containing bacilli) and Russell bodies (eosinophilic structures within plasma cells).
3. The sclerotic stage: fibrous tissue, Mikulicz's cells, and Russell bodies are difficult to see at this stage [92, 93].

Differential Diagnosis

The differential diagnosis depends greatly upon the site and extent of infection. Conditions to consider include the following: tuberculosis, actinomycosis, syphilitic gumma, leprosy, rhinosporidiosis, histoplasmosis, blastomycosis, paracoccidioidomycosis, mucocutaneous leishmaniasis, sarcoidosis, Wegener's granulomatosis, and neoplasms [92–94].

Complications

Extensive disfigurement of the face may result from erosions over the infection. Damage may be widespread enough to cause complete obstruction of the airways resulting in death [92].

Treatment

Treatment consists of prolonged antibiotic therapy. Fluoroquinolone antibiotics prove to be the most effective due to their increased penetrance. Surgical debridement or carbon dioxide laser are used to reduce symptoms of obstruction if necessary. Corticosteroids are also useful in the early stages to reduce the inflammatory symptoms [92–94].

Spirochetes

Leptospirosis

Introduction

Leptospirosis is the most common zoonosis in the world [95, 96].

Incidence and Prevalence

The majority of clinical cases occur in the tropical and subtropical areas [97]. In the USA, leptospirosis is prevalent year-round with half of the new cases occurring between July and October. Nevertheless, the incidence is unknown since leptospirosis was removed from the list of nationally reported diseases in 1994, remaining reportable only in Hawaii. Epidemics occur mostly following natural disasters such as cyclones and floods [98].

Etiology

This systemic disease is caused by various strains of the aerobe spirochetes *Leptospira* spp. bacterium. There are various species of the *Leptospira* genus, one of which, *Leptospira interrogans*, has two serovars with characteristic clinical manifestations; serotype icterohaemorrhagiae for icteric leptospirosis, and serotype autumnalis for anicteric leptospirosis. Humans most often become infected after exposure to animal urine, contaminated water or soil, or infected animal tissue. Spirochetes gain entry via wet skin, abrasions, mucous membranes, or conjunctiva [12, 96].

Clinical Features

The disease may manifest as a self-limited systemic infection, a subclinical illness followed by seroconversion, or a potentially fatal illness accompanied by multiorgan involvement. Two major clinically recognizable syndromes have been described: anicteric leptospirosis, which is the most common, and icteric leptospirosis, the most severe and potentially lethal form. After an incubation period of 1–2 weeks, each syndrome has two phases: the acute septic phase (4–7 days) and the delayed immune phase (4–30 days) [99].

Anicteric leptospirosis, also called Pretibial fever or Fort Bragg fever, has a septic phase characterized by high fevers, headaches, myalgias of the lower back and calf muscles, anorexia, nausea, vomiting, and abdominal pain. The immune phase is characterized by a more mild fever, more intense headaches, aseptic meningitis, conjunctival suffusion, uveitis, hepatosplenomegaly, and pulmonary involvement. During the immune phase, the characteristic cutaneous manifestation of non-pruritic erythematous patches or plaques on the pretibial areas can occur. Skin manifestations resolve spontaneously after a week [12, 99].

Icteric leptospirosis (Weil's syndrome) is unique in that the two phases of the illness are often continuous and indistinguishable. Initial phase starts with the sudden onset of high fever and chills, marked jaundice, hematuria, proteinuria, and azotemia. Petechiae and/or purpura may be found on the skin and mucous membranes [12].

Diagnosis

The diagnosis of leptospirosis is suspected on the basis of clinical manifestations, laboratory findings, disease course, and epidemiological features. Conjunctival suffusion, when present, is one of the most reliable distinguishing features since it rarely occurs with any infectious illness other than leptospirosis [100]. Laboratory studies of patients with *mild* disease generally reveal the following anomalies:

- Elevated erythrocyte sedimentation rate
- Leukocytosis with a left shift
- Mild elevation of aminotransferases, serum bilirubin, and alkaline phosphatase in blood
- Proteinuria, leukocytes, erythrocytes, and hyaline or granular casts in urine
- Neutrophilia, normal glucose, normal pressure, and normal or elevated protein in CSF

Laboratory studies of patients with the *severe* form of the disease exhibit:

- Mild thrombocytopenia and marked leukocytosis
- Elevated prothrombin time and creatinine phosphokinase
- Modestly elevated transaminases
- Azotemia and renal failure
- Electrocardiographic (ECG) abnormalities [95].

Since the clinical features and routine laboratory findings of leptospirosis are not specific, the organism can be cultured to arrive at a diagnosis, although, the definite diagnosis is more frequently made by serologic testing [101]. This is due to the fact that cultures may be negative if drawn too early or too late. Serologic tests include: microscopic agglutination test (MAT), macroscopic agglutination test, indirect hemagglutination, and ELISA [102, 103]. Therapy may be initiated on the basis of clinical manifestations since cultures may take several weeks to grow, and only specialized laboratories perform the serological tests, which do not yield a positive result for roughly a week after the onset of the illness [103]. *Leptospira* can be found in blood and CSF during the septic phase but are found in urine and aqueous humor during the immune phase.

Pathology

On histology, skin lesions show edema and nonspecific perivascular infiltrate [12].

Differential Diagnosis

Leptospirosis may resemble the following different infectious illnesses which share endemic areas and clinical features: dengue, malaria, scrub typhus, rickettsial diseases, salmonella typhi, ehrlichiosis, and influenza [5, 12].

Complications

Most cases of leptospirosis are self-limited, but the complications can include: uveitis, myocarditis, hemorrhage due to DIC, rhabdomyolysis that may result in renal failure, acute respiratory distress syndrome (ARDS), septic shock and multiple organ failure. Liver failure may ensue but is generally reversible [98].

Treatment

Supportive therapy along with management of hematologic, renal, hepatic, and CNS complications are essential in the treatment of leptospirosis [99]. Dialysis and blood component transfusions may be necessary. Treatment with antibiotics should be started as soon as possible since this has been proven to shorten symptom duration. For anicteric leptospirosis, doxycycline, ampicillin, or amoxicillin may be used [100]. For icteric leptospirosis, the primary therapy is penicillin G [104]. Animal vaccination has been available for years, however, these preparations were too reactogenic to be used in humans and thus have not been approved in countries other than Japan, China, and Vietnam [96]. Since no human vaccines are available yet, prophylaxis may be achieved while visiting an endemic area by administering a weekly dose of doxycycline [98].

Lyme Disease

Introduction

Lyme disease is an infectious disorder involving multiple systems when advanced, but given its classic cutaneous manifestation, this condition can be diagnosed promptly and cured effectively.

Incidence and Prevalence

Despite worldwide prevalence, the incidence of Lyme disease is highest in areas of middle Europe and the northeast and Midwest USA. In 2007, reported cases of Lyme disease in the USA totaled 27,444, with most occurring during the summer months [105].

Etiology

The symptoms of Lyme disease are due to the body's immune response to an infection with the spirochete *Borrelia burgdorferi*, transmitted by the bite of the Ixodes tick. Three serotypes of *Borrelia burgdorferi* sensu lato have been found:

- *B. burgdorferi* sensu stricto is the most common cause of Lyme disease in the USA
- *B. afzelii* and *B. garinii* are also present in Europe causing acrodermatitis chronica atrophicans and neurologic Lyme disease, respectively [106].

In addition to distinct strains manifesting with different clinical presentations, varying immune responses lead to diverse clinical scenarios and sometimes even seroconversion without the onset of symptoms [105].

Table 6 Clinical manifestations of Lyme disease

Early localized disease
Erythema migrans
Constitutional symptoms (fatigue, malaise, lethargy, headache, myalgias, arthralgias, and local lymphadenopathy)
Early disseminated disease
Cardiac involvement
AV block
Cardiomyopathy
Myopericarditis
Neurologic involvement
Cranial neuropathy (most often Bell's palsy)
Meningitis
Encephalitis
Peripheral neuropathy
Radiculoneuropathy
Musculoskeletal involvement
Migratory polyarthritis
Polyarthralgias
Myositis
Cutaneous involvement
Multiple erythema migrans lesions
Borrelial lymphocytoma (in Europe)
Lymphadenopathy
Renal involvement
Microhematuria
Proteinuria
Ocular involvement
Conjunctivitis
Iritis
Retinitis
Hepatic involvement
Hepatitis
Late/chronic disease
Musculoskeletal manifestations
Monoarticular or polyarticular arthritis
Neurologic manifestations
Encephalopathy
Encephalomyelitis
Peripheral neuropathy
Cutaneous manifestations
Acrodermatitis chronica atrophicans (in Europe)
Morphea scleroderma-like lesions (in Europe)

Clinical Features

Lyme disease is generally divided into three clinical stages: early localized, early disseminated, and late disease (described briefly in Table 6) [107–110].

Early localized disease is distinguished by the emergence of the classic skin lesion of erythema migrans (EM), which may be accompanied by constitutional symptoms. EM occurs in more than ¾ of Lyme disease patients, predominantly in the areas of the groin, axillae, and popliteal fossa [111]. The disease may start as a papule in the area of the tick bite that expands slowly to an erythematous annular plaque reaching a median size of 15 cm, and the lesion usually clears in the center creating a bull's-eye appearance (see Fig. 15) [108]. As the lesion centrifugally advances, the non-scaly edge may become crusted or vesicular. Patients do not complain of pain, but rather an occasional burning sensation. Erythema migrans is self-limited and can disappear in several weeks without treatment; however, failure to properly manage this condition may lead to systemic complications [109].

Multiple smaller disseminated EM lesions may result with spirochetemia. In addition to the multiple erythema migrans lesions, *early-disseminated disease* is characterized

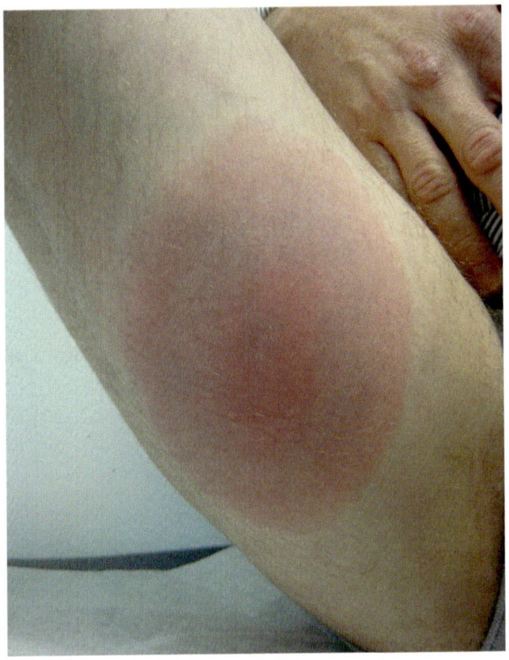

Fig. 15 Lyme disease. The disease starts as a papule in the area of the tick bite that expands slowly to an erythematous annular plaque that clears in the center creating a bull's-eye appearance known as erythema migrans

by neurologic and/or cardiac findings occurring weeks to months after the onset of infection [5, 111].

Late/Chronic Lyme disease is typically associated with arthritis involving the large joints, predominantly the knees, and/or severe neurologic problems from months up to a few years after the initial infection. In Europe, this chronic stage may present with the rare cutaneous lesions of Acrodermatitis chronica atrophicans predominantly on the extensor surfaces of hands and feet of women. It manifests as bluish-red crinkled thin skin, which progresses chronically to fibrous nodules and even to ulcerations or carcinoma [109].

Diagnosis

The most sensitive technique for the diagnosis of Lyme disease is the recognition of the skin manifestation in a patient exposed to an endemic area. If the erythema migrans (EM) is recognized early in a high-risk individual, no further laboratory test are required to arrive at a diagnosis since serology remains negative until several weeks after the onset of infection. In contrast, patients suspected of early disseminated or late disease must undergo serologic antibody detection testing by ELISA and then confirmed with western blot. PCR of CSF or synovial fluid may be performed to confirm late disease [110].

Pathology

On histology, erythema migrans (EM) may reveal spirochetes when using Warthin–Starry stain. An infiltrate of plasma cells, lymphocytes, and eosinophils may be seen in the interstitium and around vascular endothelium. Eosinophils predominate if the biopsy is taken from the center of the EM lesion [12].

Differential Diagnosis

Erythema migrans should be differentiated from fixed drug eruption, erysipelas, cellulitis, dermatitis, and other tick rashes as in Southern tick-associated rash illness (STARI). When presenting as a systemic disease: fibromyalgia, meningitis, reactive or rheumatoid arthritis, and SLE should be ruled out [5, 12].

Complications

A Jarisch–Herxheimer reaction may be experienced as an abrupt, but transient worsening of symptoms caused by the killing of spirochetes during the first hours of antibiotic treatment for early Lyme disease [107].

Treatment

A highly effective method of prevention is to inspect for ticks after outdoor activity, since the tick needs to be attached more than 24 h to transmit the disease. Nonetheless, if treated in its early stages, Lyme disease is completely curable. For early erythema migrans, 10–21 days of oral doxycycline, amoxicillin, or cefuroxime may be used; doxycycline being preferred in all patients except pregnant women or children under 8 years [112, 113]. In early disseminated disease, if the patient has isolated facial palsy, oral doxycycline for 14–21 days is enough [107]. However, if early, disseminated stage is manifested by carditis, AV block, meningitis or any other acute neurologic involvement, parenteral treatment with ceftriaxone or penicillin G for 10–28 days is necessary [113]. Patients with late disease manifested by arthritis alone may be treated with oral doxycycline therapy, but if neurologic findings with or without arthritis are present, parenteral ceftriaxone or penicillin therapy for 14–28 days is recommended [113]. Antibiotic prophylaxis in asymptomatic patients who have suffered a tick bite is very controversial. Currently, a single dose of doxycycline antibiotic is used as prophylaxis in patients who meet all of the following criteria:

- The tick has been attached ≥36 h
- The patient is within 72 h of tick removal
- The tick has been identified as *Ixodes scapularis*
- The bite occurred in an endemic area, and
- Doxycycline is not contraindicated [113, 114]

Mycobacteria

Hansen's Disease

Introduction

Hansen's disease, commonly known as Leprosy, is a chronic, disabling, and deforming infection that has been stigmatized by society for many centuries.

Incidence and Prevalence

The prevalence of leprosy at the beginning of 2008 consisted of 212,802 cases, while in the early 1980s exceeded the 12 million [115]. In the USA, its reporting began in 1824 and its incidence has never risen above 500 cases [116, 117]. Although this is certainly a positive sign of progress, the World Health Organization (WHO) has not yet reached its goal of reducing the prevalence to <1 case per 10,000 population in all endemic countries. Nepal, India, Brazil, Madagascar, Myanmar, and Indonesia have the highest rates of Leprosy contributing to more than 80% of the world's cases. Even though most of these countries are tropical or subtropical regions, it is believed that the poor hygiene and living conditions have a stronger relationship with prevalence than climate [118].

Etiology

Infection with *Mycobacterium leprae*, an obligate intracellular acid-fast bacillus with an affinity for macrophages and Schwann cells, causes leprosy. Contrary to popular belief, Leprosy is not a highly infectious disease nor is it contagious by contact with intact skin. It is principally transmitted by oral or nasal droplets from the infected individual to the exposed nasal or oral mucosa of the recipient. The incubation period can range from several months to over 40 years, with longer periods for lepromatous leprosy (LL) than for tuberculoid leprosy (TT). The areas most commonly affected are the cooler regions of the body: superficial peripheral nerves, skin (predominantly of the earlobes and nose), mucous membranes, bone, anterior chamber of the eyes, liver, and testes [115].

The clinical form of the disease, the granuloma formation, depends on the strength of the host's immune system and the development of immunologic complications (leprae reactions) rather than in the variations of the organism serotypes, as seen in Lyme disease. Hansen's disease is classified by a clinical severity spectrum with tuberculoid leprosy (TT) being the mildest form of the disease and lepromatous leprosy (LL), the most severe. The majority of the individuals exposed to *M. leprae* develop an effective immune response that is curative, while a small percentage of exposed individuals develop a chronic infection with any form within the clinical spectrum depending on immunological response. Strong cell-mediated immunity (CMI) (IFN-γ and IL-2) results in mild forms of disease (TT), with possibly only a few well-defined nerves involved and lower bacterial loads. A strong humeral response (IL-4 and IL-10) and weak CMI, results in LL with widespread lesions, extensive skin and nerve involvement, and high bacterial loads. Borderline, or "dimorphic," leprosy (BB) and the intermediary regions (BT and BL) between the two ends of the spectrum, reflect the variation of host immune response [118].

Leprae reactions are also attributed to the immunological response against leprae infection. A sudden increase in T-cell immunity is responsible for type I reversal or downgrading reactions. Type II reactions result from the activation of TNF-α, the deposition of immune complexes in tissues with neutrophilic infiltration, and complement activation in organs [119].

Clinical Features

Due to the wide spectrum of clinical findings in Leprosy, various classification protocols have been created to categorize patients within a particular zone of the spectrum and facilitate treatment directives. There are two main classifications. The Ridley–Jopling classification divides the spectrum into five groups based on the immunologic response: tuberculoid (TT) at the mild end, borderline tuberculoid (BT), borderline–borderline (BB, in the middle), borderline lepromatous (BL), and lepromatous (LL) at the severe end. Meanwhile, the WHO classification divides the gamut into three groups based on the number of cutaneous lesions: single-lesion leprosy (one skin lesion), paucibacillary leprosy (2–5 skin lesions), and multibacillary leprosy (>5 skin lesions). The Ridley–Jopling classification is more commonly used with revisions adding an Indeterminate (I) category for patients in an early stage of the disease with insufficient clinical or histological features to fulfill a definitive category. In general, Hansen's disease primarily involves the skin and nervous system. In addition to cutaneous changes in pigmentation with possible anesthesia of the lesions, peripheral nerves can become enlarged and palpable [115]. Table 7 contains a brief description of each category [115, 120] (Figs. 16–21).

Diagnosis

The diagnostic evaluation for leprosy includes a complete physical examination with thorough skin observation, neurological examination and skin smears, and/or biopsies. In 1997, the WHO Expert Committee on Leprosy established that one or more of the following three cardinal signs was enough for a diagnosis of leprae: (1) hypopigmented, erythematous, or hyperpigmented skin lesions with sensory loss, (2) nerve enlargement (predominantly great auricular nerve in the neck, median and superficial radial cutaneous nerves at the wrist, ulnar nerve at the elbow, and common peroneal nerve at the popliteal fossa), and (3) the presence of acid-fast bacilli on a skin smear [115]. At the present time,

Table 7 Characteristics of Leprosy described in Ridley–Jopling classification

Characteristics	LL	BL	BB	BT	TT	I
Cutaneous lesions	Erythematous macules that indurate into painless nodules, madarosis (hair loss of eyebrows or eyelashes), leonine facies, saddle nose, mucosal ulceration, LE ichthyosis (see Figs. 19 and 20)	Erythematous or hypopigmented macules, papules, plaques or nodules with sloping edges	Plaques with sharply demarcated central healing (punched-out lesions)	Annular, scaling erythematous infiltrated plaques	Scaling macules or infiltrated plaques, often hypopigmented with loss of hair in the lesion (see Figs. 16 and 17)	Erythematous or hypopigmented macules
Cutaneous distribution and demarcation	Multiple, symmetric, vaguely defined	Multiple, roughly symmetric, vaguely defined	Multiple, asymmetric, vaguely defined	Variable number, satellite lesions, asymmetric, well defined	One or a few (≤5) asymmetric, well-defined	One or a few, variable distribution, vaguely defined
Neuropathic changes	Early: No sensory loss, late: symmetric stocking and glove anesthesia, eye and facial nerve involvement	Slight sensory loss, minimal asymmetric peripheral involvement	Moderate sensory loss, asymmetric peripheral nerve involvement	Sensory loss, several asymmetric peripheral nerve involvement	Sensory loss, enlargement of local peripheral nerves	Slight sensory loss, no peripheral nerve enlargement, decreased sweating of affected areas
Bacilli in skin lesions[a]	≥6+ (MB)	4+ to 5+ (MB)	2+ to 3+ (MB)	Scarce (PB or MB)	None (PB)	None (PB)
Pathology	Macrophage loaded with bacilli (Virchow cells), scant lymphocytes, may have plasma cells (see Fig. 21)	Variable, in the mid range of LL and BB	Epithelioid granuloma with scanty lymphocytes	Variable, in the mid range of BB and TT	Epithelioid granuloma with dense lymphocytosis, Langerhan's giant cells, may have caseation of the nerves (see Fig. 18)	Patch of lymphocytes or macrophages that surround appendages or blood vessels
Reactions	Type II, ENL	Type I, reversal and/or type II, ENL	Type I, reversal	Type I, reversal	Rare	None

LE lower extremities, *ENL* erythema nodosum leprosum
Adapted from [115, 120]
[a]Based on average acid-fast bacilli per oil immersion field expressed as a 0 to 6+ semi-logarithmic scale

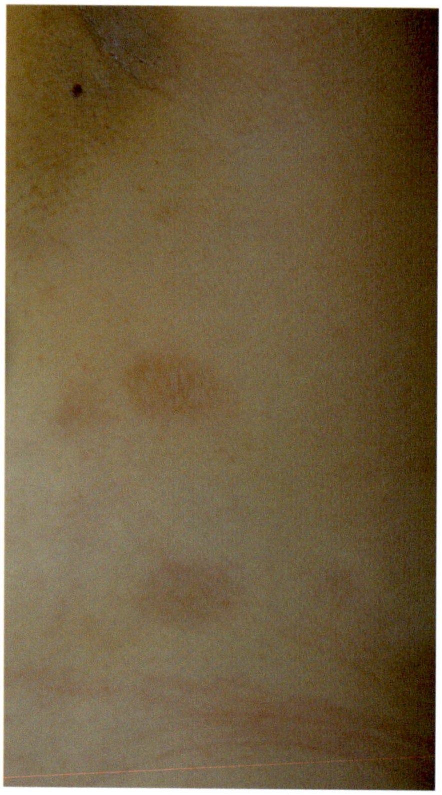

Fig. 16 Tuberculoid leprosy. Scaling patches with decreased sensation

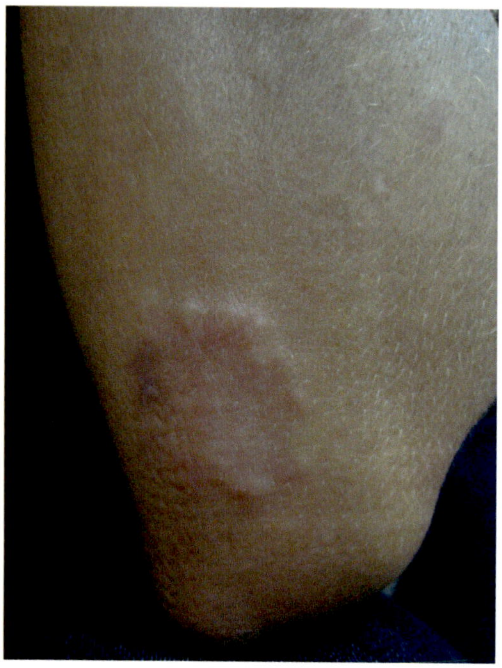

Fig. 17 Tuberculoid leprosy. Erythematous infiltrated plaque

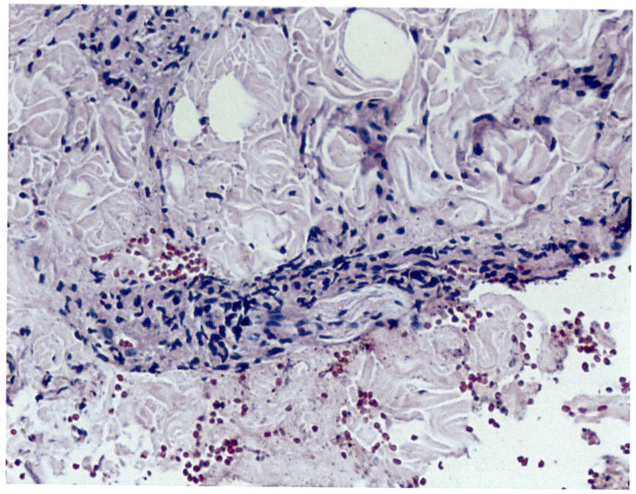

Fig. 18 Histopathological features of tuberculoid leprosy. Tuberculoid granulomas with a tendency to be linear along cutaneous nerves

diagnosis is based on clinical criteria plus skin smears or biopsy since it is known that multibacillary leprosy may not present with sensory loss and paucibacillary leprosy may be negative in skin smears [118]. Other tests (PCR, histamine, pilocarpine, and Mitsuda tests) can aid in diagnosis but are performed with less frequency due to unavailability or complexity.

Differential Diagnosis

It is important to assess sensation of the cutaneous lesions of a patient at risk of leprae since these numerous conditions in the differential diagnosis to rule out: tinea versicolor, tinea corporis, pityriasis rosea, congenital nevi, granuloma annulare, tuberculosis, sarcoidosis, psoriasis, secondary syphilis, leishmaniasis, fixed drug eruption, neurofibromatosis, and others [121]. The differential diagnosis for rare cases of isolated neural involvement (neuritic leprosy) are: diabetic neuropathy, carpal tunnel, amyloidosis, and poliomyelitis. By recognizing the specific extent of neural involvement such that leprae never involves upper motor neurons, deep tendon reflexes, proximal muscles or proprioception may the differential diagnosis be narrowed [118].

Complications

Some patients develop leprae reactions, an acute hypersensitivity to *M. leprae*. These are especially prominent during the treatment phase if a patient is pregnant or suffering from another infection. It can occur with any form of leprosy, except for the indeterminate leprosy category [118]. The clinical features of the major types of inflammatory reactions are described in Table 8 [115] (Fig. 22).

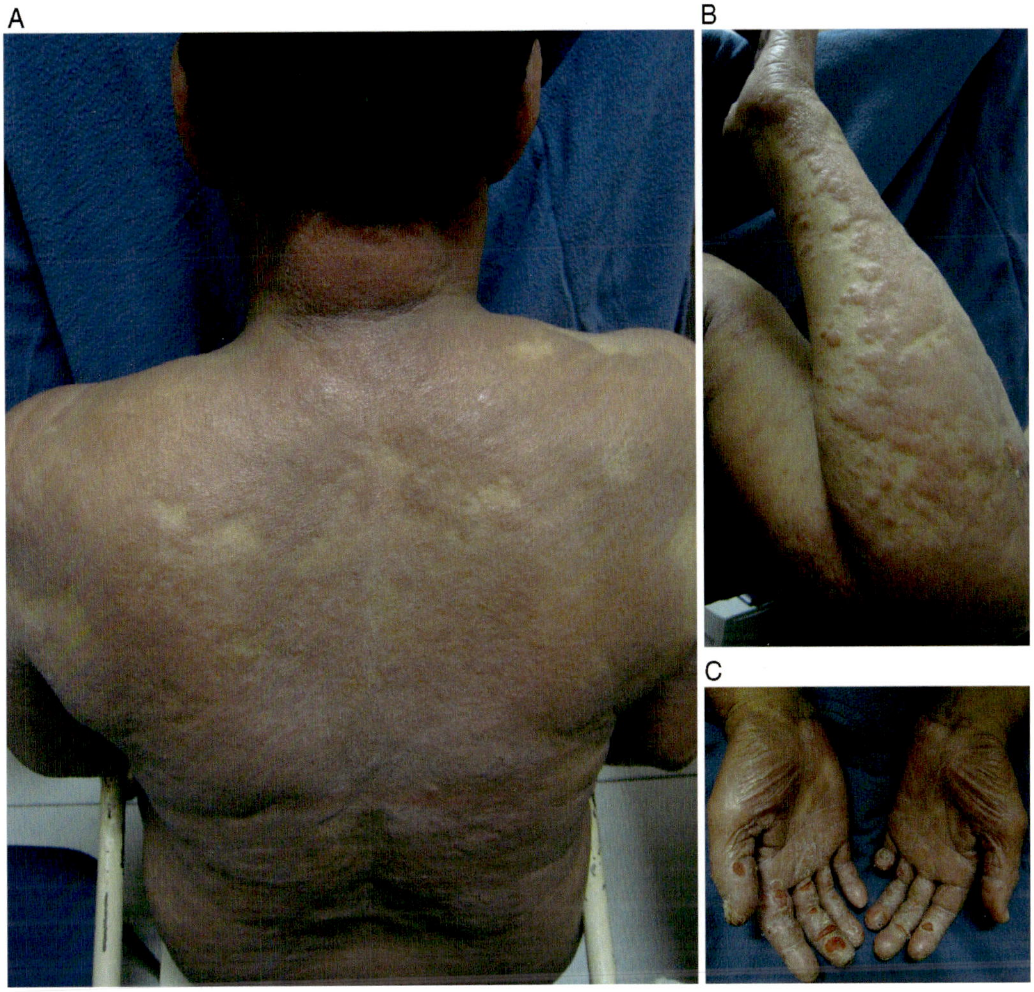

Fig. 19 Lepromatous leprosy. Erythematous plaques on the (**a**) trunk and (**b**) extremities (widespread and symmetric distribution) associated with (**c**) amyotrophy, contracture of fingers and ulcers on the hands

Treatment

Early diagnosis and treatment is the key to curing the disease effectively before it creates stigma and disability. The WHO and US treatment regimens are the two main therapeutic protocols against Leprosy, each indicated in Tables 9 and 10, respectively [118, 122]. Only the WHO has a recommended treatment for single skin lesions; nonetheless, both are multidrug therapies (MDT) that prevent dapsone resistance, eliminate contagiousness with the first dose, and reduce relapses [122].

Close follow-up is important to ensure patient compliance and monitor CBC and liver function tests, which are negatively affected by the medications. Educating patients about ways to minimize nerve damage helps prevent deformities.

Atypical Mycobacteriosis

Introduction

Mycobacteria are a family of small rod-shaped bacilli that cause a gamut of infectious conditions, of which the most notorious are *mycobacterium tuberculosis* and *mycobacterium leprae*. Nevertheless, there is a large proportion of mycobacteria that do not cause tuberculosis nor leprosy, known as atypical mycobacteria; also referred to as *Mycobacteria other than tuberculosis* (MOTT) or *Non-tuberculous mycobacteria* (NTM). To this day, a vast number of mycobacteria species have been identified and classically categorized based on the speed of growth, morphology, and pigment production, but this chapter will be limited to those with cutaneous manifestations [14]. Details on *Mycobacterium avium intracellulare* are included in the Cutaneous Manifestations of HIV Disease chapter.

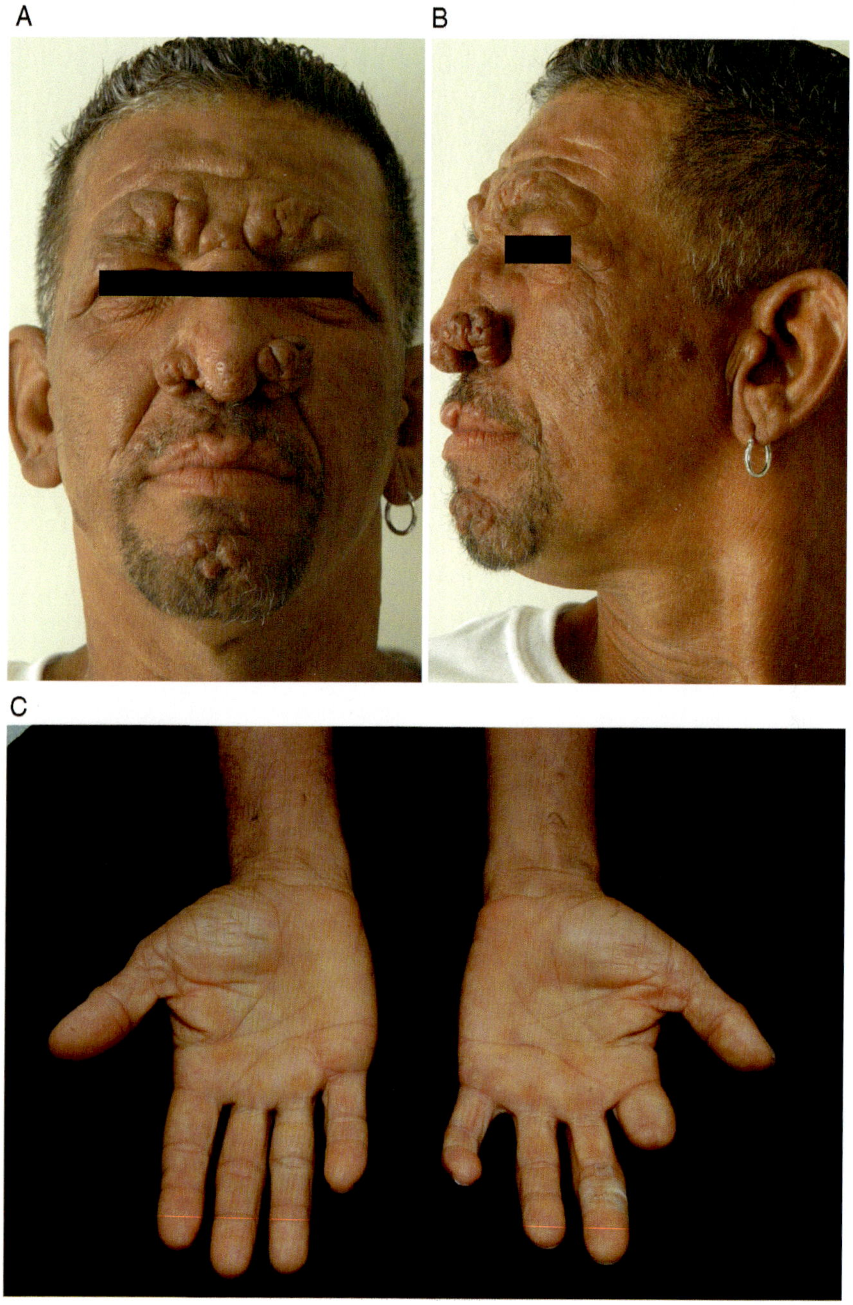

Fig. 20 Lepromatous leprosy. Diffuse infiltration of the face with leonine facies (**a**) and madarosis (**b**), "Papal hand" flexion contractures of the fourth and fifth fingers (ulnar nerve involvement) (**c**)

Incidence and Prevalence

Cutaneous infections with atypical mycobacteriosis (ATM) are rare in the USA and worldwide; however, have gained attention because the number of reported cases is increases [123]. ATM infections are more common in immunocompromised patients whom also have a greater risk of disease dissemination [13].

Etiology

These saprophytic (obtain nourishment from products of organic breakdown) organisms are found in water, soil, vegetation, and domestic and wild animals [14]. Atypical mycobacteria cannot pass through intact mucosa or skin, therefore are transmitted by inhalation, percutaneous penetration, or by ingestion [124].

Clinical Features

ATM present with variable signs and symptoms. They principally affect the lungs, lymphatics, skin, and soft tissue (see Figs. 23 and 24). See Table 11 for further details on the variable cutaneous manifestations.

Diagnosis

Because of the subtle and variable clinical presentations, cutaneous atypical mycobacterial infections are frequently misdiagnosed. They should be suspected when patients are immunosuppressed or have been exposed to a predisposing environment and present with lesions in a *sporotrichoid* pattern and/or painless ulcers, nodules, or plaques. ATM infections are confirmed by sampling the affected tissue and performing cultures at multiple temperatures (25, 37, and 42°C) to ensure growth of all possible pathogens. Infections involving the lungs, such as in *M. kansasii*, diagnosis come by examining and culturing sputum samples [124].

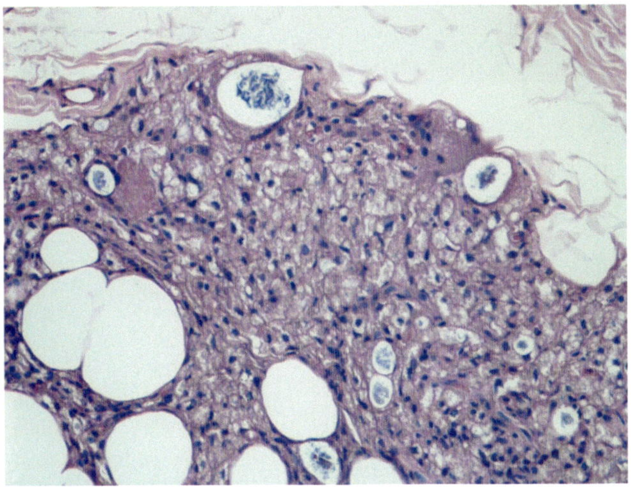

Fig. 21 Histopathologic features of Lepromatous Hansen's disease. Diffuse infiltrate of predominantly foamy histiocytes, clumps of bacilli called globi

Treatment

ATM infections cause little mortality but can lead to significant morbidity when left undiagnosed or treated poorly. Therapy varies according to the organism and extent of infection. It may require a surgical procedure and/or treatment for 3–6 months [14]. See Table 11 for more information.

Fungal Infections

Superficial Mycoses

Superficial fungal infections are the most common of all mucocutaneous infections. Many of these fungi are commensal organisms that colonize normal epithelium. Changes in the microenvironment of the skin can trigger these fungi to overgrow leading to symptomatology. These mycoses only invade the stratum corneum of the epidermis, hair, and nails thus remain superficial. Three genera are responsible for the majority of superficial mycoses: *Candida* species, *Malassezia* species, and dermatophytes. They are subdivided according to the degree of inflammation triggered when causing disease [13].

Table 8 Characteristics of leprae reactions

	Type 1: Reversal reaction	Type 2: Erythema nodosum leprosum (ENL)
Type of leprosy	Occurs in borderline leprosy (BB, BT, BL)	Occurs in borderline lepromatous and lepromatous leprosy
Pathophysiology	Type IV delayed-type hypersensitivity reaction, acute exacerbation of CMI	Antigen–antibody immune complexes formation
Clinical features	Constitutional symptoms Existent lesions become erythematous and edematous, and may ulcerate Edema of affected extremities and face Acute nerve tenderness and damage Emergence of new erythematous lesions	Constitutional symptoms Crops of erythematous tender nodules appear (extremities and face) (see Fig. 22) Edema of face, hands, and feet Orchitis Lymphadenitis Epistaxis Proteinuria Severe joint and peripheral nerve swelling Iridocyclitis
Course	Occurs during 6–18 months of treatment and persists for a few months	May occur before treatment but tends to occur after and, lasts for a few days but may recur
Treatment	Oral prednisone, NSAID's	Thalidomide, NSAID's, increase clofazimine dose

CMI cell-mediated immunity
Adapted from [115]

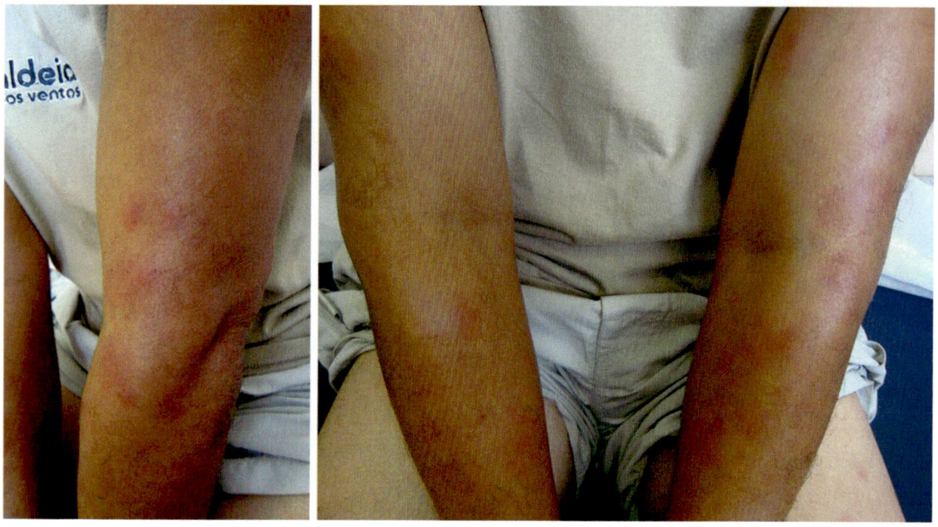

Fig. 22 Erythema nodosum leprosum (type 2 reaction). Appearance of multiple *red* papulonodules in a patient with lepromatous leprosy

Table 9 World Health Organization Recommendations for Treatment of Leprosy

WHO recommendations for treatment of leprosy
Single skin lesion: Single dose of rifampin 600 mg + ofloxacin 400 mg + minocycline 100 mg[a]
Paucibacillary: Dapsone 100 mg daily + rifampin 600 mg once a month (6 cycles in 9 months)
Multibacillary: Dapsone 100 mg daily + rifampin 600 mg once a month + clofazimine 300 mg once a month + clofazimine 50 mg daily (for 1 year)

[a]Abbreviated as ROM treatment

Table 10 United States Recommendations for treatment of Leprosy

US recommendations for treatment of leprosy
Paucibacillary: Dapsone 100 mg daily + rifampin 600 mg once a month (for 1 year)
Multibacillary: Dapsone 100 mg daily + rifampin 600 mg daily + clofazimine 50 mg daily (for 2 years)

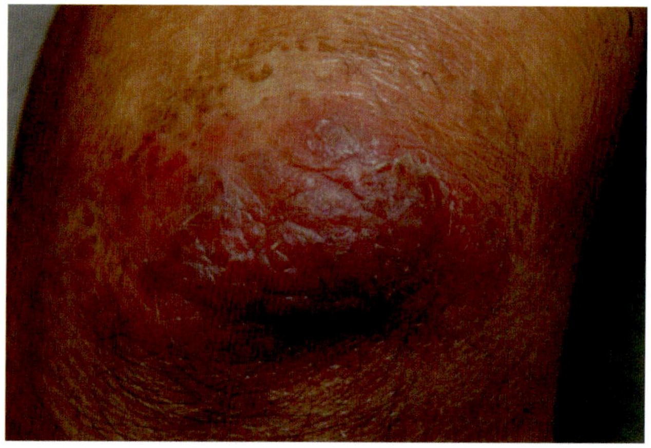

Fig. 23 Atypical mycobacteria. Erythematous violaceous indurated verrucous plaque on the elbow

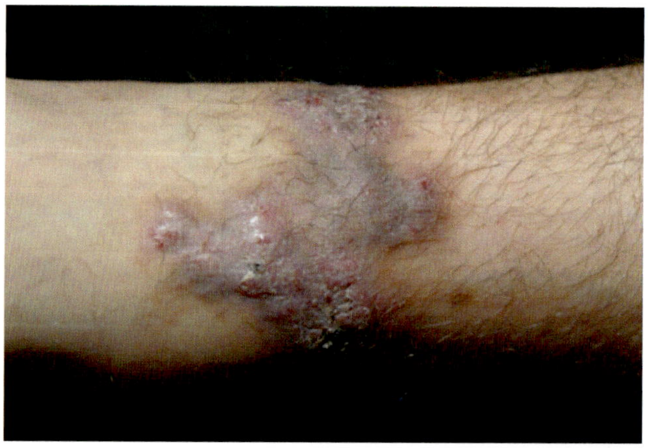

Fig. 24 Atypical mycobacteria. Irregular violaceous plaque with silvery scaling and excoriations

Inflammatory Superficial Mycoses

Dermatophytoses

Introduction

Dermatophytoses sometimes are referred by the patient as "ringworm." They are unique in that they infect tissue by metabolizing keratin. They infect skin (epidermomycosis), nails (onychomycosis), and hair (trichomycosis) producing diverse presentations named as "Tinea" followed by its location in Latin [13, 126].

Incidence and Prevalence

Dermatophyte infections are very common, accounting for over 5 million medical visits per year, with an average cost of over $200 million dollars. With the exception of tinea

Table 11 Characteristics of atypical mycobacterioses

Etiology	Epidemiology	Skin lesions	Clinical features	Pathology	Differential diagnosis	Treatment
M. marinum	Enters through breaks in the skin from contaminated fresh or salt water (also known as "swimming pool or fish tank granuloma")	Violaceous papule develops in the inoculation site, enlarges into a dark red plaque that may ulcerate or become verrucous, and suppurative, and of a sporotrichoid pattern of nodules along the lymphatics	Cutaneous lesions mostly on UE. Deeper invasion can cause septic arthritis or OM. Lesions may disseminate in immunocompromised hosts, LN uncommon	Acute and chronic inflammation, tuberculoid granulomas, fibrinoid changes and caseation necrosis may occur. Acid fast mycobacteria seen with Ziehl–Nielsen	Verruca vulgaris Sporotrichosis Tuberculosis verrucosa cutis Leishmaniasis Nocardiosis	Initial empiric treatment with clarithromycin when suspected, surgical debridement if deep tissue is involved
M. ulcerans	Enters through breaks in the skin, occurs in wetlands of tropical climates (Australia, Africa, Mexico)	Painless firm nodule, ulcerates and center becomes necrotic with undermined edges, ulcer may extend to cover entire limb	Cutaneous lesions most commonly on extensor surfaces of extremities (LE>UE), LN and systemic manifestation uncommon	Granuloma inflammation, subcutaneous fat necrosis, coagulation necrosis of dermis, and destruction of nerve, appendages, and blood vessels	Panniculitis Foreign body granuloma Fungal infections Pyoderma gangrenosum	Surgical excision, large ulcers may require skin grafts or amputation, local heating, hyperbaric oxygen
MFC: *M. fortuitum*, *M. chelonae*, *M. abscessus*	Saprophytes. Immunocompromised patients more prone to infection S/P surgery, injections (acupuncture, Botox), implants (mamoplasty), and footbaths in nail salons	Variable: most commonly erythematous subcutaneous nodules in a sporotrichoid pattern but may present as cellulitis to a sanguinolent and suppurative ulcer	May present with non-cavitary pneumonia, keratitis, endocarditis, lymph-adenitis and osteomyelitis	PMN micro-abscesses and granuloma formation with foreign body-type giant cells; necrosis may occur	Foreign body reactions Deep mycoses Osteomyelitis	*M. chelonae* and most *M. fortuitum* are sensitive to clarithromycin Excision and debridement may be required for abscesses and ulcers
M. kansasii	Acquired via minor trauma (puncture wounds), prevalent in white urban men living in temperate zones (US, UK, France), skin is involved predominantly in the immune-suppressed	Verrucous plaques, ulcers and nodules, may be arranged in a sporotrichoid pattern	Lung is the major site of infection, symptoms resemble tuberculosis	Variable: tuberculoid granulomas, dense PMN infiltrate, abscess formation or epidermal necrosis	Sporotrichosis Other atypical mycobacterial infections	Combination of antituberculous medications (Isoniazid + rifampin + ethambutol + either streptomycin or clarithromycin)

UE upper extremities, *LE* lower extremities, *OM* osteomyelitis, *LN* lymphadenopathy, *MFC Mycobacterium fortuitum complex*, *s/p* status post, *PMN* polymorphonuclear
Adapted from [5, 13, 14, 125]

capitis, which is more common in children, dermatophytoses are more common in postpubertal individuals with tinea pedis being the most common worldwide [127, 128].

Etiology

Several species of dermatophytes affect humans; these are classified into three genera: *Epidermophyton*, *Trichophyton*, and *Microsporum* [128].Contrary to the other two genera of superficial mycoses, dermatophytes are not normal flora of our skin. The infection may spread from person to person, animal to person, or soil to person. Furthermore, immunosuppression does not lead to an increased frequency of dermatophyte infection, although it increases its severity. The details of specific etiologies, clinical presentations, risk factors, and differential diagnoses can be seen in Table 12 (Figs. 25 and 26).

Diagnosis

Clinical examination is often sufficient for diagnosing dermatophytoses, however, because of its variable presentation and vast differential diagnosis, confirmatory tests are useful. Wood's light (UV light) examination is used, mainly for the diagnosis of tinea capitis. Direct microscopic examination of skin scrapings, plucked hair, or nail specimens with potassium hydroxide (KOH) can reveal hyphae. For precise identification of the species, fungal cultures are necessary [13].

Pathology

Histology is not necessary; however, biopsy findings may demonstrate spongiosis, parakeratosis, and a superficial inflammatory infiltrate in the stratum corneum. Branching hyphae are often seen in the stratum corneum. Fungal stains, such as the periodic acid Schiff (PAS) stain, aid in rapid identification. For example, infections by tinea unguium are visible with PAS staining as hyphae and/or arthroconidia in the nail plate and bed [5, 13].

Complications

The most common complication of dermatophytoses is caused by interdigital infection from tinea pedis. The fungus can produce a breach in the skin thus allowing for the inoculation of opportunistic bacteria, predisposing to cellulitis of the lower extremities. Rarely, extensive skin disease, subcutaneous abscesses, and dissemination occur in patients with impaired CMI [127].

Treatment

Preventive measures such as maintaining areas dry, frequent nail clipping, and repeated washing or discarding of fomites, help prevent and extinguish infections. The first-line therapeutic option is topical antifungals (azoles and allylamines). Systemic antifungal therapy (itraconazole, fluconazole, and terbinafine) is required to cure tinea manuum, barbae, capitis, and unguium, since topical therapy is ineffective. Systemic antifungal therapy, however, are associated with more severe and frequent side effects, this modality must be used with extreme caution. The appropriate duration of topical therapy for dermatophytic infections depends in each patient. A couple of weeks may be sufficient for dermatophytic infections of tinea corporis and cruris. However, tinea pedis may require treatment for as long as 8 weeks [129, 130].

Mucocutaneous Candidiasis

Introduction

Infection with *Candida* species has a wide spectrum of clinical presentations and ranges from local superficial mucocutaneous infections to widespread dissemination with multiorgan failure.

Etiology

The yeast *Candida albicans* is the most frequent cause of candidiasis followed by *Candida tropicalis. Candida* species may colonize the gastrointestinal tract, oropharynx, and/or vagina of healthy individuals as part of their microflora; however, it is not normal permanent flora of the skin. Colonization may turn to widespread disease when the microflora environment is altered. Some predisposing factors for mucocutaneous candidiasis include: prolonged broad-spectrum antibiotic treatment, corticosteroids use, diabetes mellitus, and other endocrinopathies, immunosuppression, obesity, xerostomia, hyperhydrosis, maceration, occlusion by clothing or dressings, indwelling catheters, oral contraceptives, and malnutrition, among others [13, 14].

Clinical Features

In immunocompetent individuals, candidiasis occurs as a localized infection of the skin or mucosal membranes, including the oral cavity, pharynx, gastrointestinal tract, urinary bladder, or genitalia. In immunocompromised individuals, the disease may infect the esophagus, tracheobronchial tree, and/or blood [14]. The most common presentations and differential diagnoses of mucocutaneous candidiasis are mentioned in Table 13 (see Fig. 27).

Diagnosis

The diagnosis is established by the presence of yeast forms and pseudohyphae on KOH direct microscopy examination of scrapings and by a positive fungal culture in a patient with symptomatology (cultures also useful to test sensitivities) [14, 131].

Treatment

The most important step in treating mucocutaneous candidiasis is the identification and mitigation of risk factors (i.e., keeping affected areas dry in intertrigo). Topical agents are frequently used as first choice to manage localized or

Table 12 Characteristics of dermatophytoses

Infection	Most common pathogens	Location	Risk factors	Clinical findings	Differential diagnosis
Tinea corporis	*T. rubrum*, *T. mentagrophytes*	Trunk and extremities excluding palms, soles, and groin	Tropical regions; outdoor work, gymnasiums, domestic animals, exposure to infected body parts or infected individuals	Mild pruritic scaly annular plaques may have pustules or vesicles in margins, enlarge peripherally producing central clearing (see Fig. 25)	Granuloma annulare Annular psoriasis Dermatitis Nummular eczema
Tinea pedis "athlete's foot"	*T. rubrum*, *T. mentagrophytes*, *E. floccosum* and *T. tonsurans* (in children)	Soles and interdigital spaces of the feet	Hot and humid weather, closed footwear, walking barefoot on contaminated floors, exposure to other tineas	Types: *Interdigital*: scaling, fissuring, maceration *Moccasin*: Erythema of sole with defined margins, hyperkeratosis *Inflammatory*: vesicle or bullaes with clear fluid *Ulcerative*: Interdigital ulcers; commonly complicated with bacteria	Psoriasis vulgaris Secondary syphilis Dermatitis Erythrasma Impetigo *Candida* intertrigo
Tinea capitis	*T. tonsurans*, *M. canis* and *M. audouinii*	Scalp	Children, black race, malnutrition, chronic disease, close contact with individuals with tinea capitis	Variable clinical. May involve posterior cervical and/or auricular LN and may cause systemic disease "*Gray patch*": dry, scaly patches of alopecia "*Blackdot*": hair breakage near the scalp "*Kerion*": severe pustular eruption with alopecia	Psoriasis Seborrheic dermatitis Alopecia areata Atopic dermatitis
Tinea cruris "jock itch"	*T. rubrum*, *E. floccosum*, and *T. mentagrophytes*	Groin and inner aspect of upper thighs but the scrotum is spared	Tropical regions, male gender, obesity, excessive perspiration, tinea pedis	Sharply demarcated circinate plaque with erythematous, scaly, and advancing border that may contain pustules or vesicles	Erythrasma *Candida* intertrigo Pityriasis versicolor Psoriasis
Tinea manum	*T. rubrum*, *T. mentagrophytes*, and *E. floccosum*	Palms and interdigital spaces of the hand	Infection with moccasin type tinea pedis of any foot or with tinea unguium of the involved hand	Predominantly unilateral, hyperkeratotic and scaly patches with well-defined margins may have papules, vesicles, or bullae	Psoriasis vulgaris Atopic dermatitis Contact dermatitis
Tinea barbae "barber's itch"	*T. mentagrophytes var mentagrophytes*, *T. verrucosum*, and *T. rubrum*	Beard areas of the face and neck	Postpubertal males, use of contaminated razors, exposure to animals (farmers)	Pustular folliculitis, scaly, erythematous patches with broken hairs, kerion, regional LN involvement, may become superinfected	Bacterial folliculitis Acne vulgaris Acne rosacea
Tinea faciei	*T. rubrum*, *T. mentagrophytes*, *T. tonsurans*, *M. audouinii*, and *T. canis*	Face	Children, animal exposure, chronic topical steroid use	Asymmetric macules or plaques with minimal scaling and well-defined borders may contain pustules (see Fig. 26)	Acne rosacea Dermatitis Acne vulgaris
Tinea unguium	*T. mentagrophytes*, *T. rubrum*, and *E. floccosum*	Toenails > fingernails	Chronic tinea pedis and trauma	Onycholytic, hyperkeratotic and yellow discoloration of multiple nails, causes discomfort and may be complicated by paronychia or cellulitis	Psoriatic nails Congenital nail dystrophy Reiter's syndrome

LN lymphadenopathy
Information extracted from [5, 13, 126, 127, 129, 130]

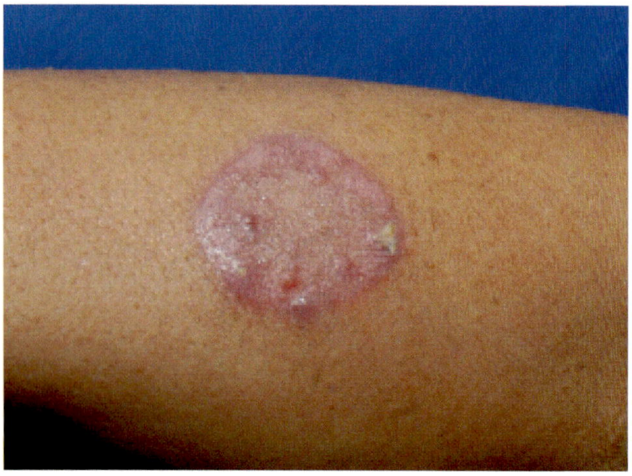

Fig. 25 Tinea profunda. Annular well-circumscribed erythematous plaque with scaling and mild central clearing

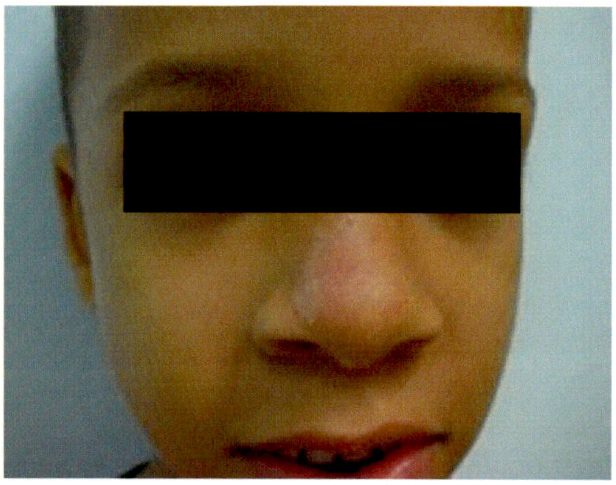

Fig. 26 Tinea faciei. Annular scaly erythematous plaque in the nose

superficial forms of candidiasis. Topical azole antifungals and topical polyenes (amphotericin B and nystatin) are the most widely used. These preparations are available as creams, troches, and vaginal suppositories or tablets. For oral therapy, azoles, especially fluconazole, are the preferred treatment [131].

Non-inflammatory Superficial Mycoses

There are three main superficial mycoses that cause disease without an inflammatory reaction: *Tinea nigra, piedra,* and *pityriasis versicolor*. Pityriasis versicolor is highly prevalent in many areas of the world and is further discussed in this section.

Pityriasis Versicolor

Introduction

Pityriasis versicolor, an asymptomatic superficial mycoses of the epidermis, is caused by a member of the normal cutaneous flora [132]. It is commonly referred to as tinea versicolor, but it is not a dermatophyte infection. This condition is very common and follows a chronic and benign course [132].

Incidence and Prevalence

The causative agent is found within the normal flora in 18% of infants and 90–100% of adults. Even though the exact prevalence remains unknown because many affected yet asymptomatic individuals do not seek medical attention, the reported prevalence is 2–8% of the general population being more prevalent in tropical climates [13].

Etiology

Malassezia furfur, also known as pityrosporum orbiculare or ovale, is responsible for causing pityriasis versicolor and has

Table 13 Clinical presentation and differential diagnosis of cutaneous candidiasis

Disease	Clinical features	Differential diagnosis
Pseudomembranous candidiasis (Thrush)	White creamy adherent plaques on any oral mucosal surface	Oral hairy leukoplakia, condyloma acuminatum, geographic tongue, lichen planus
Angular cheilitis (Perlèche)	Erythematous fissuring angles of the mouth may have underlying creamy exudate	Iron deficiency anemia, Plummer–Vinson syndrome, riboflavin or vitamin B2 deficiency, chapped lips
Intertrigo	In intertriginous zones: pustules on an erythematous base which may erode and become confluent, progresses to eroded patches with superficial pustular lesions at the periphery (satellite pustulosis)	Streptococcal intertrigo, inverse pattern psoriasis, erythrasma, dermatophytoses, pityriasis versicolor
Erosio interdigitalis blastomycetica	Maceration, erythematous fissuring of the interdigital space with underlying creamy exudates	Interdigital tinea pedis or tinea manum
Chronic paronychia	Painful, indurated and erythematous proximal nailfold, possible purulent discharge	Bacterial paronychia, trauma, cellulitis, contact dermatitis, pemphigus vulgaris, squamous cell carcinoma, Herpetic Witlow
Vulvovaginitis	Pruritus, burning, dyspareunia, erythema, and edema of vulva, white discharge, white removable plaques on vaginal walls, cottage cheese appearance	Trichomonas infection, atrophic vaginitis, bacterial vaginosis, lichen planus, lichen sclerosus et atrophicus

Information extracted from [13, 14]

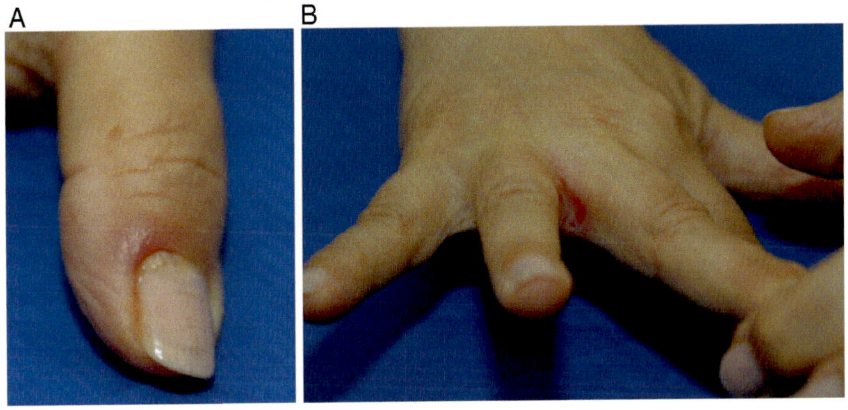

Fig. 27 Patient with paronychia by *Candida* (**a**) and erosio interdigitalis blastomycetica (**b**)

also been implicated in seborrheic dermatitis and *Malassezia* folliculitis. The condition is not contagious. Various factors may trigger its conversion to the mycelial or hyphal form associated with clinical disease; these include sun exposure, hyperhydrosis, immunosuppression, malnutrition, hot humid weather, the use of oils or oily skin, steroid treatment, and genetic predisposition, among others [132, 133].

Clinical Features

Pityriasis versicolor is usually asymptomatic causing only mild pruritus if at all, thus most patients seek medical attention merely because of cosmetic concern. *M. furfur* manifests as macules of varying size with fine scaling, especially after scrapping, however, partially treated lesions lack scales. These macules may be confluent and predominate on the upper trunk and proximal upper extremities. The term "versicolor" refers to the variety of colors present in this disease. Colors may range from hypochromic in tanned individuals to hyperchromic in the dark skinned [13, 14, 134–136].

Diagnosis

Diagnosis is mainly clinical, with confirmation from direct examination of scrapings in KOH preparations showing the classic finding of "spaghetti and meatballs" (hyphae and spores) pattern. Wood's lamp inspection of the affected skin shows positive fluorescence [13, 14].

Pathology

Budding yeast and hyphae can be detected by hematoxylin and eosin (H&E), PAS, or methenamine silver stain in the stratum corneum (see Fig. 28). The epidermis reveals mild hyperkeratosis and acanthosis with a possible chronic inflammatory infiltrate [134].

Differential Diagnosis

The differential diagnosis can be divided by the changes in pigmentation and scaling, and these include: vitiligo, pityriasis alba, post-inflammatory hyperpigmentation, tuberculoid leprosy, secondary syphilis, tinea corporis, seborrheic dermatitis, nummular eczema, guttate psoriasis, and pityriasis rosea [13].

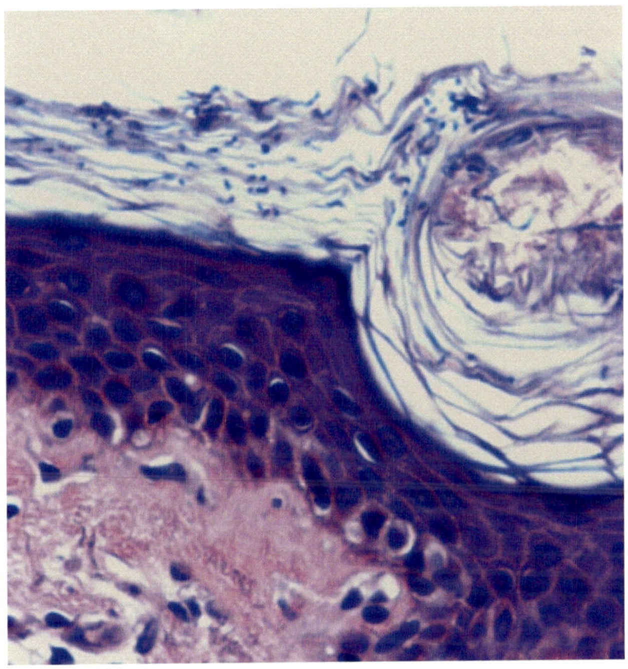

Fig. 28 Pityriasis versicolor. Numerous budding yeasts and short hyphae are present in the stratum corneum

Treatment

In patients with limited and localized disease, 2 weeks of topical antifungal therapy is the treatment of choice. These include (1) selenium sulfide 2.5% shampoo or lotion, (2) azoles, and (3) terbinafine 1% solution [135].

For patients with extensive disease, oral medications are more convenient and effective. Most oral antifungal agents (itraconazole, ketoconazole, and fluconazole) may be used, with the exception of griseofulvin and terbinafine with a duration of days to weeks depending on the agent used.

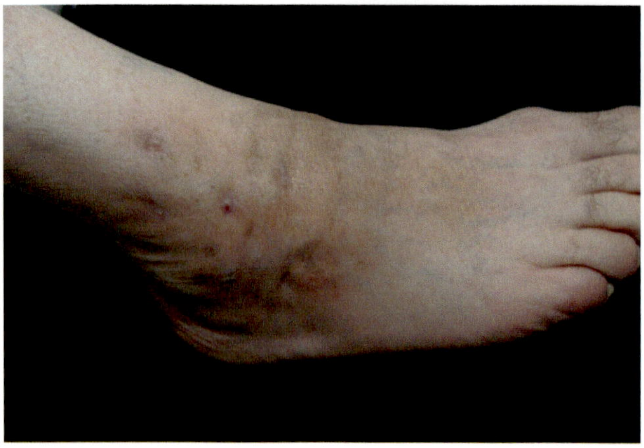

Fig. 29 Mycetoma, also known as Madura foot, is a indolent localized suppurating chronic infection characterized by the presence of grains in the purulent drainage [13, 14]

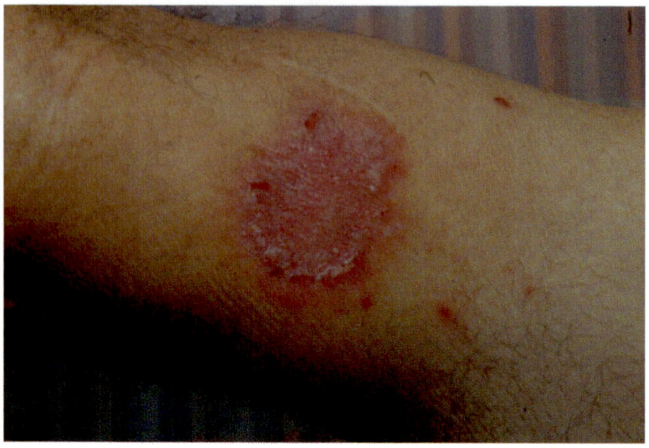

Fig. 30 Chromomycosis, also known as chromoblastomycosis, is a chronic indolent localized infection characterized by a verrucous plaque that developed from papules that coalesce usually on the lower extremities

For example, ketoconazole for 5 days is a typical regimen for this condition [135, 137].

Recurrence is common [137]. Patients who experience frequent recurrences can use topical or oral therapy, particularly during the warm weather months to prevent even more relapses. Prophylaxis with topical selenium sulfide solution 2.5% applied to the entire body for 10 min every 2–3 weeks, which is just as effective as oral ketoconazole or itraconazole once a month [135].

Subcutaneous Mycoses

Subcutaneous mycoses are invasive fungal infections caused by numerous organisms that generally originate as localized cutaneous infections, but extend deeper when the integrity of the skin is breached. They rarely disseminate or produce systemic disease [12]. These include: mycetoma (see Fig. 29), chromomycosis (chromoblastomycosis) (see Figs. 30 and 31), sporotrichosis, lobomycosis, rhinosporidiosis, zygomycosis, and phaeohyphomycosis. In the following section, sporotrichosis will be discussed.

Sporotrichosis

Introduction

Also known as Rose gardener's disease, sporotrichosis is a granulomatous infection that usually involves the skin and superficial lymph nodes.

Incidence and Prevalence

Sporotrichosis incidence has not been properly established. Although the causative agent is present in the soil throughout the world, this infection is endemic to Mexico, Central and South America, South Africa, and rarely occurring in Europe. In the USA, it is most commonly found in the Missouri and Mississippi River Valleys. All age groups are affected, but it is more common in adults [138].

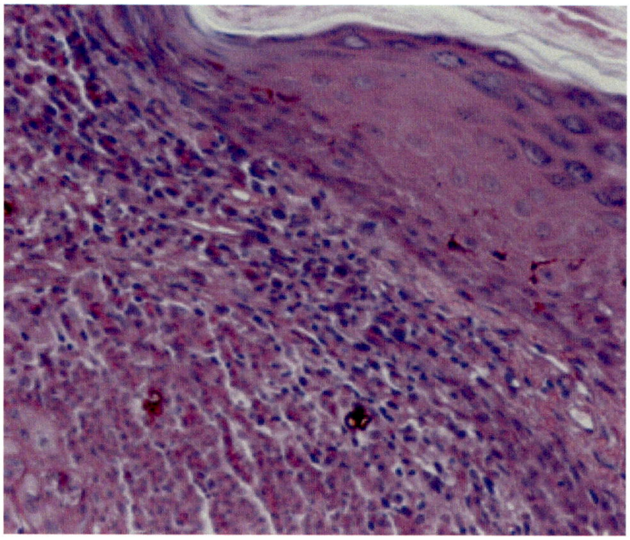

Fig. 31 Chromomycosis. *Round golden brown* cells (medlar bodies) can be seen in a suppurative granulomatous process in the dermis

Etiology

This infection is caused by the fungus *Sporothrix schenckii*, which is found in soil, sphagnum moss, certain animals, and thorny plants. It is most commonly acquired from cutaneous inoculation. As a result, farmers, gardeners, florists, and some animal handlers are at greatest risk [139].

Clinical Features

Sporotrichosis may present with various types of clinical manifestations depending mostly on the host immune response. Cutaneous sporotrichosis limited to the site of inoculation is commonly referred to as plaque sporotrichosis (see Fig. 32). The most common cutaneous manifestation (80% of cases) is a lymphocutaneous or "sporotrichoid" pattern, in other words, a lesion at the primary inoculation site with a direct spread of the infection along the lymphatic drainage creating a visible linear pattern (see Fig. 33). Plaque sporotrichosis is more common on the hands and face, whereas lymphocutaneous sporotrichosis is more common on the arms and upper extremities since they contain the majority of the lymphatic vessels. Extensive cutaneous disease with or without systemic involvement is also possible in the immunocompromised host [140].

The initial presentation of plaque sporotrichosis is a painless papule, pustule, or nodule at the location of injury several weeks after inoculation. The lesion rapidly ulcerates, becoming erythematous and indurated, yet remains painless. The lesion continues localized but draining lymph nodes may become inflamed and suppurative. In the lymphocutaneous pattern, additional lesions appear as dermal and subcutaneous nodules and ulcers along the path of lymphatic drainage [139, 140].

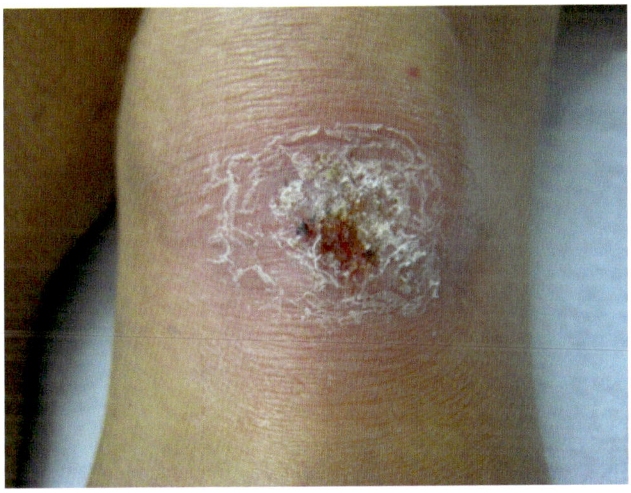

Fig. 32 Plaque sporotrichosis. Initial presentation is a painless papule, pustule, or nodule at the location of inoculation which rapidly ulcerates, becoming erythematous, indurated, and may scale; yet remains painless and localized

Diagnosis

The condition may be diagnosed clinically, if there is a strong suspicion from the history and physical examination. Contrary to many other fungal infections, *Sporothrix schenckii* organisms are not usually seen by KOH; therefore, cultures taken from tissue or secretions in Sabouraud's medium are often required for confirmation. At the present time, the use of PCR assay for diagnosis is increasing [139].

Pathology

On histology, sporotrichosis is a mixed granulomatous and pyogenic process. Granulomatous Langhans-type giant cell and microabscesses are visualized. In immunocompetent individuals, organisms are not seen under the microscope while, on the contrary, the immunosuppressed present with numerous organisms, often as cigar-shaped forms of yeast [13].

Differential Diagnosis

The differential diagnosis for the sporotrichoid pattern includes: atypical mycobacterial infection (i.e., *M. marinum*), leishmaniasis, cat-scratch disease, and *Nocardia*. While the differential diagnosis of plaque sporotrichosis includes: cutaneous tuberculosis, atypical mycobacterioses, tularemia, foreign body granulomas, and other infectious or inflammatory granulomatous diseases [13].

Treatment

Itraconazole for 3–6 months is the treatment of choice for lymphocutaneous or local cutaneous sporotrichosis. Fluconazole is the second choice since ketoconazole has been shown less effective. A saturated solution of potassium iodide was commonly used in the past because of its low

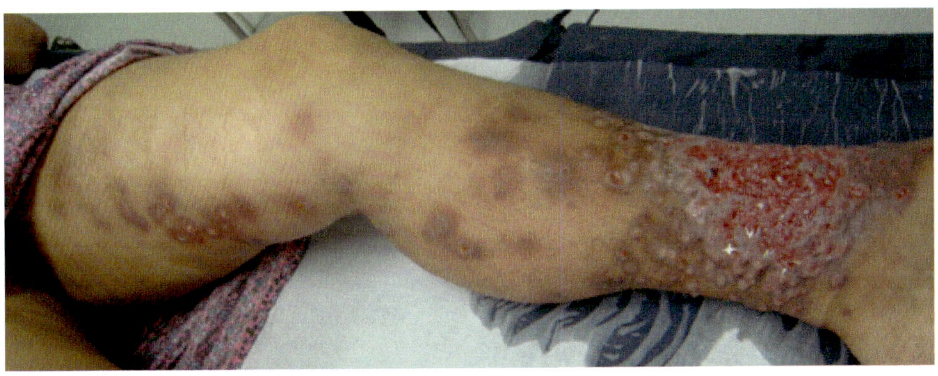

Fig. 33 Sporotrichoid pattern. Lesions appear as dermal and subcutaneous nodules and ulcers along the path of lymphatic drainage

cost, but has been found less effective than the oral antifungal agents [141]. Amphotericin B may be used in disseminated disease.

Systemic Mycoses

Systemic mycoses are fungal infections that originate within deep tissue and organs which then disseminate throughout the body causing widespread symptomatology. Many of these systemic mycoses have cutaneous manifestations and will be discussed further in this section. They can be classified into two main groups: endemic respiratory infections (true fungal pathogens) and opportunistic infections. The former can cause infection in immunocompetent individuals, while the latter in an immunocompromised host [12] (Table 14 and Figs. 34–37).

Endemic respiratory infections:

- *Histoplasma capsulatum* (histoplasmosis)
- *Coccidioides immitis* (coccidioidomycosis)
- *Blastomyces dermatitidis* (blastomycosis)
- *Paracoccidioides brasiliensis* (paracoccidioidomycosis)

Opportunistic infections

- *Candida* species (candidiasis)
- *Aspergillus* species (aspergillosis)
- *Cryptococcus* (cryptococcosis)
- *Zygomycetes* (zygomycosis)

Diagnosis

All systemic mycoses can be diagnosed via direct examination (with KOH or Calcofluor) of dermal samples and/or cultures of infected tissue, pus, or bodily fluids. In some systemic mycoses (i.e., coccidioidomycosis and histoplasmosis), serologic testing, exoantigen testing, and PCR assays can also help in the diagnosis [14].

Treatment Histoplasmosis

Intravenous Amphotericin B should be used for severe or life-threatening histoplasmosis. In mild or moderate localized disease, itraconazole is the preferred treatment, but ketoconazole can also be used. In some asymptomatic cases, the disease may be self-limited and treatment may not be necessary [142].

Treatment Coccidioidomycosis

Similar to histoplasmosis, amphotericin B is required for severe or disseminated coccidioidomycosis. The only azole approved by the FDA for non-life-threatening coccidioidomycosis is ketoconazole; however, itraconazole and fluconazole are commonly used by clinicians especially with skeletal or meningeal involvement, respectively [143].

Treatment Blastomycosis

Amphotericin B is the treatment of choice when blastomycosis is severe or progressive. In mild-to-moderate disease not involving the central nervous system, itraconazole is the treatment of choice with ketoconazole and fluconazole as alternative medications [142].

Treatment Paracoccidioidomycosis

Paracoccidioidomycosis requires prolonged therapy with the same antifungals used for the systemic mycoses previously mentioned with the addition of sulfonamides among the treatment options. In disseminated disease, systemic therapy with amphotericin B is indicated. Itraconazole is the preferred treatment for non-life-threatening paracoccidioidomycosis [144].

Viral Infections

Varicella-Zoster Virus

Introduction

Varicella-zoster virus (VZV) infection causes two distinct forms of disease: varicella (chickenpox) and herpes zoster (shingles). The latter is the reactivation of latent varicella infection.

Incidence and Prevalence

Varicella is prevalent worldwide with the peak incidence during the spring. Varicella most commonly occurs during childhood. Vaccination against varicella began in 1995. This brought down the four million cases of chickenpox that occurred annually in the USA and that affected 90% of children by the time they reached 10 years [145]. There is a 20% lifetime chance of developing herpes zoster in individuals with a past history of varicella. In the USA, nearly one million individuals per year develop shingles, although this number is expected to diminish since the varicella vaccine will also alter the incidence of herpes zoster [146]. The severity and the incidence of shingles increase significantly with age.

Etiology

Varicella is highly contagious and is transmitted through airborne droplets or contact with cutaneous lesions. The patient is contagious starting 4 days prior to the cutaneous manifestations until all lesions have crusted. In addition to invading the skin, VZV infects dorsal root ganglion cell bodies, where it becomes dormant for a lifetime or until stress, trauma, or immunosuppression permit its reactivation into herpes zoster. A patient with herpes zoster can infect a susceptible person with varicella, but a person with varicella cannot infect someone with herpes zoster [14].

Table 14 Characteristics of systemic mycoses

Etiology	Epidemiology	Cutaneous lesions	Non-cutaneous involvement	Pathology
Histoplasma capsulatum	Soil in warm humid climates (southeastern and central US, Central America, South America, Africa, and Asia), bird and bat droppings, inhalation or direct skin inoculation	Acute disease: May cause erythema multiforme, erythema nodosum Disseminated disease: *Immunocompromised*: Mucocutaneous erosions, multiple erythematous necrotic hyperkeratotic papules, or nodules, panniculitis, erythroderma (see Fig. 34) *Immunocompetent*: Oral ulcers, less frequent skin nodules	Lung and the reticuloendothelial system: spleen, bone marrow, lymph nodes, and liver may present with meningitis	Intracellular yeast forms surrounded by a rim of clearing, histiocytes, and giant cells (see Fig. 35)
Coccidioides immitis	Inhaled via dust, rarely by direct inoculation into the skin, summer and fall in southwest USA, Philipino race, immuno-suppression, and pregnancy predispose to disseminated disease	*Acute disease*: Toxic erythema, erythema multiforme, and erythema nodosum *Disseminated disease*: Central face is predominant site, papules progress to pustules, plaques, abscesses, and multiple sinus tracts, or subcutaneous cellulitis	Primary asymptomatic lung infection or flu-like syndrome with pleuritic chest pain; osteomyelitis and meningitis occurs in the immuno-suppressed	Endospore-containing spherules with surrounding granulomatous inflammation with histiocytes, lymphocytes, and giant cells
Blastomyces dermatitidis	Inhaled via soil, rarely inoculates the skin, southeastern USA, men are more prone to systemic disease	*Acute disease*: Erythema multiforme, erythema nodosum *Disseminated disease*: On exposed skin; mucosal involvement; verrucous plaques with crusted borders progressing to central healing are the most common findings	Primary pulmonary infection usually subclinical, bone involvement (osteomyelitis) with extension to muscle or joints, rarely genitourinary involvement	Round yeast with broad-based budding and thick, double walls within giant cells and microabscesses, pseudo-epitheliomatous hyperplasia
Paracoccidioides brasiliensis	Inhaled via soil, trauma from chewing or rarely through skin; most common in males; endemic of Venezuela, Columbia, Ecuador, Argentina, and Brazil	*Primary pulmonary*: Predominates on the face and nasal and oral mucosa; painful ulcerative or verrucous lesions; "moriform stomatitis" *Primary mucocutaneous*: Intraoral and perioral distribution due to trauma from chewing contaminated flora *Primary cutaneous*: Single verrucous papule, plaque or ulcer at the skin inoculation site	Primary pulmonary disease is subclinical to mild, but may disseminate to skin and/or mucous membranes, spleen, adrenal glands, GI tract, and lymph nodes (especially cervical)	Narrow-based buds resemble a "mariner's wheel," yeast forms are found within giant cells, pseudo-epitheliomatous hyperplasia, cutaneous granulomatous inflammation
Aspergillus species	Neutropenia, steroid therapy, solid organ, or BM transplant patients, HIV, broad spectrum antibiotics	Single or multiple papules that enlarge into ulcers with a necrotic base and surrounding erythematous halo, propensity to blood vessel invasion (see Fig. 36)	Lungs and sinuses are the major sites of infection may affect skin by dissemination, skin lesions may spread to musculoskeletal system	Septate hyphae with acute branching (see Fig. 37)

BM bone marrow, *GI* gastrointestinal
Created from information of [12, 13]

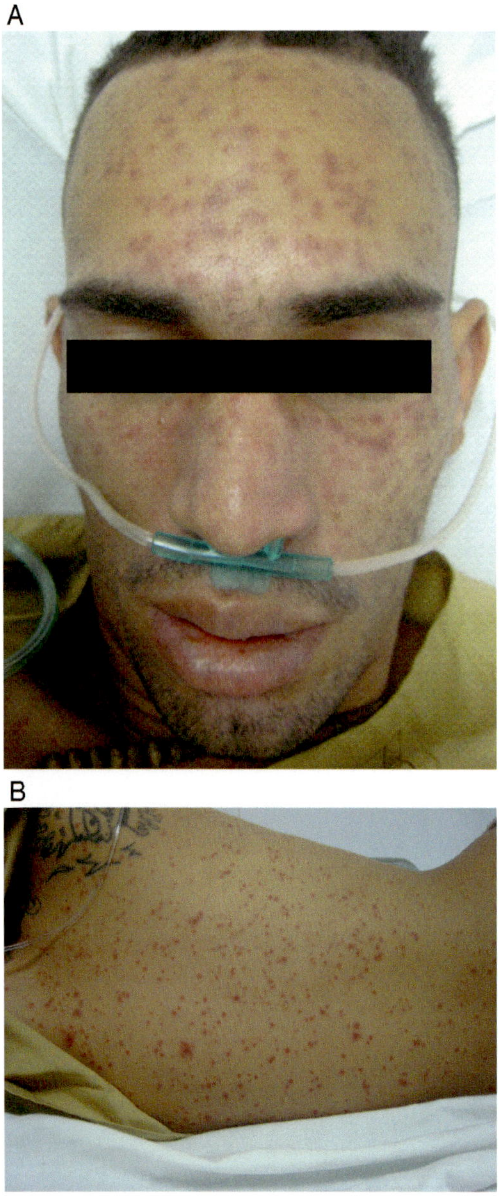

Fig. 34 Disseminated histoplasmosis. In immunocompromised patients histoplasmosis manifests as mucocutaneous erosions, multiple erythematous necrotic hyperkeratotic papules, or nodules as seen here in face (**a**) and trunk (**b**)

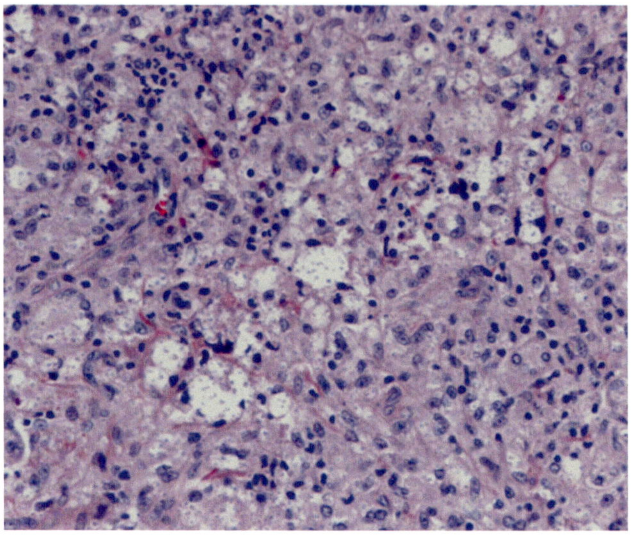

Fig. 35 Histopathological features of histoplasmosis. Diffuse mixed dermal infiltrate composed of neutrophils, lymphocytes, and histiocytes. Numerous small spores surrounded by a clear space (pseudocapsule)

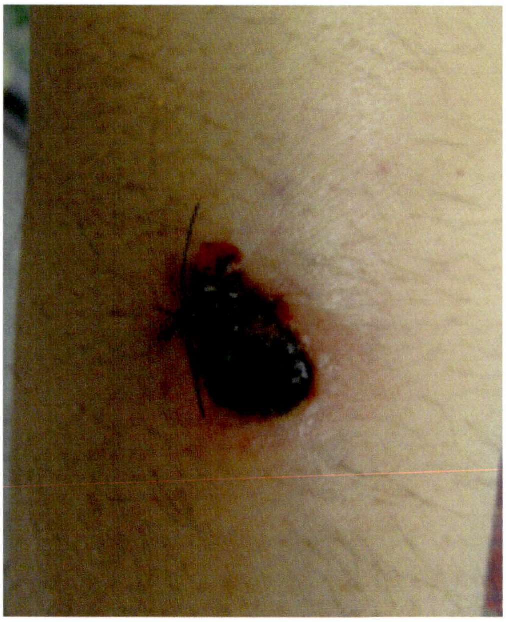

Fig. 36 Disseminated aspergillosis. In immunocompromised patients *Aspergillus* affects the skin by forming papules that enlarge into ulcers with necrotic base and surrounding erythematous halo, it has propensity to invade blood vessels

Clinical Features: Varicella

Symptoms begin approximately 10–20 days after the patient has been exposed to varicella [147]. Mild fever, malaise, muscle pain, and/or pharyngitis usually herald the cutaneous eruption that starts on the scalp, face, and oral mucosa and then spreads caudally. Crops of diffuse, pruritic, and erythematous macules and papules rapidly evolve into serous fluid containing vesicles with an erythematous base. The vesicles progress into pustules and crusted erosions. Lesions in all stages of development can present at the same time [14, 147] (see Fig. 38).

Clinical Features: Herpes Zoster

A cutaneous eruption following a unilateral dermatomal distribution in an individual with a past history of primary varicella is considered herpes zoster until proven otherwise. The painful, pruritic, and erythematous papules rapidly evolve into crops of vesicles or bullae that occasionally become hemorrhagic. Herpes zoster often begins with a prodrome of intense pain and hyperesthesia over the affected area [148].

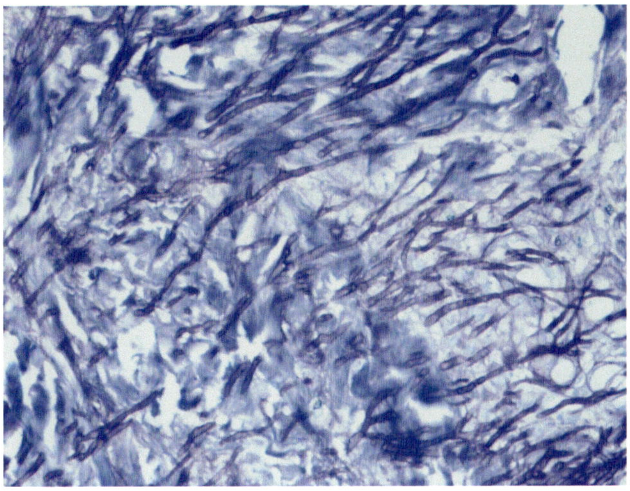

Fig. 37 Aspergillosis. Numerous septate hyphae with branching at acute angles in the dermis (PAS stain)

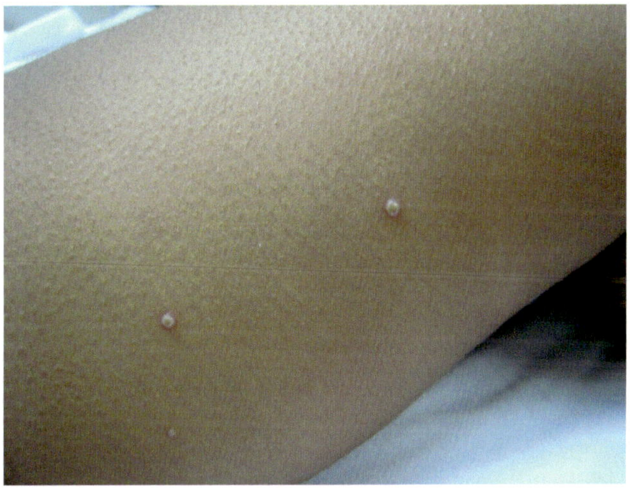

Fig. 38 Varicella. Serous fluid-filled vesicles in an erythematous base progress to pustules and crusted erosions. Typically, varicella lesions are at different stages

The most common areas involved are the thoracic dermatomes followed by the facial dermatomes, a distribution of the first branch of the trigeminal nerve [146] (see Fig. 39). In some patients, multiple adjacent dermatomes may be involved, but generally do not cross the midline. In immunocompetent hosts, the entire course takes approximately 2 weeks with lesions no longer contagious by the end of the first week. Therefore, if the patient presents with new lesions after a week, an underlying immunodeficiency should be suspected [148]. Contrary to varicella, herpes zoster may recur in 5% of patients and most often affects the same dermatome [14].

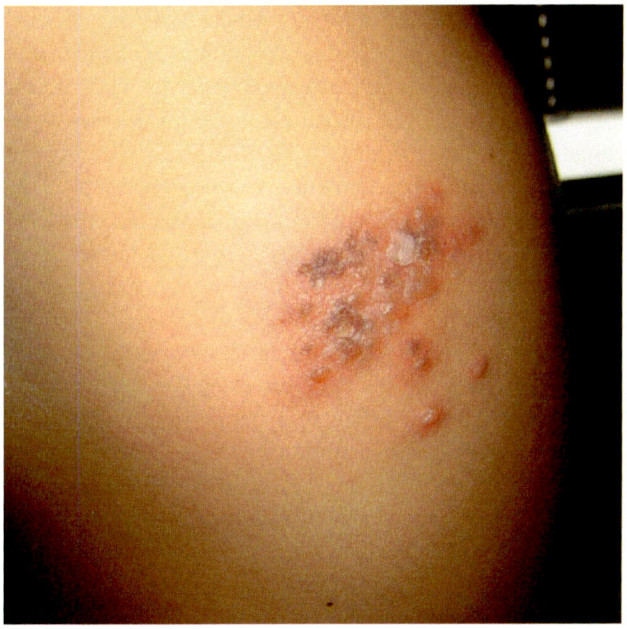

Fig. 39 Herpes zoster. Erythematous papules develop into clusters of vesicles or bullae that could turn hemorrhagic. Most commonly, affects thoracic dermatomes, as we see in this patient

Diagnosis

The history and physical exams are generally enough to make the diagnosis. When a diagnosis is uncertain, however, a Tzanck smear or direct fluorescent antibody (DFA) test can be performed. DFA is more specific, thus permits distinction from Herpes simplex virus (HSV). Lesion biopsy, immunohistochemical staining, viral cultures, serology, and PCR are techniques also available for making the diagnosis [149].

Differential Diagnosis

The differential diagnoses of varicella includes: other vesicular viral exanthems (i.e., *cocksackie virus*), disseminated HSV infection, *pityriasis lichenoides et varioliformis acuta* (PLEVA), rickettsial pox, bullous impetigo, drug eruptions, contact dermatitis, and insect bites [5].

If severe enough, the pain of the prodromal stage of herpes zoster can be misdiagnosed as a migraine, myocardial infarction, pleural disease, or acute abdomen, depending on its location. The cutaneous manifestation must be differentiated from *zosteriform HSV*, erysipelas, cellulitis, bullous impetigo, and localized contact dermatitis [5, 13].

Complications

In children, varicella is usually self-limited. The most common complication is secondary bacterial infection of the lesions. Scarring, Reye's syndrome, encephalitis, and acute cerebellar ataxia can also occur [70].

When varicella occurs in adults, especially those immunosuppressed, the severity and complications increase and may involve other body systems. Adults have an increased number of lesions, greater dissemination, and can develop, although rare, pneumonia, glomerulonephritis, optic neuritis, arthritis, myocarditis, pancreatitis, orchitis, hepatitis, and vasculitis [147]. In pregnant women, especially during the first trimester, the infection can pass through the placenta and lead to congenital varicella infection. The infected fetus will suffer from low birth weight, scarring skin lesions, ocular abnormalities, cortical atrophy, psychomotor retardation, and hypoplastic limbs [5].

Herpes zoster is also a self-limited disease in immunocompetent individuals but with increasing age and diminishing immunity, the probability of complications increases. The most common complication of herpes zoster is postherpetic neuralgia, which as defined by the FDA is pain that has not resolved 30 days after disease onset [149, 150]. Other complications include: scarring, changes in pigmentation, secondary bacterial infection, zoster ophthalmicus, acute retinal necrosis, aseptic meningitis, encephalitis, Ramsay–Hunt syndrome, pneumonitis, and hepatitis. An immunocompromised host can have lesions that persist or recur multiple times and then disseminated cutaneous disease (defined as more than 20 vesicles outside the area of the primary or adjacent dermatomes) may ensue [5, 13, 149, 150].

Treatment

The best management modality for varicella is prevention. Live attenuated VZV vaccine is highly recommended for children, adults who live or work in settings where transmission of VZV is probable, and women of childbearing age who are not pregnant [70]. The vaccine has been proven highly effective in decreasing the severity of the disease, and fairly effective in preventing its occurrence. Passive protection with varicella zoster immunoglobulin (VIG) is also available for immunosuppressed patients, pregnant women exposed to VZV and for newborns of infected mothers shortly before birth [148]. VIG should be administered within 96 h of exposure and provides protection for approximately 3 weeks [5].

Once infected, children <12 years old should be treated symptomatically with calamine lotion, antihistamines and frequent baths to alleviate the pruritus. If the patient is febrile, acetaminophen rather than aspirin should be given as needed since aspirin use in viral infections increases the risk of Reye's syndrome. Acyclovir, given within 72 h of symptom onset, has been approved by the FDA to lessen the severity and duration of varicella in immunosuppressed children, children >12 years old, and all adults [70, 150–152]. Intravenous administration of acyclovir is recommended in immunosuppressed and complicated cases of varicella and herpes zoster.

Acyclovir, valacyclovir, and famciclovir, within 72 h of symptom onset, are all FDA approved for the treatment of herpes zoster to decrease the duration and pain. Although controversial, systemic corticosteroids within 72 h have been demonstrated to improve the quality of life of patients by accelerating healing and decreasing acute pain [150]. The FDA has also recently approved the varicella zoster vaccine as prophylaxis for herpes zoster in patient's ≥60 years old with a past history of varicella but no prior episode of shingles [146].

References

1. Stevens DL. Chapter 9: Cellulitis, pyoderma, absces and other skin and subcutaneous infection. In: Cohen and Powderly, editors. Infectious diseases, 2nd ed. Elsevier 2004.
2. Feaster T, Stinger J. Topical therapies for impetigo. Pediatr Emerg Care. 2010;26:222–31.
3. Stulberg D, Penrod M, Blatny R. Common bacterial skin infections. Am Fam Physician. 2002;66:119–24.
4. Luelmo-Aguilar J, Santandreu M. Folliculitis: recognition and management. Am J Clin Dermatol. 2004;5:301–10.
5. Bolognia J, Jorizzo J, Rapini R. Dermatology. 2nd ed. St. Louis: Mosby; 2008.
6. Chiller K, Selkin B, Murakawa G. Skin microflora and bacterial infections of the skin. J Investig Dermatol Symp Proc. 2001; 6(3):170–4.
7. Rhody C. Bacterial infections of the skin. Prim Care. 2000;27(2):459–73.
8. Zichichi L, Asta G, Noto G. Pseudomonas aeruginosa folliculitis after shower/bath. Int J Dermatol. 2000;39(4):270–3.
9. Sadick N. Current aspects of bacterial infections of the skin. Dermatol Clin. 1997;15:341–9.
10. Arnold H, Odom R, James W. Bacterial infections. In: Arnold H, Odom R, James W, editors. Diseases of the skin. 9th ed. Philadelphia: WB Saunders; 2000. p. 332.
11. Dong H, Duncan L. Cytologic findings in Demodex folliculitis: a case report and review of the literature. Diagn Cytopathol. 2006;34(3):232–4.
12. James W, Berger T, Elston D. Andrews' diseases of the skin clinical dermatology. 10th ed. Philadelphia: Saunders; 2005.
13. Wolff K, Johnson R, Suurmond D. Fitzpatrick's color atlas and synopsis of clinical dermatology. 5th ed. New York: McGraw-Hill; 2005.
14. Fitzpatrick J. Dermatology secrets in color. 5th ed. Philadelphia: Hanley & Belfus; 2007.
15. McNamara D et al. Incidence of lower-extremity cellulitis: a population-based study in Olmsted County, Minnesota. Mayo Clin Proc. 2007;82(7):817–21.
16. Leppard B et al. The value of bacteriology and serology in the diagnosis of cellulitis and erysipelas. Br J Dermatol. 1985;112(5): 559–67.
17. Bernard P et al. Streptococcal cause of erysipelas and cellulitis in adults. A microbiologic study using a direct immunofluorescence technique. Arch Dermatol. 1989;125(6):779–82.
18. Bjornsdottir S et al. Risk factors for acute cellulitis of the lower limb: a prospective case-control study. Clin Infect Dis. 2005;41(10):1416–22.
19. Randall G et al. Facial cellulitis in childhood: a changing spectrum. South Med J. 2002;95(7):672–4.
20. Perkins R, Morgan S. Poisoning, envenomation, and trauma from marine creatures. Am Fam Physician. 2004;69(4):885–90.
21. Haburchak D. Aeromonas hydrophila: an underappreciated danger to fisherman. Infect Med. 1996;13(10):893–6.

22. Brooke C, Riley T. Erysipelothrix rhusiopathiae: bacteriology, epidemiology and clinical manifestations of an occupational pathogen. J Med Microbiol. 1999;48(9):789–99.
23. Ellis S et al. Cellulitis incidence in a defined population. Epidemiol Infect. 2006;134(2):293–9.
24. Schmid M, Kossmann T, Duewell S. Differentiation of necrotizing fasciitis and cellulitis using MR imaging. Am J Roentgenol. 1998;170(3):615–20.
25. Falagas M, Vergidis P. Narrative review: diseases that masquerade as infectious cellulitis. Ann Intern Med. 2005;142(1):47–57.
26. Madaras K, Arbogast R, Jue S. Increased therapeutic failure for cephalexin versus comparator antibiotics in the treatment of uncomplicated outpatient cellulitis. Pharmacotherapy. 2000;20(2): 199–205.
27. Gilbert D, Moellering R, Sande M. The Sanford guide to antimicrobial therapy 2000. 30th ed. Hyde Park: Antimicrobial Therapy; 2000. p. 39.
28. Swartz M. Clinical practice. Cellulitis. N Engl J Med. 2004; 350(9):904–12.
29. Stevens D, Bisno A, Chambers H, et al. Practice guidelines for the diagnosis and management of skin and soft-tissue infections. Clin Infect Dis. 2005;41:1373.
30. Elston D. Community-acquired methicillin-resistant Staphylococcus aureus. J Am Acad Dermatol. 2007;56:1–16.
31. Wisplinghoff H, Bischoff T, Tallent S, et al. Nosocomial bloodstream infections in US hospitals. Analysis of 24,179 cases from a prospective nationwide surveillance study. Clin Infect Dis. 2004;39:309.
32. Hersh A, Chambers H, Maselli J, Gonzalez R. National trends in ambulatory visits and antibiotic prescribing for skin and soft-tissue infections. Arch Intern Med. 2008;168:1585.
33. Odell C. Current opinion in community pediatric-associated methicillin resistant Staphylococcus aureus (CA-MRSA) skin infections. Curr Opin Pediatr. 2010;22:273–7.
34. Heymann W. Community-acquired methicillin-resistant Staphylococcus aureus. J Am Acad Dermatol. 2005;53:318–9.
35. Lee M, Rios A, Aten M, et al. Management and outcome of children with skin and soft tissue abscesses caused by community-acquired methicillin-resistant Staphylococcus aureus. Pediatr Infect Dis J. 2004;23:123.
36. Chartier C, Grosshans E. Erysipelas. Int J Dermatol. 1990;29: 458–67.
37. Schmitt J. Erysipelas and necrotizing cellulitis. Ann Dermatol Venereol. 2001;128:334–7.
38. Bonnetblanc J, Bedane C. Erysipelas: recognition and management. Am J Clin Dermatol. 2003;4(3):157–63.
39. Jorup-Ronstrom C et al. The course, costs and complications of oral versus intravenous therapy of erysipelas. Infection. 1984;12:390–4.
40. Facinelli B, Spinaci C, Magi G, et al. Association between erythromycin resistance and ability to enter human respiratory cells in group A streptococci. Lancet. 2001;358:30.
41. Sjoblom A, Eriksson B, Jorup-Ronstrom C. Antibiotic prophylaxis in recurrent erysipelas. Infection. 1993;6:390–4.
42. Carroll J. Common bacterial pyodermas. Postgrad Med. 1996;100:311–22.
43. Dagan R. Impetigo in childhood: changing epidemiology and new treatments. Pediatr Ann. 1993;22(4):235–40.
44. Kelly C, Taplin D, Allen A. Streptococcal ecthyma. Treatment with benzathine penicillin G. Arch Dermatol. 1971;103(3): 306–10.
45. Dagan R, Bar-David Y. Double-blind study comparing erythromycin and mupirocin for treatment of impetigo in children: implications of a high prevalence of erythromycin-resistant Staphylococcus aureus strains. Antimicrob Agents Chemother. 1992;36(2): 287–90.
46. Epstein M, Amodio-Groton M, Sadick N. Antimicrobial agents for the dermatologist. I. Beta-lactam antibiotics and related compounds. J Am Acad Dermatol. 1997;37(149–65):166–8.
47. Vidal F, Mensa J, Almela M, Martínez J, Marco F, Casals C, et al. Epidemiology and outcome of Pseudomonas aeruginosa bacteremia, with special emphasis on the influence of antibiotic treatment. Analysis of 189 episodes. Arch Intern Med. 1996;156(18): 2121–6.
48. Reich H et al. Nonpseudomonal ecthyma gangrenosum. J Am Acad Dermatol. 2004;50(5):S114–7.
49. Leslie K, McCann B, Levell N. Candidal ecthyma gangrenosum in a patient with malnutrition. Br J Dermatol. 2005;153(4):847–8.
50. Dorff G, Geimer N, Rosenthal D, Rytel M. Pseudomonas septicemia. Illustrated evolution of its skin lesion. Arch Intern Med. 1971;128(4):591–5.
51. Ghosheh F, Kathuria S. Bilateral periorbital ecthyma gangrenosum. Ophthal Plast Reconstr Surg. 2006;22(6):492–3.
52. Halpern A, Heymann W. Bacterial diseases. In: Bolognia J, Jorizzo J, Rapini R, editors. Dermatology, vol. 1. 2nd ed. Spain: Elsevier; 2008. Ch 73.
53. Greene S, Su W, Muller S. Ecthyma gangrenosum: report of clinical, histopathologic, and bacteriologic aspects of eight cases. J Am Acad Dermatol. 1984;11(5 Pt 1):781–7.
54. Painter D, Trevillion N. Staphylococcal scalded skin syndrome. Emerg Nurse. 2007;14(10):20–1.
55. Nishifuji K et al. Staphylococcal exfoliative toxins: "Molecular scissors" of bacteria that attack the cutaneous defense barrier in mammals. J Dermatol Science. 2008;49:21–31.
56. Amagai M et al. Staphylococcal exfoliative toxin B specifically cleaves desmoglein 1. J Invest Dermatol. 2002;118:845–50.
57. Simpson C. The management of staphylococcal scalded skin syndrome in infants. Nurs Times. 2003;42:26–30.
58. Helali N et al. Nosocomial outbreak of staphylococcal scalded skin syndrome in neonates; epidemiological investigation and control. J Hosp Infect. 2005;61(2):121–38.
59. Davis M et al. Toxic shock syndrome: epidemiologic features, recurrence, risk factors and prevention. N Engl J Med. 1980;303:1429–35.
60. Hajjeh R, Reingold A, Weil A, Shutt K, Schuchat A, Perkins B. Toxic shock syndrome in the United States: surveillance update, 1979–1996. Emerg Infect Dis. 1999;5(6):807–10.
61. McCormick J, Yarwood J, Schlievert P. Toxic shock syndrome and bacterial superantigen: an update. Ann Rev Microbiol. 2001;55: 77–104.
62. Stevens D. The toxic shock syndromes. Infect Dis Clin North Am. 1996;10(4):727–46.
63. Hibralova V. Streptococcus pyogenes and the toxic shock syndrome. Ann Intern Med. 1988;108:772.
64. Bohach G, Fast D, Nelson R, Schlievert P. Staphylococcal and streptococcal pyrogenic toxins involved in toxic shock syndrome and related illnesses. Crit Rev Microbiol. 1990;17:251–72.
65. Schlievert P, Jablonski L, Roggiani M, Sadler I, Callantine S, et al. Pyrogenic toxin superantigen site specificity in TSS and food poisoning in animals. Infect Immun. 2000;68:3630–4.
66. Cone L, Woodard D, Schlievert P, Tomory G. Clinical and bacteriologic observations of a toxic shock-like syndrome due to Streptococcus pyogenes. N Engl J Med. 1987;317:146–9.
67. Begovac J et al. Group A beta-hemolytic streptococci toxic shock-like syndrome. Pediatr Infect Dis J. 1990;9:369–70.
68. Bisno A, Stevens D. Streptococcal infections of skin and soft tissues. N Engl J Med. 1996;334:240–5.
69. Bach M. Dermatologic signs in toxic shock syndromes-clues to diagnosis. J Am Acad Dermatol. 1983;8:343–7.
70. Centers for Disease Control and Prevention. Case definitions for infectious conditions under public health surveillance. MMWR Morb Mortal Wkly Rep. 1997;46(RR-10):39.

71. Darenberg J, Soderquist B, Normark BH, Norrby-Teglund A. Differences in potency of intravenous polyspecific immunoglobulin G against streptococcal and staphylococcal superantigens: implications for therapy of toxic shock syndrome. Clin Infect Dis. 2004;38(6):836–42.
72. Norcross M, Mitchell D. Blistering distal dactylitis caused by Staphylococcus aureus. Cutis. 1993;51:353–4.
73. Parras F, Ezpeleta C, Romero J, Sendagorta E, Buzon L. Blistering distal dactylitis in an adult. Cutis. 1988;41:127–8.
74. Scheinfeld N. Is blistering distal dactylitis a variant of bullous impetigo? Clin Exp Dermatol. 2007;32(3):3314–6.
75. Urschel J. Necrotizing soft tissue infections. Postgrad Med J. 1999;75:645–50.
76. McDonel J. Clostridium perfringens toxins. Pharmacol Ther. 1980;10:617–55.
77. Headley A. Necrotizing soft-tissue infections: a primary care review. Am Fam Physician. 2003;68(2):323–8.
78. Schwartz M, Pasternack M. Cellulitis and subcutaneous tissue infections. In: Mandell G, Bennett J, Dolin R, editors. Principles and practice of infectious diseases. 6th ed. Philadelphia: Churchill Livingstone; 2005. p. 1172.
79. O'Loughlin R, Roberson A, Cieslak P, et al. The epidemiology of invasive group A streptococcal infection and potential vaccine implications: United States, 2000–2004. Clin Infect Dis. 2007;45:853.
80. Morgan MS. Diagnosis and management of necrotizing fasciitis a multiparametric approach. J Hosp Infect. 2010;75:249–57.
81. Aronoff D, Bloch K. Assessing the relationship between the use of nonsteroidal antiinflammatory drugs and necrotizing fasciitis caused by group A streptococcus. Medicine. 2003;82:225.
82. Wong C, Chang H, Pasupathy S, et al. Necrotizing fasciitis: clinical presentation, microbiology, and determinants of mortality. J Bone Joint Surg Am. 2003;85-A:1454.
83. Gozal D, Ziser A, Shupak A, et al. Necrotizing fasciitis. Arch Surg. 1986;121:233.
84. Bosshardt T, Henderson V, Organ C. Necrotizing soft-tissue infections. Arch Surg. 1996;131:846–52.
85. Simonart T, Simonart J, Derdelinckx I, et al. Value of standard laboratory tests for the early recognition of group A beta-hemolytic streptococcal necrotizing fasciitis. Clin Infect Dis. 2001;32:E9.
86. Anaya D, Patchen E. Necrotizing soft-tissue infection: diagnosis and management. Clin Infect Dis. 2007;44:705.
87. Schmid M, Kossmann T, Duewell S. Differentiation of necrotizing fasciitis and cellulitis using MR imaging. Am J Roentgenol. 1998;170:615.
88. Darenberg J, Luca-Harari B, Jasir A, et al. Molecular and clinical characteristics of invasive group A streptococcal infection in Sweden. Clin Infect Dis. 2007;45:450.
89. Stevens DL, Gibbons AE, Bergstrom R, Winn V. The Eagle effect revisited: efficacy of clindamycin, erythromycin, and penicillin in the treatment of streptococcal myositis. J Infect Dis. 1988;158:23.
90. Rudge F. The role of hyperbaric oxygenation in the treatment of clostridial myonecrosis. Mil Med. 1993;158:80–3.
91. Van Rhenterghem L et al. Scleroma and rhinoscleroma, a difficult diagnosis: a review of the literature. Cahier d'Otol Rhinol Larynghol. 1993;10:419–24.
92. Hart C. Rhinoscleroma. J Med Microbiol. 1990;48:395–6.
93. Simons M et al. Rhinoscleroma: case report. Rev Bras Otorrinolaringol. 2006;72(4):568–71.
94. Al Serhani A, Al Qahtani A, Arafa M. Association of rhinoscleroma with rhinosporidiosis. Rhinology. 1998;36(1):43–5.
95. Palaniappan R, Ramanujam S, Chang Y. Leptospirosis: pathogenesis, immunity, and diagnosis. Curr Opin Infect Dis. 2007;20(3):284–92.
96. Adler B, De La Pena Moctezuma A. Leptospira and leptospirosis. Vet Microbiol. 2010;140:287–96.
97. Sehgal S. Epidemiological patterns of leptospirosis. Indian J Med Microbiol. 2006;24:310–1.
98. Kobayashi Y. Human leptospirosis: management and prognosis. J Postgrad Med. 2005;51:201–4.
99. Farr RW. Leptospirosis. Clin Infect Dis. 1995;21:1–8.
100. Karande S, Gandhi D, Kulkarni M, et al. Concurrent outbreak of leptospirosis and dengue in Mumbai, India, 2002. J Trop Pediatr. 2005;51:174.
101. Bajani M, Ashford D, Bragg S, et al. Evaluation of four commercially available rapid serologic tests for diagnosis of leptospirosis. J Clin Microbiol. 2003;41(2):803–9.
102. Levett P, Whittington C. Evaluation of the indirect hemagglutination assay for diagnosis of acute leptospirosis. J Clin Microbiol. 1998;36:11.
103. Ahmad S, Shah S, Ahmad F. Laboratory diagnosis of leptospirosis. J Postgrad Med. 2005;51:195–200.
104. Watt G, Tuazon M, Santiago E, et al. Placebo-controlled trial of intravenous penicillin for severe and late leptospirosis. Lancet. 1988;1:433.
105. Extracted from DVBID: Statistics | CDC Lyme Disease. http://www.cdc.gov/ncidod/dvbid/lyme/ld_statistics.htm.
106. Burgdorfer W et al. Lyme disease: a tick-borne spirochetosis? Science. 1982;216:1317.
107. Steere A. Lyme disease. N Engl J Med. 1989;321:586.
108. Hengge U et al. Lyme borreliosis. Lancet Infect Dis. 2003;3:489.
109. Stanek G, Strle F. Lyme borreliosis. Lancet. 2003;362:1639.
110. Nowakowski J et al. Laboratory diagnostic techniques for patients with early Lyme disease associated with erythema migrans: a comparison of different techniques. Clin Infect Dis. 2001;33:2023.
111. Steere A, Sikand V. The presenting manifestations of Lyme disease and the outcomes of treatment. N Engl J Med. 2003;348:2472.
112. Wormser G, Ramanathan R, Nowakowski J, et al. Duration of antibiotic therapy for early Lyme disease. A randomized, double-blind, placebo-controlled trial. Ann Intern Med. 2003;138:697.
113. Wormser G, Dattwyler R, Shapiro E, et al. The clinical assessment, treatment, and prevention of Lyme disease, human granulocytic anaplasmosis, and babesiosis: clinical practice guidelines by the Infectious Diseases Society of America. Clin Infect Dis. 2006;43:1089.
114. Nadelman R, Nowakowski J, Fish D, et al. Prophylaxis with single-dose doxycycline for the prevention of Lyme disease after an Ixodes scapularis tick bite. N Engl J Med. 2001;345(2):79–84.
115. Moschella S. An update on the diagnosis and treatment of leprosy. J Am Acad Dermatol. 2004;5(3):417–26.
116. National Hansen's Disease Program. Number of Hansen's Disease Cases By Year. http://www.hrsa.gov/hansens/data/uscases1824.htm. Extracted from The World Wide Web on 18 Dec 2010.
117. White C. Déjà vu: leprosy and immigration discourse in the twenty-first century United States. Lepr Rev. 2010;81:17–26.
118. Yoder L, Guerra I. Hansen's disease: a guide to management in the United States. 2nd ed. Carville: Hansen's Disease Foundation; 2001. p. 1–43.
119. McInturff J, Modlin R, Kim J. The role of toll-like receptors in the pathogenesis and treatment of dermatological disease. J Invest Dermatol. 2005;125(1):1–8.
120. World Health Organization. A guide to leprosy control. 2nd ed. Geneva: World Health Organization; 1988. p. 28.
121. WHO recommended MDT regimens. World Health Organization. http://www.who.int/lep/mdt/regimens/en/.
122. Leiker D. Leprosy: classification and differential diagnosis. AIFO, Italy. 2004. http://www.aifo.it/english/resources/online/courses/lepdd/lepdd1.htm.
123. Horsburgh C. Epidemiology of disease caused by nontuberculous mycobacteria. Semin Respir Infect. 1996;11(4):244–51.

124. Sungkanuparph S et al. Rapidly growing mycobacterial infections: spectrum of diseases, antimicrobial susceptibility, pathology and treatment outcomes. J Med Assoc. 2003;86(8):772–80.
125. Dodiuk-Gad R, Dyachenko P, Ziv M, et al. Nontuberculous mycobacterial infections of the skin: a retrospective study of 25 cases. J Am Acad Dermatol. 2007;57(3):413–20.
126. Gupta A, Sibbald R, Lynde C, et al. Onychomycosis in children: prevalence and treatment strategies. J Am Acad Dermatol. 1997;36(3 Pt 1):395–402.
127. Smith E, Fleischer A, Feldman S, Williford P. Characteristics of office-based physician visits for cutaneous fungal infections: an analysis of 1990 to 1994 National Ambulatory Medical Care Survey Data. Cutis. 2002;69:191.
128. Warnock D. Superficial Fungal Infections. In: Cohen and Powderly, editors. Infectious diseases, 2nd ed. Elsevier 2004.
129. Gupta A, Sauder D, Shear N. Antifungal agents: an overview. Part I. J Am Acad Dermatol. 1994;30(5 Pt 1):677–700.
130. Gupta A, Sauder D, Shear N. Antifungal agents: an overview. Part II. J Am Acad Dermatol. 1994;30(6):911–33.
131. Pappas P, Rex J, Sobel J, et al. Guidelines for treatment of candidiasis. Clin Infect Dis. 2004;38(2):161–89.
132. Mendez-Tovar L. Pathogenesis of dermatophytosis and tinea versicolor. Clin Dermatol. 2010;28:185–9.
133. Faergemann J. Pityriasis versicolor. Semin Dermatol. 1993;12:276.
134. Janaki C, Sentamilselvi G, Janaki V, Boopalraj J. Unusual observations in the histology of Pityriasis versicolor. Mycopathologia. 1997;139(2):71–4.
135. Leeming J, Sansom J, Burton J. Susceptibility of Malassezia furfur subgroups to terbinafine. Br J Dermatol. 1997;137:764.
136. Faergemann J, Gupta A, Al Mofadi A, et al. Efficacy of itraconazole in the prophylactic treatment of pityriasis (tinea) versicolor. Arch Dermatol. 2002;138:69.
137. Hu S, Bigby M. Pityriasis versicolor: a systematic review of interventions. Arch Dermatol. 2010;146(10):1132–40.
138. Da Rosa A, Scroferneker M, Vettorato R, et al. Epidemiology of sporotrichosis: a study of 304 cases in Brazil. J Am Acad Dermatol. 2005;52:451.
139. Kauffman C. Sporotrichosis. Clin Infect Dis. 1999;29:231.
140. De Araujo T, Marques A, Kerdel F. Sporotrichosis. Int J Dermatol. 2001;40:737–42.
141. Kauffman C. Old and new therapies for sporotrichosis. Clin Infect Dis. 1995;21:981.
142. Bradsher R. Histoplasmosis and blastomycosis. Clin Infect Dis. 1996;22 Suppl 2:S102.
143. Galgiani J, Ampel N, Blair A, et al. Coccidioidomycosis. Clin Infect Dis. 2005;41:1217.
144. Brummer E, Castaneda E, Restrepo A. Paracoccidioidomycosis: an update. Clin Microbiol Rev. 1993;6(2):89–117.
145. CDC. Decline in annual incidence of varicella, 1990–2001. MMWR Morb Mortal Wkly Rep. 2003;52:884.
146. Yawn B, Saddier P, Wollan P, et al. A population-based study of the incidence and complication rates of herpes zoster before zoster vaccine introduction. Mayo Clin Proc. 2007;82:1341.
147. Straus S, Ostrove J, Inchauspe G, et al. NIH conference. Varicella-zoster virus infections. Biology, natural history, treatment, and prevention. Ann Intern Med. 1988;108:221.
148. Dworkin R, Johnson R, Breuer J, et al. Recommendations for the management of herpes zoster. Clin Infect Dis. 2007;44 Suppl 1:S1–6.
149. Gnann J, Whitley R. Herpes zoster. N Engl J Med. 2002;347:340.
150. Whitley R et al. Management of herpes zoster and post-herpetic neuralgia now and in the future. J Clin Virol. 2010;48(S1):520–8.
151. Centers for Disease Control and Prevention. Prevention of varicella: update recommendations of the advisory committee on immunization practices. MMWR Morb Mortal Wkly Rep. 1999;48(RR-6):1.
152. Feder H. Treatment of adult chickenpox with oral acyclovir. Arch Intern Med. 1990;150:2061.

Cutaneous Manifestations of HIV Disease

Humberto M. Guiot, Carlos G. Sánchez Sergenton, Carlos J. Sánchez Rivera, and Rosbel González Rivera

HIV is an enveloped RNA retrovirus that can lead to the acquired immunodeficiency syndrome (AIDS), a condition characterized by the depletion of T-lymphocyte (CD4+) cells, leading to life-threatening opportunistic infections. Since it was first recognized in 1981, it has taken a toll of more than 25 million deaths. It is estimated that about 0.6% of the world's living population is infected with HIV [1].

Patients with human immunodeficiency virus (HIV) are prone to a variety of cutaneous abnormalities, including inflammatory conditions, infections, and neoplastic processes. Their manifestations can be different when compared with normal hosts due to the loss of T-lymphocyte (CD4+) cells of the immune system. The frequency and distribution of skin complications in persons affected by HIV, or its late stage AIDS, can vary widely. Certain skin conditions, namely bacillary angiomatosis, diffuse interstitial lymphocytosis syndrome, Kaposi's sarcoma, and proximal white subungual onychomycosis, are characteristic of HIV infection. Other conditions are not specific, but occur with an increased prevalence. These include bacterial and viral infections such as staphylococcus, herpes simplex virus (HSV), human papillomavirus (HPV), varicella-zoster virus (VZV), and molluscum contagiosum. Psoriasis vulgaris, seborrheic dermatitis, vitiligo, alopecia, lymphoma and dermatofibromas, among many others are also prevalent although not specific.

This chapter reviews some of the most common and characteristic skin lesions in this population, including the exanthem of primary HIV infection, bacillary angiomatosis, VZV, seborrheic dermatitis, oral hairy leukoplakia, mucocutaneous candidiasis, onychomycosis, Kaposi's sarcoma, and molluscum contagiosum.

H.M. Guiot (✉) • C.G. Sánchez Sergenton • C.J. Sánchez Rivera
Department of Medicine, University of Puerto Rico School of Medicine, Medical Sciences Campus, San Juan, Puerto Rico
e-mail: humberto@guiot.com

R. González Rivera
Department of Dermatology, University of Puerto Rico School of Medicine, Medical Sciences Campus, San Juan, Puerto Rico

Exanthem of Primary HIV Infection (Acute Retroviral Syndrome)

The exanthem of primary HIV infection is defined as the cutaneous eruption that occurs due to HIV viremia before one can detect HIV antibodies by ELISA. Cutaneous manifestations occur in up to 70% of the cases of HIV during the acute retroviral syndrome phase. The exanthem is an eruption of erythematous macules and papules that may become confluent. Occasionally, the eruption progresses into papules and vesicles. This exanthem typically involves the trunk, but there can be involvement of the palms, soles, oral mucosa, and genital mucosa [2]. The histology is generally nonspecific, and is not helpful in establishing the diagnosis. It shows normal epidermis and a sparse perivascular, lymphocytic/histiocytic infiltrate around vessels of the superficial plexus [3]. Although rarely seen in clinical practice, it is imperative to be familiar with the acute retroviral syndrome to establish the diagnosis.

Bacillary Angiomatosis

Bacillary angiomatosis (BA) is a bacterial skin and visceral infection caused by either *Bartonella henselae* or *Bartonella quintana*. *Bartonella* species are usually vector born, but can also be transmitted by animal scratches or bites [4]. Bacillary angiomatosis is most commonly seen in patients with AIDS (CD4+ < 100 cells/μL), and a history of a cat scratch or bite. A cat carrying *B. henselae* may be asymptomatic, yet be bacteremic for weeks to years. Infection is more common in young cats.

Cutaneous bacillary angiomatosis (BA) presents as single or multiple lesions on or under the skin. These may be papules or nodules which are red-purple, globular, and non-blanching, with a vascular appearance, or they can appear as a violaceous plaque. Although vascular proliferation can be similar to

N.P. Sánchez (ed.), *Atlas of Dermatology in Internal Medicine*,
DOI 10.1007/978-1-4614-0688-4_8, © Springer Science+Business Media, LLC 2012

Kaposi's sarcoma, angiosarcoma or pyogenic granuloma, the diagnosis of *Bartonella*-associated infections can be confirmed by histopathology analysis of biopsy specimens, culture of tissue samples, blood culture, and serology [5]. However, its diagnosis is complicated as the organism needs to be cultured for at least 21 days, and serology studies are often unreliable, requiring confirmation of diagnosis through histologic staining with the Warthin–Starry stain [6]. The classic histologic presentation of bacillary angiomatosis involves three components: a lobular proliferation of capillaries with enlarged endothelial cells, neutrophilic debris, and clumps of finely granular material identified as bacteria with staining techniques [7]. The Warthin–Starry stain demonstrates clumps of bacilli.

Bacillary angiomatosis may be fatal, as it can affect bones and viscera [8]. But the organism can be effectively eradicated by the use of antibiotics such as erythromycin, azithromycin, ciprofloxacin, doxycycline, tetracycline, or minocycline.

Varicella-Zoster Virus

The VZV is a virus belonging to the Herpesviridae family. Primary VZV infection results in chickenpox and may reactivate later, producing a disease known as herpes zoster or shingles. It may occur at any stage in an HIV-infected patient as well as in immunocompetent persons. HIV-infected children are more likely to suffer from complications, such as pneumonia, than non-HIV-infected individuals. Herpes zoster is common in the early stages of HIV infection and may be the first clue of HIV infection in an otherwise young, healthy adult.

The clinical appearance of herpes zoster among HIV positive individuals does not differ from those of HIV negative individuals. The lesions are usually unilateral and in a dermatomal distribution; they may be crusting, erythematous, pustular, or vesicular depending on the stage of disease (Fig. 1). Multidermatomal lesions are more frequent in advanced HIV disease (Fig. 2). Interestingly, herpes zoster may develop during the immune reconstitution syndrome, as the CD4+ count rises to 300 cells/μL. However, based on incidence-rate data from studies on the incidence of VZV during pre- and post-HAART therapy periods, others argue that this occurrence may be better explained by a depressed level of VZV-specific cell-mediated immunity and not due to an immune reconstitution syndrome, as the depression of VZV-specific immune responses and not increased responses determines VZV reactivation [9].

The initial test of choice for diagnosis is a Tzanck smear, where characteristic multinucleated epithelial giant cells are observed under light microscopy (Fig. 3). A skin biopsy will demonstrate epidermal necrosis, enlarged and pale keratinocytes (ballooning), acantholysis, and multinucleated keratinocytes (Fig. 4). Viral culture is the most specific test but not the most sensitive.

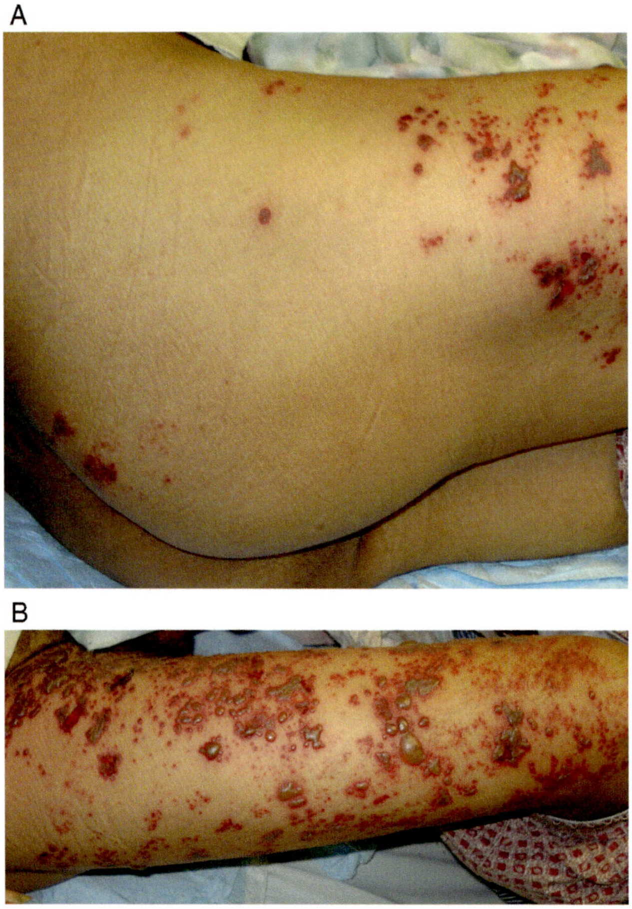

Fig. 1 (**a**, **b**) Presentation of herpes-zoster in a dermatomal distribution

Ophthalmic zoster is a severe complication with 20–70% developing associated ocular disease including blindness (Fig. 5). Those patients that develop herpes zoster ophthalmicus usually present with periorbital vesicular rash distributed according to the affected dermatome, while a minority of them may also develop conjunctivitis, keratitis, uveitis, and ocular cranial-nerve palsies [10]. Coexisting infection with HIV should be suspected in a young patient with ophthalmic zoster, if multiple dermatoses are affected and if there is a presence of peripheral retinal perivasculitis, chronic dendritic infection, serious neurologic disease, or ocular disease sine herpete (ophthalmic zoster without its characteristic cutaneous manifestations) [11].

Treatment of VZV in uncomplicated cases is done with oral acyclovir (800 mg five times/day). In the disseminated infection, or when intraocular involvement occurs, intravenous acyclovir (10 mg/kg/day) is the preferred treatment. A live attenuated VZV Oka/Merck strain vaccine is now available [12]. The live varicella virus vaccine (Varivax) has been proven to be effective in preventing varicella infection in healthy individuals, and when breakthrough infections do occur illness is typically mild [13]. There is also a live

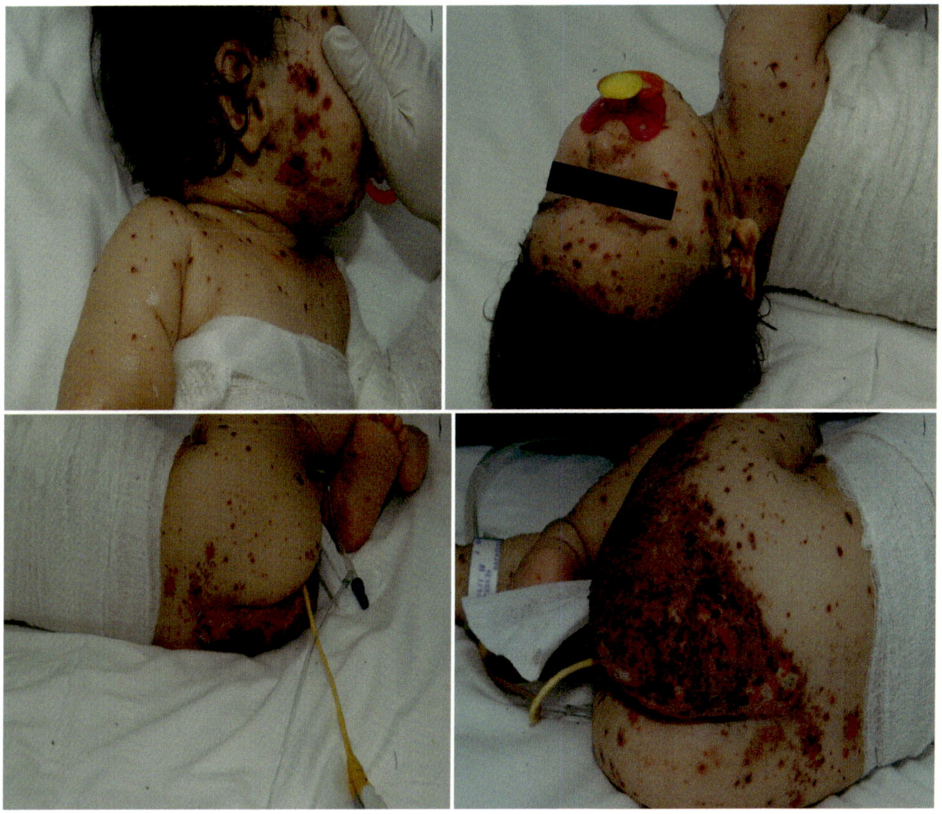

Fig. 2 Varicella-zoster virus. Disseminated form of herpes-zoster in child-infected with HIV

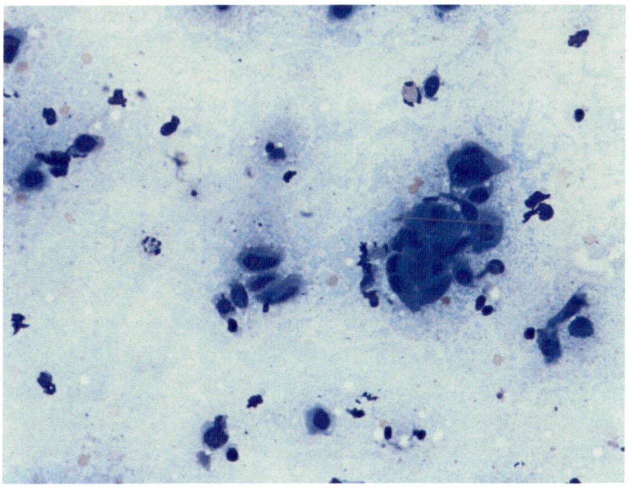

Fig. 3 Tzanck smear showing multinucleated epithelial giant cells

vaccine for the prevention of shingles, called Zostavax, designed to elicit an immune response in the elderly whose immunity to VZV wanes with advancing age [14]. Inactivated vaccines are generally safe and are beneficial for HIV-infected patients. However, live vaccines should be used with caution since some of the vaccines may be harmful to patients with severe immunologic suppression [15].

Seborrheic Dermatitis

Seborrheic dermatitis is a skin disorder affecting the scalp, central areas of the face, and trunk. It usually causes scaly, flaky, pruritic, and erythematous patches, and plaques that waxes and wanes. It occurs in up to 3% of the general population and up to 50% of the HIV-infected population. The prevalence and severity increases as the CD4+ cell count declines. The cause of seborrheic dermatitis is not completely understood. The yeast known as *Malassezia furfur* (formerly *Pityrosporum ovale*) is thought to play a role, but the causative factor has not been successfully elucidated with firm evidence [16].

Flare-ups of this condition often occur when the afflicted individual is recovering from a severe illness. It responds quickly to low-mid-potency topical corticosteroid therapy. Chronic treatment with topical corticosteroids may lead to permanent skin changes, such as atrophy and telangiectasias [17]. Although it is clear that seborrheic dermatitis is not diagnosed exclusively in patients with HIV, it occurs with such frequency in patients with this condition that some investigators have even found an association between seborrheic dermatitis and the advanced progression of HIV disease [18].

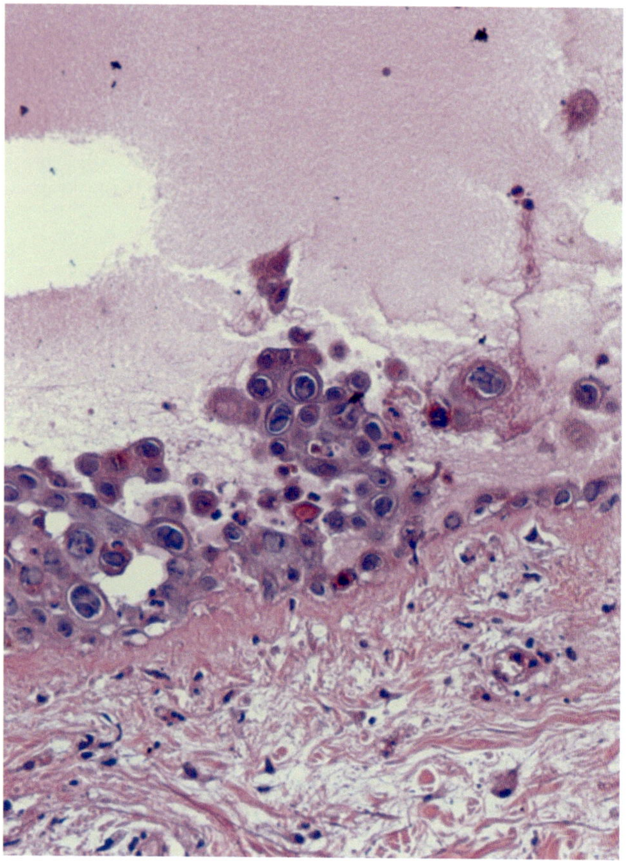

Fig. 4 A biopsy of a varicella-zoster lesion showing characteristic multinucleated epithelial giant cells and epidermal necrosis

Oral Hairy Leukoplakia

Oral hairy leukoplakia (OHL) is a disease of the mucosa first described in 1984 that involves the formation of white leathery spots on the mucous membranes of the tongue and inside of the mouth. It affects less than 1% of the population and is most common in adults within the 50 to 70-year-old age group. It is not a specific entity and may cause lesions similar in appearance to oral candidiasis and lichen planus.

It is associated with Epstein–Barr virus (EBV) and occurs mostly in people with HIV. The cause in most cases is unknown, but it is thought to be related to chronic factors of irritation [19]. OHL associated with HIV does not appear to place patients at increased risk of developing oral cancer.

Mucocutaneous Candidiasis

Oral Thrush

Oral candidiasis is an infection caused by *Candida*, usually *C. albicans*, in the mucous membranes of the mouth. It appears as thick white or cream-color plaques (Fig. 6). Angular cheilitis may also accompany the thrush. Underlying the deposits, the mucosa of the mouth may appear inflamed. It is one of the most common forms of yeast infections in HIV patients. Treatment includes eliminating the pathogenic organism. Antifungals are the treatment of choice and include clotrimazole troches for oral thrush, and anticandidal creams for the affected lips. Other common antifungal agents include nystatin oral suspension. Patients who are immunocompromised may often require systemic treatment with orally or intravenously administered antifungal (fluconazole, itraconazole, amphotericin B, or caspofungin) depending on the

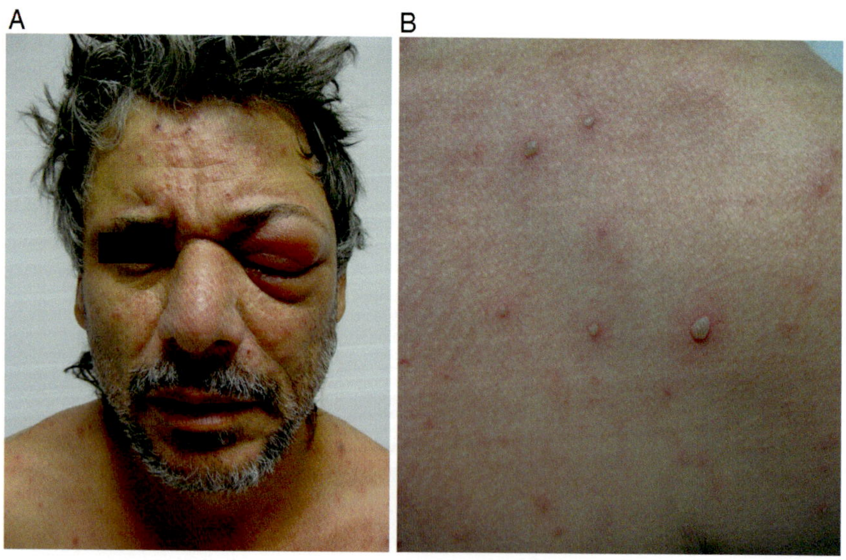

Fig. 5 (**a**, **b**) The initial presentation of ophthalmic herpes-zoster (**a**) that rapidly disseminated (**b**), in an immunocompromised patient

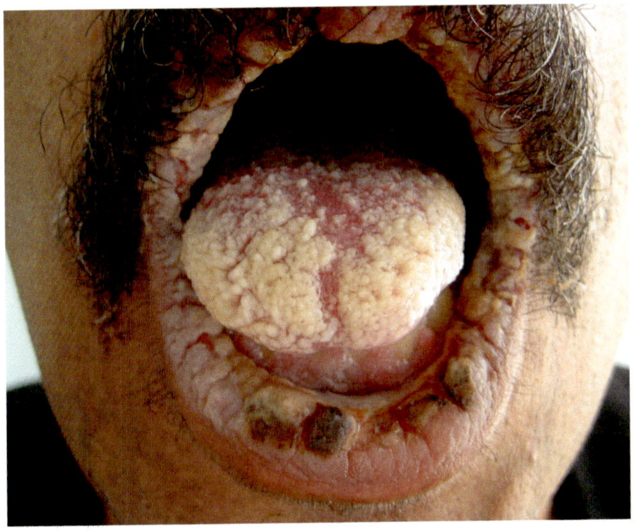

Fig. 6 Oral candidiasis (thrush). Thick, white plaques on the dorsum of the tongue in an immunocompromised patient

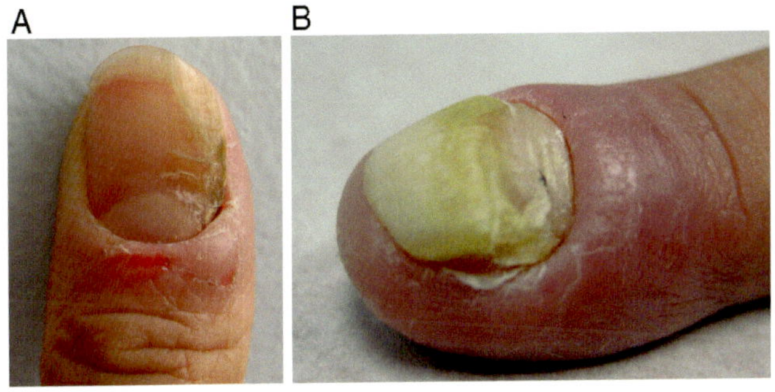

Fig. 7 (**a**, **b**) Candidal paronychia. Inflammation of the nailfold producing redness, edema, and tenderness associated with thickening and *yellow-brownish* discoloration of the nail plate

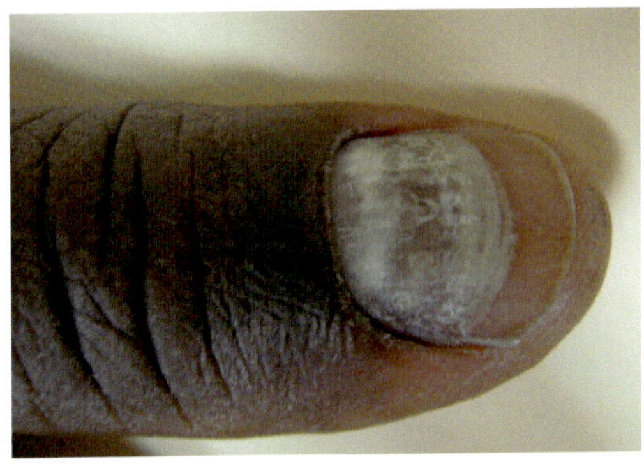

Fig. 8 Proximal subungual onychomycosis in a patient with HIV

severity of disease [20]. In patients with AIDS, treatment of the underlying HIV infection with highly aggressive antiretroviral therapy (HAART) is critical for preventing and managing these infections.

Intertriginous Infections

Infections of the skin folds may be caused by either *Candida* or *Tinea*. These usually involve the axillary, groin, or inframammary areas. In these areas, candidiasis presents as a bright red, vesicopustules, which enlarge and rupture, causing maceration and fissuring in the depths of the folds. Small pustules may appear, especially at the edges of the rash. The surface is wrinkled and a white membrane may coat the eroded surface. A hallmark of this rash is scattered satellite pustules extending out from the central eroded areas. Diagnosis of skin infection by *Candida* is based upon the clinical presentation and demonstration of budding yeast and psuedohyphae on potassium hydroxide preparation or culture.

Onychomycosis (Tinea Unguium)

Onychomycosis is defined as a fungal infection of the nails, commonly caused by dermatophytes, such as *Trichophyton rubrum*. It may also be caused by non-dermatophyte yeasts such as *Candida*.

Candida frequently affects the tissue around the fingernails, presenting as a paronychia (inflammation of the tissues surrounding the nail). Symptoms include tenderness, erythema, and bogginess of the proximal nail fold (Fig. 7). This type of infection tends to be chronic, in which case the cuticle is lost, and the nail plate may become ridged or dystrophic. Onycholysis, loosening of the exposed portion of the nail from the nail bed, may also occur. The nail plate itself is usually not invaded but nail plate thickening and opacity may be present. Candidal paronychia has been associated to frequent immersion of the hands in water, such as in dishwashers and laundry workers. There is also a higher incidence of paronychia among diabetics and immunocompromised people [21].

Proximal subungual onychomycosis is an uncommon form of onychomycosis that usually reflects a state of immunosuppression, most commonly HIV infection (Fig. 8). It results from a direct invasion under the proximal nail fold, most commonly caused by *T. rubrum*.

Kaposi's Sarcoma

Kaposi's sarcoma (KS) is a neoplasm of endothelial cells involving the skin and internal organs and is associated to the human herpesvirus 8 (HHV-8) [22]. This condition became more widely known as one of the AIDS defining illnesses in the 1980s. While in Africa, (where HHV-8 virus is endemic), men, women and children are all commonly affected, in western countries HIV-related KS is primarily a

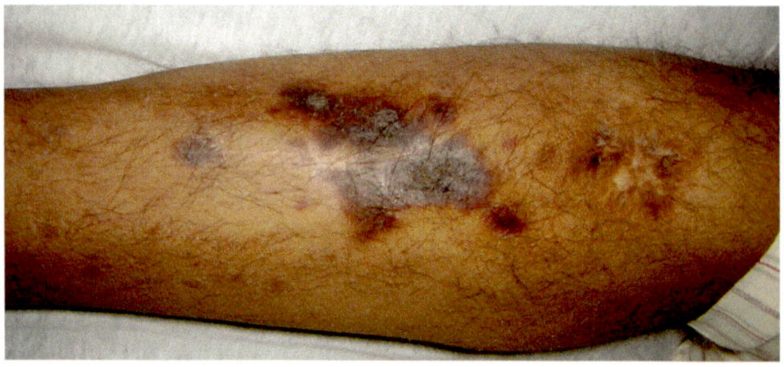

Fig. 9 Kaposi's sarcoma. Violaceous plaques on the extremities in a patient with AIDS

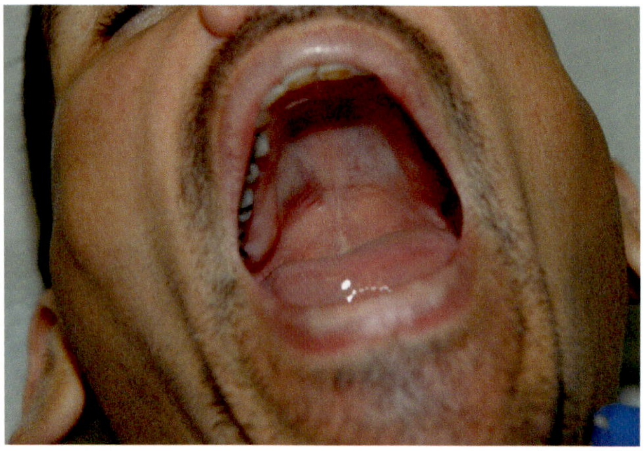

Fig. 10 Kaposi sarcoma. *Red-violet* plaques on the palate

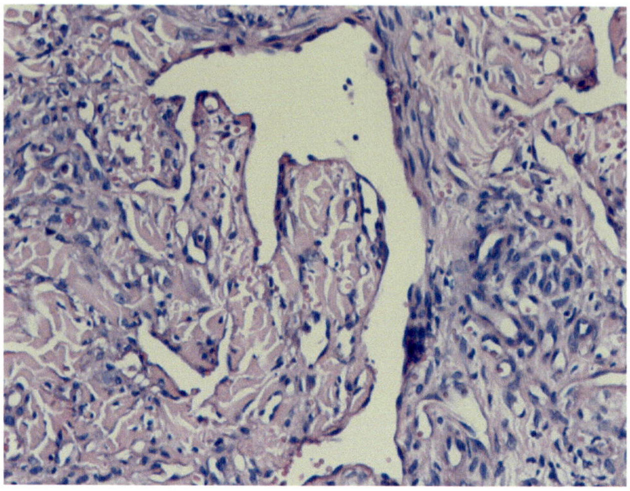

Fig. 11 Histopathology of Kaposi sarcoma. A dermal vascular proliferation: slit-like vascular spaces lined by spindled endothelial cells. Promontory sign may be present (small blood vessel projecting like a promontory into a vascular space)

disease of homosexual men [8]. However, most people infected with HHV-8 do not get Kaposi sarcoma, and those who are most likely to develop Kaposi sarcoma are immunocompromised [23].

It initially appears as red-purple macules that can progress to papular nodules; the color can vary from red, purple, and brown to black (Fig. 9). The skin lesions most commonly affect the lower limbs, face, mouth, and genitalia. The mouth is involved in about 30% of cases, especially the hard palate and gums (Fig. 10). Visceral involvement tends to occur in patients with advanced HIV disease and Kaposi's sarcoma, most often affecting the gastrointestinal tract and lungs [24–26]. The gastrointestinal lesions may be silent or cause weight loss, pain, nausea, vomiting, diarrhea, bleeding, malabsorption, or intestinal obstruction [27]. Histopathology demonstrates a dermal vascular proliferation of slit-like vessels (Fig. 11).

Treatment for epidemic Kaposi sarcoma combines treatment for Kaposi sarcoma with treatment for AIDS. There are four types of standard treatment for Kaposi sarcoma: radiation therapy, surgery, chemotherapy, and biologic therapy. The evolution in the treatment of AIDS has influenced the incidence of KS, which has decreased significantly over the years. A recent study has described a decrease of 87% in the 5-year cumulative incidence of Kaposi sarcoma in AIDS patients for the years 1996–2006 (HAART era), when compared with those diagnosed in the 1980s, time at which HIV was first described [28].

Molluscum Contagiosum

Molluscum contagiosum (MC) is a superficial cutaneous viral infection caused by the molluscum contagiosum virus (MCV) that usually presents as flesh-colored umbilicated papules. Characteristically, a faint whitish core is at the center of each papule, causing it to have an umbilicated appearance. It may affect any area, except the palms and soles. In children, lesions occur mainly on the trunk and proximal extremities. In adults, lesions occur on the trunk, genital areas, and inner thighs. In HIV patients, lesions tend to occur along the beard lines in males, or anywhere on the face [29]. The diagnosis of MC is typically made by its clinical appearance and can be confirmed by histological demonstration of intracytoplasmic eosinophilic inclusions in the epidermis (Fig. 12); however, the virus cannot routinely be cultured [30].

The lesions tend to persist for 2 months and then spontaneously resolve when the host develops resistance to the virus. However, the disease usually persists for 6–9 months, and may persist in individuals with impaired cell-mediated immunity, such as HIV patients [29]. It occurs in approximately 5–18% of HIV-infected persons, and once the CD4+ counts fall below 200 cells/μL, the molluscum contagiosum lesions tend to proliferate [29]. They often grow in numbers greater than 100. Extensive molluscum contagiosum disease is a cutaneous marker of advanced HIV (CD4+ < 100 cells/μL) [31, 32].

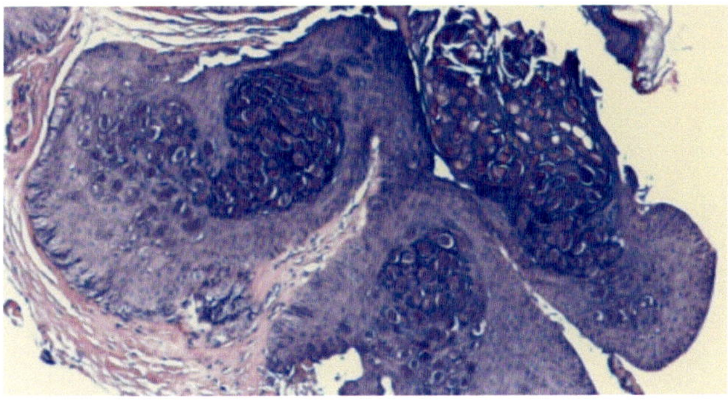

Fig. 12 Characteristic histopathological findings of molluscum contagiosum: Henderson–Paterson or molluscum contagiosum bodies (intracytoplasmic inclusions)

Summary

In summary, patients with HIV are prone to a multitude of dermatological problems. These include viral, fungal, and bacterial infections, inflammatory conditions and malignancies. Noninfectious cutaneous manifestations are not prognostic of rapid progression of immunosuppression, but they may be specific markers of the stage of HIV disease. These cutaneous changes may be the initial signs of immunosuppression, and recognition of HIV-related skin changes can lead to an early diagnosis and initiation of the appropriate therapy.

References

1. Joint United Nations Programme on HIV/AIDS. Overview of the global AIDS epidemic. 2006 Report on the global AIDS epidemic, Geneva; 2006.
2. Bratzke B, Eichhorn R, Höffken G, et al. Acute primary phase as an indicator of HIV-1 infection. The general symptoms and polymorphic exanthema with mouth mucosal involvement 2 to 6 weeks before seroconversion. Dtsch Med Wochenschr. 1988;113:1312–6.
3. Balslev E, Thomsen HK, Weismann K. Histopathology of acute human immunodeficiency virus exanthema. J Clin Pathol. 1990;43:201–2.
4. Maguina C, Guerra H, Ventosilla P. Bartonellosis. Clin Dermatol. 2009;27:271–80.
5. Spach DH, Dowhler JE. Bartonella-associated infections. Infect Dis Clin North Am. 1998;12:137–55.
6. Grilo N, Modi D, Barrow P. Cutaneous bacillary angiomatosis: a marker of systemic disease in HIV. S Afr Med J. 2009;99: 220–1.
7. Amsbaugh S, Huiras E, Wang NS, et al. Bacillary angiomatosis associated with pseudoepitheliomatous hyperplasia. Am J Dermatopathol. 2006;28:32–5.
8. Amerson EH, Maurer TA. Dermatologic manifestations of HIV in Africa. Top HIV Med. 2010;18:16–22.
9. Levin MJ, Anderson JP, Seage 3rd GR, Williams PL. Short-term and long-term effects of highly active antiretroviral therapy on the incidence of herpes zoster in HIV-infected children. J Acquir Immune Defic Syndr. 2009;50:182–91.
10. Shaikh S, Ta CN. Evaluation and management of herpes zoster ophthalmicus. Am Fam Physician. 2002;66:1723–30.
11. Saxena R, Phuljhele S, Aalok L, Sinha A, Menon V, Sharma P, et al. A rare case of orbital apex syndrome with herpes zoster ophthalmicus in a human immunodeficiency virus-positive patient. Indian J Ophthalmol. 2009;58:527–30.
12. Arvin AM. Varicella-zoster virus. Clin Microbiol Rev. 1996;9:361–81.
13. Centers for Disease Control and Prevention (CDC). Prevention of varicella: recommendations of the Advisory Committee on Immunization Practices (ACIP). MMWR 1996;45(No.RR-11).
14. Poland G. The growing paradigm of preventing disease. Ann Intern Med. 2005;143:539–41.
15. Pancharoen C, Ananworanich J, Thisyakorn U. Immunization for persons infected with human immunodeficiency virus. Curr HIV Res. 2004;2:293–9.
16. Johnson BA, Nunley JR. Treatment of seborrheic dermatitis. Am Fam Physician. 2000;61:2703–10, 2713–4.
17. Scheinfeld N. Seborrheic dermatitis. Skinmed. 2005;4:49–50.
18. Ippolito F, Passi S, Di Carlo A. Is seborrhoeic dermatitis a clinical marker of HIV disease? Minerva Ginecol. 2000;52:54–8.
19. Hille JJ, Webster-Cyriaque J, Palefski JM, Raab-Traub N. Mechanisms of expression of HHV8, EBV and HPV in selected HIV-associated oral lesions. Oral Dis. 2002;8 Suppl 2:161–8.
20. Pappas PG et al. Guidelines for the treatment of candidiasis. Clin Infect Dis. 2004;38:161–89.
21. Mandell GL, Bennett JE, Dolin R. Principles and practice of infectious diseases. Edwards JE Candida Species. 2005;6:2938–57.
22. Moore PS, Chang Y. Detection of herpes-virus like DNA sequences in AIDS-associated Kaposi's sarcoma. Science. 1995;266:1865.
23. General information about Kaposi sarcoma. National Cancer Institute. http://www.cancer.gov/cancertopics/pdq/treatment/kaposis/Patient/page1. Accessed 28 Apr 2008.
24. Miranda AM, Gomes MH, Marques R, et al. Kaposi sarcoma associated with HIV infection. Acta Med Port. 1999;12:357–66.
25. Lemlich G, Schwam L, Lebwohl M. Kaposi's sarcoma and acquired immunodeficiency syndrome. Postmortem findings in twenty-four cases. J Am Acad Dermatol. 1987;16:319–25.
26. Dhrif AS, Kilani B, Ammari L, et al. AIDS-associated Kaposi's sarcoma: 22 cases. Tunis Med. 2007;85:494–9.
27. Danzig JB. Gastrointestinal malignancy in patients with AIDS. Am J Gastroenterol. 1991;86:715–8.
28. Simard EP, Pfeiffer RM, Engels EA. Cumulative incidence of cancer among individuals with acquired immunodeficiency syndrome in the United States. Cancer. 2011;117(5):1089–96.
29. Mandell GL, Bennett JE, Dolin R. Principles and practice of infectious diseases. Damon I other Poxvirus that Infect Humans. 2005;6:1753–56.
30. Wang F. Harrison's Principles of Internal Medicine. Molluscum contagiosum and other poxviruses. 16th ed. New York: McGraw-Hill. 2005;16:1053–54.
31. Alan C. Jung, Douglas S Paauw. Diagnosing HIV-related disease: using the CD4 count as a guide. J Gen Intern Med. 1998;13:131–6.
32. Waugh MA. Molluscum contagiosum. Dermatol Clin. 1998;16: 839–41.

Cutaneous Disorders in the Intensive Care Unit

Tania M. González Santiago
and Jacobo M. Orenstein Cardona

Cutaneous disorders in the intensive care unit (ICU) may develop as a consequence of life-threatening diseases or as complications from treatment regimens. Few studies report the prevalence of cutaneous conditions in ICUs. According to current data available, the most common dermatological disorders in this setting are: pathogen-related (35%), peripheral vascular disease-related (27%), and drug reaction-related (21%). The objective of this chapter is to provide a practical pathophysiological and clinical overview of the most common dermatological conditions observed in the ICU. Further research needs to be conducted to study the prevalence, manifestations, and complications of skin disorders in the ICU in a prospective manner, in a larger number of hospitals, and in different geographical locations.

Introduction

The skin is often affected by many pathological processes, including life-threatening diseases that lead to hospitalization in intensive care units (ICUs). Skin disorders also arise frequently as a complication in patients undergoing treatment in ICUs [1]. Few studies, however, analyze the prevalence of cutaneous conditions in the ICU, engage in prospective studies, or provide guidelines for their diagnosis and management [1–4]. Badia et al., in a 2-year prospective study of dermatological conditions in patients (of all ages) in an ICU, determined that the overall prevalence of dermatoses was 10.4% [1]. The study also found that critically ill patients with cutaneous disorders had a higher degree of severity and a longer ICU stay than critically ill patients without dermatological conditions. Despite the significant prevalence, the higher degree of severity, and the associated longer hospitalization time of ICU patients with dermatological conditions, skin disorders often go unrecognized and untreated in ICUs [1].

This practical overview of the most common dermatological disorders observed in the ICU will provide epidemiologic information, common presentations, and course of illness, etiology, diagnostic signs, symptoms, and tests, possible differential diagnoses, current management options, prognoses, risk factors, potential complications, and related factors to patient monitoring. This chapter is ultimately intended to introduce medical professionals to current principles regarding the diagnosis and management of skin disorders in the ICU based on a wide revision of literature.

The prevalence of the cutaneous conditions is principally obtained from the work by Badia et al., who classifies the dermatoses according to etiology. In this study, the most common dermatological disorders in ICUs were pathogen-related (35%), peripheral vascular disease-related (27%), and drug reaction-related (21%). Skin disorders associated with allergic contact dermatitis (10%) or pre-existing dermatological conditions not associated to the cause of admission (6%) were not discussed. Of note, Badia et al. excluded pressure ulcers, burns, and other dermatological conditions because they were considered irrelevant in the context of the patient and are not discussed in this chapter either. Nonetheless, these skin conditions contribute to overall patient morbidity and mortality and should be taken into account in the comprehensive treatment of critically ill patients.

Among the pathogen-related skin disorders, most common conditions include dermatomycosis due to *Candida* and pyoderma due to impetigo. Of the peripheral vascular disease-related dermatoses observed in the ICU, the two most frequent, both of which are due to underlying systemic infections, are meningococcal septicemia and ecthyma gangrenosum [1]. In the category of drug reaction-related cutaneous disorders, the three most prevalent and, coincidentally, the most severe manifestations include: hypersensitivity syndrome, also known as Drug Reaction with eosinophilia and Systemic Symptoms (DRESS), Steven–Johnson syndrome and toxic

T.M. González Santiago (✉)
Mayo Clinic Department of Dermatology Residency, Rochester, MN
e-mail: tania2009@gmail.com

J.M. Orenstein Cardona
Candidate Center for Translational Science Activities,
Mayo Clinic Rochester, MN

N.P. Sánchez (ed.), *Atlas of Dermatology in Internal Medicine*,
DOI 10.1007/978-1-4614-0688-4_9, © Springer Science+Business Media, LLC 2012

epidermal necrolysis (SJS and TEN, respectively), and hypersensitivity vasculitis, also known as leukocytoclastic vasculitis (LCV).

Pathogen-Related Skin Disorders

The most common cause of cutaneous disorders in the ICU is direct infections of the skin by fungi, bacteria, and viruses, of which we consider the two most common in this section: fungal and bacterial infections [2]. Viral pathogens, although not discussed in this chapter, usually elicit cutaneous manifestations via viral reactivation, most commonly herpes simplex 1 and 2, and varicella zoster.

Dermatomycoses: Mucocutaneous Candidiasis

Candida is the most common type of dermatomycosis. In a prospective study, dermatomycoses comprised 20% of all ICU dermatological disorders, of which *Candida* was the causative fungal agent in 100% of the cases detected. According to recent studies, *Candida* is the fourth most common nosocomial bloodstream isolate in the USA, with slightly more than half of the cases occurring in the ICU [5].

Candida infections affect skin, mucosa, and appendages. The most common pathogenic form in humans is the albicans species. In humans, *Candida* species are part of the endogenous flora of the gastrointestinal and genitourinary tracts, however, in states of altered physiological environments, *Candida* can colonize the skin or appendages pathologically. *Candida* typically becomes pathogenic in three circumstances: increased colonization, due to the use of broad spectrum antibiotics; normal mucosal and skin barrier breakdown by the use of chronic indwelling devices, recent surgery or trauma; and immune system dysfunction, usually neutropenia [5]. These conditions are commonly found in critically ill patients and can lead to invasive candidiasis, with widespread dissemination. The conversion of *Candida* from its commensal to its pathogenic form in critically ill patients is favored by local factors such as humidity, maceration, and high temperatures and by systemic factors such as diabetes, leukemia, AIDS, and the use of corticosteroids [1]. In the general population, neonates and immunocompromised patients are considered high-risk groups for candidiasis. The frequency of infection is rising due to HIV infection and increased resistance to antifungal agents [6, 7].

The most frequent locations of mucocutaneous candidiasis infections arise in the intertriginous regions (submammary, genitocrural, and subaxillary regions) [1] (Fig. 1). Pustules are formed which are quickly macerated by opposing skin layers, thus presenting as red papules with intact, non-macerated pustules extending just beyond these areas. Candidal skin lesions may also present within intertriginous regions as confluent erythematous, macerated, glistening plaques, with long, well-delimited borders. The classic, diagnostically useful "satellite lesions" of cutaneous candidiasis consists of pinpoint pustules located just beyond the borders of these plaques. The intertriginous lesions commonly develop painful fissures [8]. The differential diagnosis includes dermatophytosis, pityriasis versicolor, psoriasis, and erythrasma.

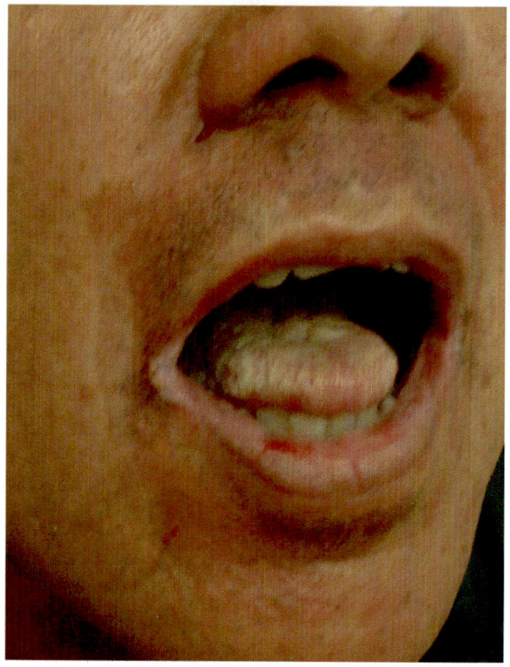

Fig. 1 Oral candidiasis (trush) and Angular cheilitis (perlèche), *grayish-white* membranous plaque on the tongue, and maceration and transverse fissuring of the oral commissures

In immunocompromised patients, such as patients receiving cancer treatment or steroids, or with diseases such as AIDS or leukemia, *Candida* can disseminate and become life-threatening. Organs that may be affected are the blood, brain, eye, kidney, heart, and less commonly, the lungs, liver, and spleen. *Candida*, for example, is the leading cause of esophagitis in people with AIDS [9]. The use of devices that penetrate the skin, such as urinary catheters, IV ports, and IV drug injections, provide an access point for the entry of *Candida*, and should be minimized to decrease the risk for infection.

Cutaneous candidiasis may be diagnosed by obtaining a sample from an infected region and observing the classic nonseptate hyphae and pseudohyphae in a 10% potassium hydroxide (KOH) microscope slide preparation. Cultures should also be done. *Candida* esophagitis can be diagnosed by endoscopy, by the identification of fistulas or the classic "cobblestone" appearance of the esophageal mucosa, and more definitively, by endoscopic biopsy [10].

Primary intertriginous lesions are treated by maintaining the infected area dry, and using topical azoles and polyenes, including clotrimazole, miconazole, and nystatin. Invasive candidiasis can be treated with IV caspofungin, amphotericin B, fluconazole (IV or oral), or fluconazole combined with amphotericin B. More severe infections are treated with flucytosine and amphotericin B [11].

Pyoderma: Impetigo

Impetigo is the most common type of pyoderma. It is a common, contagious, bacterial infection of the superficial epidermis. In one series, pyodermal infections represented 8% of all ICU dermatological disorders, and *Staphylococcus aureus* was the causative agent in every case [1]. Like the dermatomycoses, bacterial infections of the skin are also promoted by both local and systemic factors commonly found in critically ill patients in the ICU. In the general population, impetigo is most common in children aged 2–5 years [12]. It presents in two forms: bullous and nonbullous impetigo, the latter of which is also known as impetigo contagiosa. Nonbullous impetigo represents approximately 70% of all cases. Its causative agents are either *S. aureus* or *Streptococcus pyogenes*, although coinfection is relatively common. The causative agent of all bullous impetigo infections and of the majority of nonbullous infections is *S. aureus*. In nonbullous impetigo, *S. pyogenes*, which in the past was believed to be the principal infectious agent, is present alone, or in combination with *S. aureus* [13]. Methicillin-resistant *S. aureus* (MRSA), whether hospital or community acquired, is an alarmingly increasing cause of impetigo [14, 15]. Patients with nonbullous impetigo commonly spread the infection by excoriation of infected skin lesions. The peak incidence of bullous impetigo is in the summer, and it is more prevalent in warm climates, areas with poor hygiene, and in crowded living conditions [13]. In patients in the ICU, impetigo appears in areas of pressure zones and skin folds, or in patients with broken skin due to prior lesions or indwelling devices.

Nonbullous impetigo lesions begin as a single, erythematous macule or papule. The initial lesions quickly develop into a vesicle, which easily rupture and dry out, producing firmly attached, occasionally pruritic, characteristic "honey-colored" crusts (Fig. 2). In the immunocompetent host, the lesions typically resolve without scarring in a few weeks without treatment. A subtype of nonbullous impetigo, called "common," "impetiginous," or "secondary" impetigo develops in areas of skin breakage due to, for example, varicella or herpes simplex virus infections, which can have the same presentation as that of nonbullous impetigo [13].

Bullous impetigo lesions are caused by toxin-producing *S. aureus* and are considered to be a localized form of staphylococcal scalded skin syndrome (SSSS) [16]. Bullous impetigo begins as vesicles and pustules near a hair follicle, arising between the corneal and granulosum layers of the epidermis [1]. The lesions first appear over intact skin as vesicles which rapidly progress to flaccid, enlarging bullae with well-demarcated margins and without surrounding erythema. The clear content of the bullae tend to turn cloudy and then collapse, releasing a yellowish exudate, while retaining fluid at the rim of the lesions.

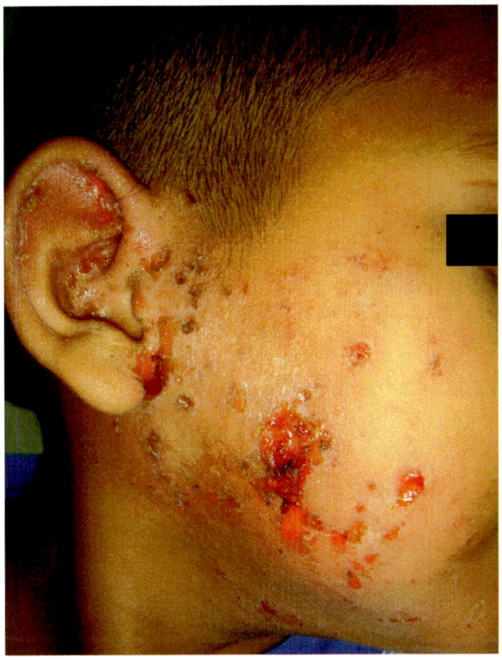

Fig. 2 Nonbullous impetigo. Eroded plaques with honey-colored crusts

The center of ruptured bullae can develop a thin, flat, and "honey-colored" or "varnish-like" crust, which if removed, displays an erythematous, inflamed, oozing, and moist base. The surrounding fluid-filled rim usually transforms into the pathognomonic "collarette" of scale, or "tinea-like scaling border." The surrounding scales link forming contiguous, enlarged lesions. Non-ruptured bullae display a negative nikolsky sign. This contrasts with the lesions of pemphigus vulgaris, in which the epidermal layers above the basal layer can be separated and rubbed off by pressing the lesions with a sliding motion (positive nikolsky sign) [8, 13].

In the ICU, the pathogens responsible for impetigo are mainly transmitted through direct hand contact or fomites, entering through broken skin due to prior skin infections, burns, surgery, trauma, or radiation therapy. It also arises in this setting in those patients on immunosuppressive drug therapy, such as systemic corticosteroids, oral retinoids, or chemotherapy or those patients with systemic diseases, such as HIV, diabetes mellitus, or dialysis [1].

A deeply ulcerated form of impetigo is termed "ecthyma." This ulcerative pyoderma of the skin extends into the dermis and is caused by group A beta-hemolytic streptococci. It may be the result of a direct inoculation by the bacteria or a secondary infection of a preexisting wound.

Impetigo is chiefly diagnosed based on history and clinical presentation. Cultures reveal the usual causative agents but are rarely performed. Gram stains of sampled vesicles reveal gram-positive cocci [8]. Anti-streptolysin O titers are usually low in streptococcal impetigo, but anti-DNAse B levels have been found to be consistently elevated [17]. Streptococcal antibody assays may be used to confirm recent streptococcal infection in patients suspected of having poststreptococcal glomerulonephritis, a rare complication of nonbullous impetigo characterized by a sudden onset of edema, hypertension, hematuria, and/or proteinuria. Acute poststreptococcal glomerulonephritis affects between 1 and 5% of patients with nonbullous impetigo and cannot be prevented by antibiotic therapy. Other rare complications include sepsis, osteomyelitis, arthritis, endocarditis, pneumonia, cellulitis, lymphangitis or lymphadenitis, guttate psoriasis, toxic shock syndrome, and SSSS [13]. Rheumatic fever, commonly associated *S. pyogenes* infections, is not a significant consequence of nonbullous impetigo.

Since *S. aureus* is the causative agent of bullous impetigo, as well as of the majority of cases of nonbullous impetigo, treatment should include penicillinase-resistant penicillins, or first-generation cephalosporins [17]. MRSA infections may be treated according to a reported empiric antibiotic therapy schema with antibacterials such as vancomycin, clindamycin, co-trimoxazole, linezolid, minocycline, ordaptomycin, while results of bacterial cultures are pending. Erythromycin, which in the past was the drug of choice for treating impetigo, is no longer recommended due to a high prevalence of erythromycin-resistant strains of *S. aureus* [17].

Peripheral Vascular Disease-Related Skin Disorders

In patients presenting to the ICU with a systemic infectious disease, skin vasculature may be affected by direct injury or via hypersensitivity reactions. These reactions produce characteristic cutaneous lesions that are useful aids in the early diagnosis of the underlying disease. The etiological treatment usually leads to the improvement of the skin lesions [1].

Meningococcal Septicemia

The most common cause of skin disorder in the ICU is meningococcal septicemia. In one study, meningococcal septicemia represented up to 24% of all ICU dermatological disorders, and 86% of all ICU skin lesions attributable to an underlying systemic infection [1].

Meningococcal septicemia, or meningococcemia, is defined as the presence of *Neisseria meningitidis*, a gram-negative diplococcal bacterium, in the bloodstream. Acute meningococcemia kills faster than any other known infection. Chronic meningococcemia presents with arthritis and dermatitis, similar to gonococcemia, but is a rare presentation [8]. Infection with *N. meningitidis* usually presents in four clinical situations: (1) asymptomatic nasopharyngeal colonization, (2) asymptomatic benign bacteremia, (3) meningitis, and (4) meningococcemia. Asymptomatic nasopharyngeal colonization is the most common form, present in 5–10% of the population in the USA. Asymptomatic benign bacteremia usually represents a stage of clinical improvement, following an untreated infection that still yields positive blood cultures. Meningitis is associated with the classic findings of fever, headache, and nuchal rigidity, with a 5% mortality rate in children less than 5 years, and a 10–15% mortality rate in adults, despite adequate medical treatment. Meningococcemia is the most severe clinical manifestation, characterized by a petechial or purpural rash, hypotension, anorexia, disseminated intravascular coagulation (DIC), and multiorgan system failure, which if untreated, can lead to a fulminant death in as little as 12–24 hours [18, 19]. The most common and feared clinically relevant presentations of meningococcal disease are meningitis and meningococcemia.

The incidence of meningococcal disease in the general population of the USA is between 2,500 and 3,000 cases per year. The prevalence of the disease varies according to age groups: rates are high in young infants, drop in infancy, increase in adolescence and early adulthood, and once again drop after early adulthood. However, the highest rates have been observed to occur in people aged 23–64 years [20]. In the ICU, meningococcemia is the most common systemic infectious disorder that can lead to cutaneous lesions. Skin lesions in meningococcemia are highly conspicuous and aid in establishing a prompt diagnosis. Immediate medical intervention is life-saving thus high-index suspicion is crucial [1, 19].

N. meningitidis is transmitted via respiratory secretions and can enter the bloodstream following a viral infection. Flu-like symptoms or a mild upper respiratory illness are possible prodromal manifestations [18]. *N. meningitidis* invades the endothelium of small blood vessels using specialized pili, the release of a unique lipooligosaccharide endotoxin and other antigens, and autolysis by the induction of endothelial cells, monocytes, and macrophages to release inflammatory cytokines [20]. The release of inflammatory cytokines can initiate a pathophysiological cascade of severe hypotension, lowered cardiac output, decreased endothelial permeability, organ hypoperfusion, and massive DIC, which can ultimately end in multiple organ failure, shock, and death. This pathogenic chain of events incorporates decreased endothelial permeability and thrombosis resulting in cutaneous infarction, manifesting cutaneously as irregular patterns of small areas of purpura or the larger purpura fulminans, characterized by ecchymoses [8] (Fig. 3). Less conspicuous, non-hemorrhagic cutaneous

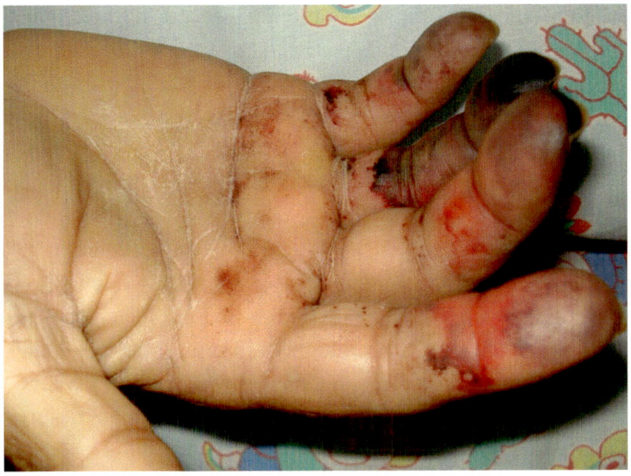

Fig. 3 Disseminated intravascular coagulation (DIC). Sudden appearance of large ecchymotic areas which progressed to acral hemorrhagic skin necrosis. Lesions followed an acute infectious process

lesions are a late sign of meningococcal disease most prevalent in children with meningococcemia and can consist of purpuric lesions (60%), erythematous papules (32%), faint pink macules (28%), or conjunctival petechiae (10%) [21–23]. The classic presenting petechial or purpural rash in pediatric patients with meningococcal meningitis is composed of 1–2 mm, non-blanchable, macular lesions occurring on the mucous membranes, trunk, legs, and areas of increased pressure, such as beneath waistbands. Larger numbers of petechiae correlate with increased severity of disease [18].

The majority of patients with meningococcal disease have a left shift on laboratory findings. Additional laboratory findings, which vary according to the severity of the infection, are metabolic acidosis, proteinuria, elevated urine specific gravity, cerebrospinal fluid (CSF) white blood cell counts of more than 90% segmented neutrophils, elevated levels of CSF protein, and CSF glucose <60 mg/dl or less than half of the patient's normal blood glucose level. A gram stain of lesion samples can identify the encapsulated gram-negative causative agent, but has a low specificity. The definitive diagnosis of meningococcal disease depends on culture isolation and identification of *N. meningitidis* from blood or CSF [18]. Additional diagnostic techniques involve commercial kits to identify antigens in CSF, serologic testing with enzyme-linked immunosorbent assays, and polymerase chain reaction (PCR), which can detect serogroup-specific strains of *N. meningitidis* DNA [20]. The differential diagnosis includes Rocky Mountain spotted fever, echovirus and coxsackie virus infections, toxic shock syndrome, gonococcemia, Henoch–Schönlein purpura, and LCV [8].

Meningococcal disease is considered a medical emergency due its high risks of severe illness and death, and thus, antibiotics should be administered to patients with suspected infection without delay [19]. Treatment with penicillin is the recommended first-line therapy for identified meningococcal infections, despite reports outside of the USA of specific strains with intermediate resistance to penicillin. However, within the USA, penicillin is rarely used as the initial treatment of a patient presenting with meningitis or sepsis. Rather, empirical therapy is initiated with third-generation cephalosporins, mainly cefotaxime or ceftriaxone, due to the high prevalence of penicillin-resistant *Streptococcus pneumoniae*, particularly in children [20]. Supportive care, to manage the possibility of septic shock, includes the continuous monitoring of vital signs and urine output, ready intervention with ventilatory equipment, inotropic agents, intravenous fluids, fresh frozen plasma in cases of DIC, and debridement or skin grafting in the case of cutaneous and tissue complications [8, 18]. Health care workers must be aware of the possibility of the deadly complication Waterhouse–Friderichsen syndrome, which is massive, usually bilateral, adrenal hemorrhage [20].

Risk factors for the development of meningococcemia are: deficiencies of complements (C5–C8), functional or anatomical asplenia, a deficiency of properdin, and HIV infection [20]. Prophylaxis with rifampin, ciprofloxacin, or ceftriaxone is recommended for household and close contacts of patients with meningococcal disease. A relatively new meningococcal conjugate vaccine containing serogroups A, C, Y, and W-135 is recommended for 11 to 12-year-old adolescents, adolescents beginning high school, freshmen students living in college dormitories, and persons 11–55 years who belong to high-risk groups, such as recruits in training centers and travelers [24].

Ecthyma Gangrenosum

Ecthyma gangrenosum (EG) is a less common, but equally feared, cutaneous manifestation associated with systemic infections. In one series, only one patient presented with EG, representing 7% of all ICU skin lesions attributable to an underlying systemic infection [1]. The patient was admitted to the ICU for neutropenia and septic shock of unknown etiology. The progression of the patient's skin lesions revealed early signs of *Pseudomonas aeruginosa* septicemia and alerted the medical staff as to the nature of his condition: multiple purple macules located in the trunk and gluteal regions, which subsequently evolved to necrotic nodules with a central black crust.

EG has a classic skin manifestation and is considered to be pathognomic for *P. aeruginosa* septicemia [25]. Less commonly EG may be due to infection with *Klebsiella pneumoniae, Pseudomonasmaltophilia and Burkholderia cepacia complex* [26]. EG may also arise without an initial bacteremia, via direct inoculation of *P. aeruginosa* into the skin.

Inadequate treatment of skin lesions in this scenario, however, may lead to secondary invasion into the bloodstream [25]. EG occurs in 1.3–6% of patients with *P. aeruginosa* septicemia, and much less frequently if no bacteremia is present [8]. *P. aeruginosa* septicemia is an alarmingly lethal condition, with mortality rates ranging from 20 to 70%. The non-septicemic presentation of EG has mortality rates that range from 7 to 15% [27]. Fortunately, prompt diagnosis and immediate treatment with appropriate antibiotics can be life-saving [28].

EG presents acutely, progresses rapidly, and occurs principally in patients with neutropenia. It also presents in immunocompromised patients due to neoplasia, leukemia, HIV, immunosuppressive treatment, grafts, malnutrition, diabetes, burns, or patients previously treated with penicillin (decreased natural inhibitory effect of gram-positive cocci present in endogenous bacterial flora) [8, 25–27]. The emergence of HIV has significantly impacted the epidemiology and mortality of *P. aeruginosa* bacteremia. In one study, infection with HIV was identified as the most common underlying disease (15%) and the second most fatal risk factor (mortality rate of 32%) for patients with *P. aeruginosa* septicemia [29]. Clearly, knowledge about EG is essential for the management of patients in the ICU with such predisposing conditions.

Skin lesions in EG begin as isolated, painless and red or purpuric macules, usually numbering less than 10, that subsequently indurate, enlarge, and elevate to become vesicular lesions. In as little as 12 hours, they can progress into hemorrhagic papules or bullae, which can remain localized or, more commonly, extend over several centimeters. The central regions of the lesions proceed to rupture and become necrotic. Lastly, the lesions slough and acquire their characteristic appearance: multiple noncontiguous or solitary gangrenous ulcers with a "gray-black eschar" surrounded by an "erythematous halo" [8, 25–28]. Patients with septicemia simultaneously present with high temperatures, chills, hypotension, tachycardia, and tachypnea [8]. EG lesions can appear anywhere on the body, but the initial presentation is usually on the gluteal or perineal regions (57%), and it subsequently metastasizes to the extremities (30%), trunk (6%), and face (6%) [8, 26].

The pathogenesis of the skin lesions in EG is not completely understood. Colonization by *P. aeruginosa* starts in the gastrointestinal tract and then spreads to moist cutaneous sites such as the axilla and perineum [30]. Pathophysiological theories include a vasculitis caused by bacilli within the vessel wall, circulating immune complexes, and/or the effect of bacterial exotoxins or endotoxins [8]. The vasculitic mechanism postulates that bacterial multiplication in the walls of cutaneous vessels at sites of involvement result in arterial and venous thrombi which lead to dermal necrosis [30]. The bacterial toxin mechanism proposes that EG skin lesions represent sites where numerous *P. aeruginosa* bacteria aggregate in the walls of underlying cutaneous blood vessels, dissolve the vessel's elastic lamina using elastase, enter into and proliferate in the adjacent subcutaneous tissue, and finally, produce exotoxin A and proteases which result in the hemorrhagic, ulcerative lesions surrounded by reactive erythema [31].

P. aeruginosa is a well-known opportunistic pathogen that can thrive in water, resist temperature extremes, and resist antiseptics, and is thus a common nosocomial pathogen [30]. This gram-negative aerobic rod prefers humid environments, and only transiently forms part of the endogenous flora of human skin. In immunocompromised and hospitalized patients, *P. aeruginosa* gains access to the body when it circumvents normal mechanical barriers: via skin fissures and erosions, venipuncture sites, nasogastric and endotracheal tubes, and urinary catheters [8]. Sites of infection exude and produce a classic "fruity odor." Recommendations for the diagnosis of EG include: (a) a deep skin biopsy (4–5 mm) and histopathologic studies for tissue infections; (b) a more superficial biopsy and culture for skin lesions, or a needle aspiration and Gram stain if a rapid diagnosis is warranted; and (c) blood culture, particularly during fever spikes, for suspected cases of septicemia [8]. The differential diagnosis of EG are infections by organisms that can give rise to EG-like lesions: bacterial pathogens such as *S. aureus, Serratia marcescens, Klebsiella species, Escherichia coli, N. meningitidis, Aeromonas hydrophila, Stenotrophomonas maltophilia*, and fungal agents such as *Aspergillus, Candida, Fusarium*, and *Rhizopus species* [30] (Fig. 4).

Treatment of the septicemic form of EG can include use of a fluoroquinolone, such as ciprofloxacin, an aminoglycoside in combination with an antipseudomonal penicillin, ceftazidime, or imipenem. The nonsepticemic form of EG can be treated with topical therapy, such as 5% silver nitrate, 5% acetic acid, or silver sulfadiazine cream. Incision and drainage of subcutaneous abscesses may be indicated, if skin lesions persist [8, 27]. Skin lesions take an average of 4 weeks to heal [8]. There exists controversy regarding factors associated to poor prognosis. Studies suggest that a poor prognosis is associated with severe underlying disease, surgery, pneumonia, and sepsis but not with neutropenia [29]. Another study, however, reports that neutropenia does correlate with clinical outcome where the majority of patients died if their absolute neutrophil count was less than 500/mm^3, despite receiving the appropriate therapy [32].

Drug Reaction-Related Skin Disorders

Cutaneous reactions are considered the most common adverse reactions to drugs. Sevensson et al. found that among hospitalized patients the incidence of these skin reactions ranges from 1 to 3% [33]. Recognition of the cutaneous manifestations of reactions to drugs is of great importance due to

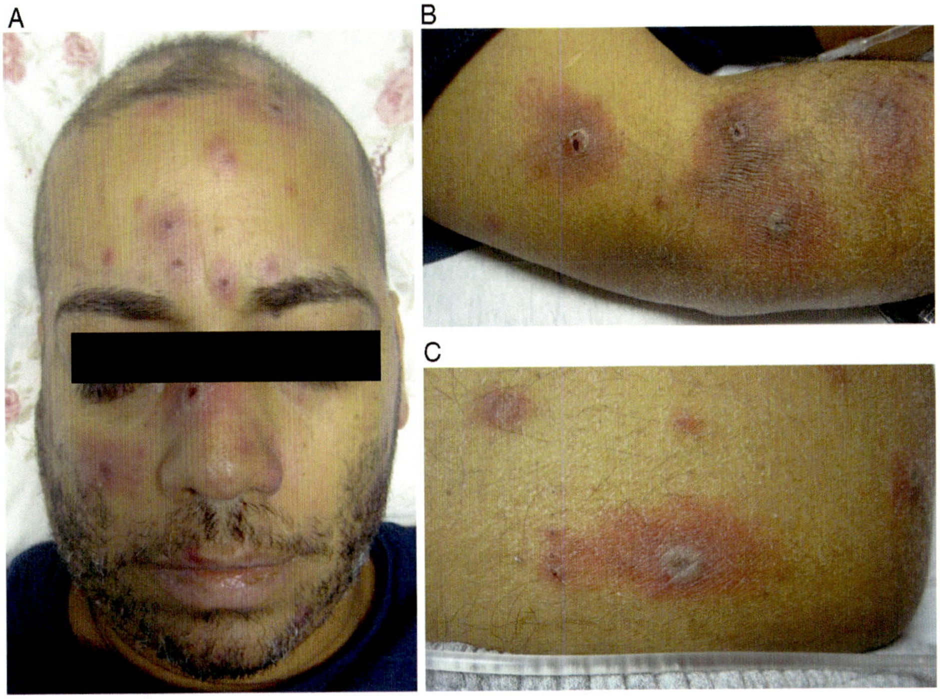

Fig. 4 (**a**–**c**) An immunocompromised patient with disseminated *Fusarium* infection. He presented with erythematous areas that developed necrotic centers. Ecthyma gangrenosum and other fungal infections can produce similar lesions

the large degree of variation of its consequences: from mild discomfort to life-threatening situations. Drug reactions commonly initiate cutaneously as a result of metabolic and immunologic activity of the skin. Assessment of drug allergy must start with a precise and exhaustive history, including clinical symptoms and their timing and duration in relation to the contact with the drug. Most of the time, there is no specific treatment for these allergic reactions, other than symptomatic relief. Most reactions are self-limited, and, therefore, prompt recognition of the distinctive skin manifestations and early withdrawal of all suspected drugs are the most important preliminary measures.

Hypersensitivity Syndrome or Drug Reaction with Eosinophilia and Systemic Symptoms

Most cutaneous manifestations to drugs are caused by a variety of hypersensitivity reactions. DRESS syndrome refers to a distinct, severe, unexpected and multi-systemic reaction 1–8 weeks after the drug exposure [34] (Table 1). Hematological abnormalities, especially eosinophilia and atypical lymphocytosis are common consequences. Despite the fact that in most cases total recovery is possible, DRESS syndrome is a potentially life-threatening disease, with a mortality rate of approximately 10% [35] (Table 1).

Table 1 Time intervals from the exposure to onset of symptoms and mortality rates of DRESS and SJS/TEN

Disease	Time interval from exposure to onset	Mortality (%)
DRESS	15–40 days	10
SJS/TEN	7–21 days	5, SJS; 30, TEN

DRESS syndrome is characterized by the clinical triad of fever, rash, and internal organ involvement, which may include the liver, heart, kidneys, or lungs. After exposure to the offending agent, the patient may present with a high fever and facial edema. This usually precedes a widespread papulopustular or erythematous skin eruption that often progresses to an exfoliative dermatitis (Fig. 5). Internal organ damage may remain asymptomatic or be life-threatening. Eosinophilia and atypical lymphocytosis are common, occurring in up to 30% of cases. Due to its risk for mortality in 10% of patients, those presenting with these symptoms should be further assessed with a complete blood test, liver function tests, serum creatinine level and urinalysis [35].

Although a role of viral co-infection is often suspected, by definition drugs are the causal agents [36]. The pathogenesis of DRESS syndrome involves accumulation of the reactive drug metabolites [34]. Among the most common drugs to cause DRESS syndrome are aromatic anticonvulsants and the sulfonamide group of antibiotics. For phenytoin, carbamazepine,

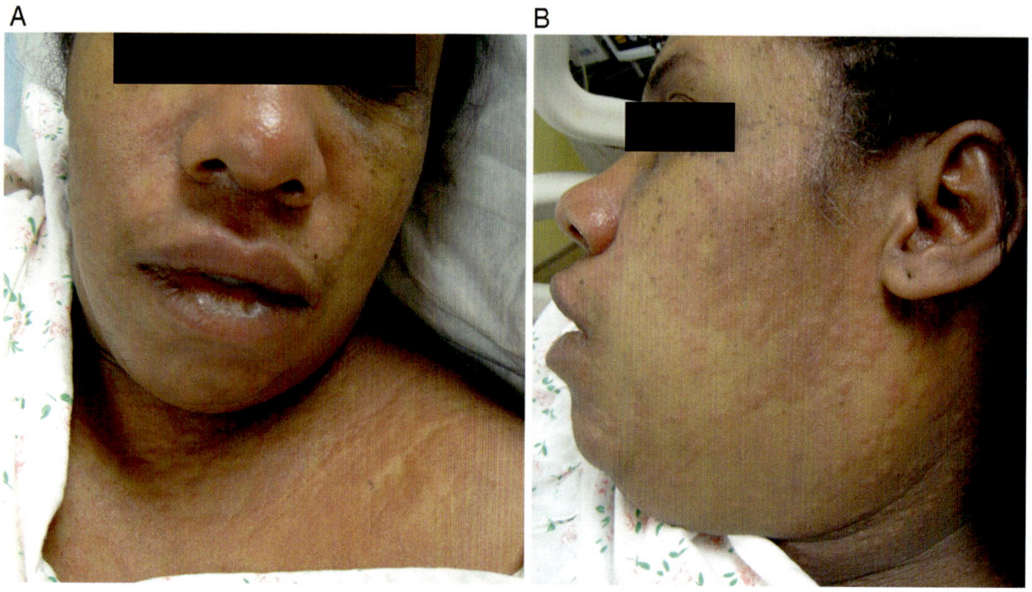

Fig. 5 (**a**, **b**) Drug reaction with eosinophilia and systemic symptoms (DRESS) syndrome. Characterized by facial edema and confluent, edematous, and erythematous papules and accompanied by elevated liver enzymes

and phenobarbital, the incidence of this reaction has been estimated to be one reaction per 5,000–10,000 exposures [37]. The disease, however, is not limited exclusively to these drugs. A variety of other drugs commonly used in the ICU have also been implicated, include: allopurinol, nonsteroidal anti-inflammatory drugs (NSAIDs), captopril, calcium channel blockers, metronidazole, mexiletine, fluoxetine, dapsone, and antiretroviral drugs.

The most common differential diagnoses for DRESS syndrome includes Steven–Johnson syndrome (SJS), toxic epidermal necrolysis (TEN), Kawasaki disease, and systemic onset juvenile rheumatoid arthritis. Cutaneous features of DRESS syndrome are distinguishable among these other conditions. DRESS syndrome is characterized by facial edema, widespread papulopustular or erythematous skin eruption, exfoliative dermatitis, and thigh blisters. Kawasaki disease is characterized by conjunctival infection, palmar erythema, polymorphous exanthema, and strawberry tongue [38]. Systemic onset juvenile rheumatoid arthritis also known as Still's disease, presents with intermittent fever, a salmon-colored rash, and inflammation of the joints. Neither in Still's disease nor in Kawasaki disease do patients have a previous history of drug exposure attributable to their respective manifestations. SJS/TEN is characterized by blisters and mucocutaneous eruptions that will be described later in this chapter.

The only way to treat DRESS syndrome is the prompt withdrawal of the offending drug, or, if unknown, of all suspected drugs. In the case of delayed diagnosis, supportive therapy and therapies aimed at accelerating the elimination of the causative drug should be initiated. Skin care should include the use of topical steroids to alleviate and improve symptoms [8]. If exfoliative dermatitis has occurred, the main therapy should include: warming the patient to prevent hypothermia, the use of local moisturizing ointments and/or lotions, correction of electrolyte imbalances, high caloric intake, and measures to prevent secondary infections and sepsis. Antipyretics should be prescribed to reduce the effects of fever. Systemic steroids are reserved for patients with life-threatening visceral manifestations, such as interstitial pneumonitis or nephritis, for which they should be initiated as soon as the diagnosis of DRESS syndrome is confirmed; otherwise it may have no benefit. Caution should be taken, if the patient has septic manifestations, since systemic corticosteroids can elicit further complications in patients with sepsis [39].

According to Sullivan et al., genetic factors are suspected in DRESS syndrome. First-degree relatives should be alerted to their elevated risk of developing hypersensitivity reactions to the same drugs. Also, cross-hypersensitivity reactions are common between the three main aromatic anticonvulsants: phenytoin, carbamazepine, and phenobarbital [39]. Therefore, these drugs must be avoided in patients who have experienced DRESS syndrome with any one of these medications. Cross-reactions may also occur with nonsteroidal anti-inflammatory agents. Patients should be monitored closely for systemic complications such as renal failure, liver failure, pulmonary fibrosis, and endomyocardial damage and should be treated accordingly if these complications develop [34].

Steven–Johnson Syndrome and Toxic Epidermal Necrolysis

SJS, also known by some as erythema multiforme major, is an immune-mediated hypersensitivity disorder that may be caused by many drugs, viral infections, and malignancies. SJS and TEN are considered by many authors as different parts of a spectrum of the same disease. For this reason, many refer to the entity as SJS/TEN. SJS/TEN is a serious systemic disorder with the potential for severe morbidity and even death. Differentiation between cases of SJS and TEN depends on the extent of body area involvement. The initial manifestations are similar, starting with a prodrome of malaise and fever, followed by the rapid onset of erythematous or purpuric macules and plaques. Although similar skin manifestations are present between SJS and TEN, SJS is characterized by epidermal detachment involving less than 10% of the total body skin area, while TEN is defined by epidermal detachment greater than 30%. Based on case registries and observational studies, the incidence of SJS is one to three cases per million inhabitants per year [40, 41]. The incidence of TEN is estimated to be 1–1.4 cases per million inhabitants per year [40]. TEN is considered to be a more dangerous disease that may include all organs, leading to potentially life-threatening processes. The total mortality rates observed by Bastuji-Garin et al. were found to be 5% in SJS and 30% for overlap SJS/TEN [42] (Table 1).

Several signs and symptoms following exposure to a drug or drug regimen can alert the physician to a potentially serious skin manifestation that may progress to SJS/TEN. These symptoms include confluent erythema, facial edema, skin pain, palpable purpura, skin necrosis, blisters, urticaria, tongue swelling, and/or mucous membrane erosions. The skin lesions usually appear days after unspecific symptoms of fever, odynophagia, and eye discomfort [41]. Cutaneous manifestations begin most of the time as ill-defined, erythematous macules with purpuric centers distributed symmetrically on the face and thorax before spreading to other areas. Vesicles and flaccid bullae then form, which spread laterally with pressure. The skin sloughs off rapidly within days, but typically ceases after 2–3 days. Skin pain may be prominent and out of proportion to medical findings, especially in TEN. In SJS, the skin lesions progress to epidermal necrosis and sloughing that is limited to less than 10% of the body surface. TEN leads to full-thickness epidermal necrosis and sloughing involving a total surface area greater than 30%. The ultimate appearance of the skin in TEN has been described as similar to that of widespread thermal injury. Mucosal membranes in SJS are affected in 92–100% of patients, while TEN involves mucous membranes in nearly all cases. Most commonly, mucosal involvement usually occurs at two of three distinct sites which may include ocular, oral, and genital areas [41, 43] (Fig. 6).

Although few cases have been caused by infections or remain unexplained, SJS/TEN is essentially a drug-induced reaction [44]. Medications cause 30–50% of cases of SJS and up to 80% of cases of TEN. The most common imputable drugs for SJS/TEN are antibacterial sulfonamides, anticonvulsant agents, NSAIDS, and allopurinol, but may also be caused by quinolones, cephalosporins, and penicillins [39, 41]. Immunosupression and HIV infection increases the

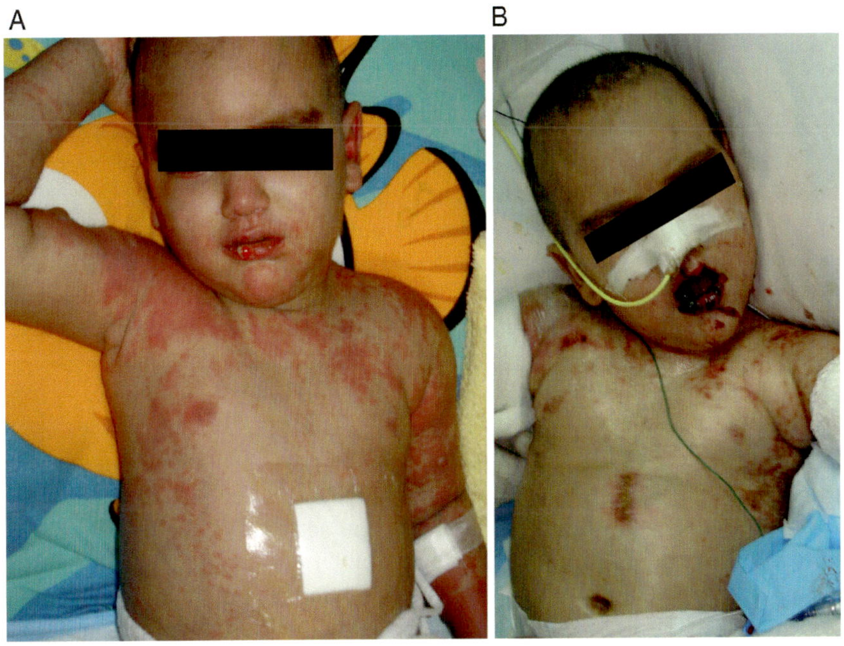

Fig. 6 (**a**, **b**) Skin and mucosal involvement in Steven-Johnson syndrome induced by phenytoin, which evolved from (**a**) to (**b**) over a 24 hour period

risk for SJS/TEN. Autoimmune disorders, such as systemic lupus erythematosus, and an HLA-linked genetic susceptibility have also been implicated as possible etiological conditions and as risk factors for the development of SJS/TEN [41, 45].

The differential diagnosis for SJS/TEN may include a long list of dermatological diseases manifesting with blistering, skin sloughing, and mucosal involvement. Among the most common diseases that could be confused with SJS/TEN are: erythema multiforme, DRESS syndrome, pemphigus diseases, SSSS, toxic shock syndrome (TSS), acute generalized exanthematous pustulosis (AGEP), and disseminated fixed bullous drug eruption [41]. Erythema multiforme is associated with a viral infection in more than 50% of cases, and although it may be due to the same pathological process as SJS/TEN, its minimal mucosal involvement, as well as less than 10% epidermal detachment, distinguishes it from SJS/TEN [46].

Pemphigus vulgaris is an autoimmune disease causing blistering of the skin and the oral mucosa. Patients often present with flaccid bullae and erosions on the face and trunk that usually are not associated with recent ingestion of drugs. This produces painful, raw areas of the skin and mucous membranes that will not heal. In some cases, these sores can cover a significant area of the skin. The definitive diagnosis of pemphigus vulgaris is made with skin biopsy [47]. DRESS syndrome is characterized by the previously described clinical triad of fever, rash, and internal organ involvement. SSSS is caused by epidermolytic toxins produced by certain strains of Staphylococci, which presents clinically with fever, irritability, and a generalized, erythematous, micromacular to maculopapular rash. SSSS usually affects newborns and children, but adults are less commonly affected due to improved renal function which allows elimination of the toxins from the body. SSSS is best differentiated from SJS/TEN by the lack of history of drug exposure and the skin biopsy revealing only limited thickness epidermal sloughing and minimal keratinocyte necrosis [47]. Similarly, TSS, a disease caused by *S. aureus* that develops acutely in individuals without an identified disease also lack a previous history of drug exposure. The clinical manifestations of TSS, such as fever, hypotension, and skin manifestations, are caused by the activation of a large number of T lymphocytes by bacterial toxins that act as super-antigens [48]. In comparison to SJS/TEN, TSS presents with more involvement of multiple organ systems which include diarrhea, vomiting, mental status changes, and elevations of creatinine phosphokinase, transaminases, and creatinine [48]. Despite the strong association of SJS/TEN with drug ingestion, eosinophilia is unusual. Patients with TEN commonly present with anemia and lymphopenia. Neutropenia is noted in about one-third of patients and is correlated with a poor prognosis. Mild elevations in serum aminotransferase levels occur in one-half of patients, while overt hepatitis occurs in just 10% of patients [49].

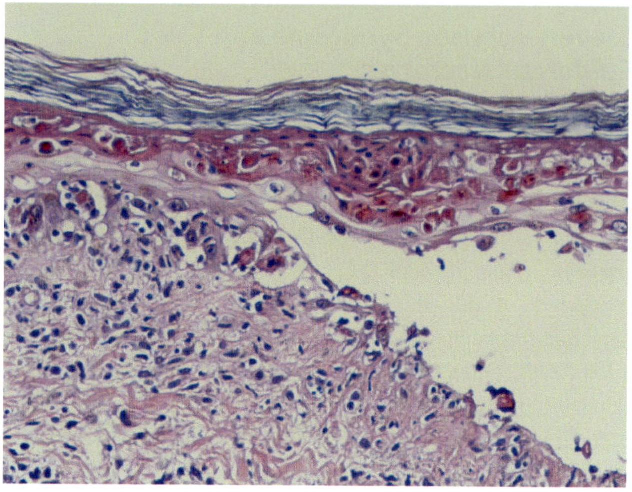

Fig. 7 In this histopathologic specimen of TEN, one can see that there is impending formation of a subepidermal blister. The epidermis contains multiple necrotic keratinocytes. The stratum corneum exhibits some parakeratosis, but for the most part has maintained its normal pattern

SJS and TEN are clinical diagnoses supported by histopathologic findings. Early lesions on skin biopsy show a superficial and perivascular lymphocyticinfiltrate associated with edema along the dermoepidermal junction. These lesions are closely associated with degenerating necrotic keratinocytes. As the lesions progress, discrete and confluent zones of epidermal necrosis occur with connecting blister formation. The stratum corneum may exhibit some parakeratosis, but for the most part has maintained its normal pattern [50] (Fig. 7). Once the diagnosis of SJS/TEN has been confirmed by skin biopsy, internal organ involvement should be ruled out by complete blood count tests, liver enzyme tests, and chest radiographs [43].

The only definitive treatment is the discontinuation of the offending drug, followed by supportive measures [8]. Patients who have developed SJS/TEN should not be rechallenged with the suspected causative drug, nor should they undergo desensitization to the medication [39, 42]. When epidermal detachment and fluid losses are extensive, electrolyte imbalances can result. Therefore, fluid and nutritional replacement are essential in managing SJS/TEN complications. Further systemic complications can include superinfection, which can lead to sepsis. Signs of infection include sudden decreases in temperature, rapid clinical deterioration, positive cultures, and increased quantities of bacteria from cultured skin, catheters, or gastric and urinary tubes. Sterile techniques and wound care are essential [39]. Prophylactic antibiotics are not usually employed, but topical antibiotics may be beneficial in preventing sepsis. Because of the strong association of sulfonamide antibiotics with SJS/TEN, these must be avoided and prescriptions should be specified according to laboratory culture result [51].

Table 2 (**a**, **b**) SCORTEN scoring system designed by Bastuji-Garin et al. [40]

SCORTEN parameter	Score
(**a**)	
Age > 40 years	Yes = 1, no = 0
Malignancy	Yes = 1, no = 0
Tachycardia > 120/min	Yes = 1, no = 0
Initial surface of epidermal detachment > 10%	Yes = 1, no = 0
Serum urea > 10 mmol/l	Yes = 1, no = 0
Serum glucose > 14 mmol/l	Yes = 1, no = 0
Bicarbonate < 20 mmol/l	Yes = 1, no = 0
SCORTEN (sum of scores)	Predicted mortality (%)
(**b**)	
0–1	3.2
2	12.1
3	35.8
4	58.3
≥5	90

Because of the highly morbid complications associated with mucous involvement, medical consultations and attentive care is essential. Involvement of tracheobronchial epithelium and less often, gastrointestinal epithelium causes high morbidity. When the trachea and bronchi are involved, intubation and mechanical ventilation are recommended [39]. Additionally, antacids may be used to reduce the incidence of gastric bleeding. The use of corticosteroids in SJS/TEN is controversial since no randomized trials support this, or any other, treatment modality [52].

There are no established scoring systems for prognosis estimation. However, a specific score, SCORTEN, developed by Sylvie Bastuji-Garin et al. has been recently elaborated and validated, which can be applied to all TEN patients, based on variables available upon patient admission [42] (Table 2). The variables indicative of a poor prognosis are: greater than 40 years of age, presence of malignancy, heart rate greater than 120 beats per minute, initial percentage of epidermal detachment greater than 10%, BUN levels greater than 10 mg/dl, serum glucose levels greater than 14 mmol/l, and bicarbonate levels lesser than 20 mmol/l. Patients with a SCORTEN score of 0–1, greater or equal to 2, greater or equal to 3, greater or equal to 4, and totaling 5 or more, have a 3.2%, 12.1%, 35.3%, 58.3%, and a greater than 90% increased rate of mortality, respectively (Table 2). Ophthalmologic complications are the most feared. They progress from months to years and follow-up is mandatory to monitor for the development of sicca syndrome, keratitis, corneal lesions, and severe impairment of vision. Patients who survive SJS/TEN should not be reexposed or desensitized to the medication [39, 42].

Hypersensitivity Vasculitis or Leukocytoclastic Vasculitis

Hypersensitivity vasculitis, or LCV, is the most common vasculitis encountered in clinical practice. Due to a great inconsistency of definitions among physicians, the American College of Rheumatology proposed in 1990 the following five criteria for the classification of hypersensitivity vasculitis: (1) age should be greater than 16 years, (2) use of a possible offending drug in temporal relation to the symptoms, (3) presence of palpable purpura, (4) maculopapular rash, and (5) biopsy of a skin lesion showing neutrophils around an arteriole or a venule. The presence of three of these criteria has sensitivity and specificity of 71%, but when more than three criteria are met, the sensitivity and specificity increases to 84%. It is important to recall that these criteria do not distinguish hypersensitivity vasculitis from Henoch–Schönlein purpura, a systemic vasculitis characterized by the deposition of IgA in skin lesions [53]. Hypersensitivity vasculitis represents an immune complex process. Evidence for circulating immune complex formation includes: the recognition of soluble complexes, hypocomplementemia, and the deposition of immunereactants in vessels. Immune complexes are detected more frequently in early, rather than late, lesions [51].

In most patients, the associated signs and symptoms begin 7–10 days after antigen exposure. This amount of time is necessary to produce a sufficient quantity of antigen–antibody complexes. Once these immune complexes have formed, palpable purpura is the most common presentation of small vessel vasculitis [53]. Lesions are commonly round, measuring approximately 1–3 mm in diameter. These lesions may coalesce to form plaques and can eventually ulcerate. The legs are most commonly involved but any cutaneous surface can be affected (Fig. 8). In addition to skin manifestations, patients can present with fever, urticaria, arthralgias, and/or lymphadenopathy [39]. Biopsy of the lesions demonstrates inflammation of the small blood vessels that is most prominent in the postcapillary venules. The change is limited to infiltration with neutrophils. The nuclei of the neutrophil's become fragmented as they follow the vessel wall and exhibit "nuclear dust." There is fibrinization of the walls of venules [50] (Fig. 9). Internal organ involvement is not often observed, but can be severe. In most cases, the assessment of noncutaneous organ involvement is difficult [45]. Glomerulonephritis, interstitial nephritis, and varying degrees of hepatocellular injury have all been described. Involvement of the lung, heart, or central nervous system has been rarely reported.

When a physician encounters a clinical scenario of hypersensitivity vasculitis, it is important to remember that more

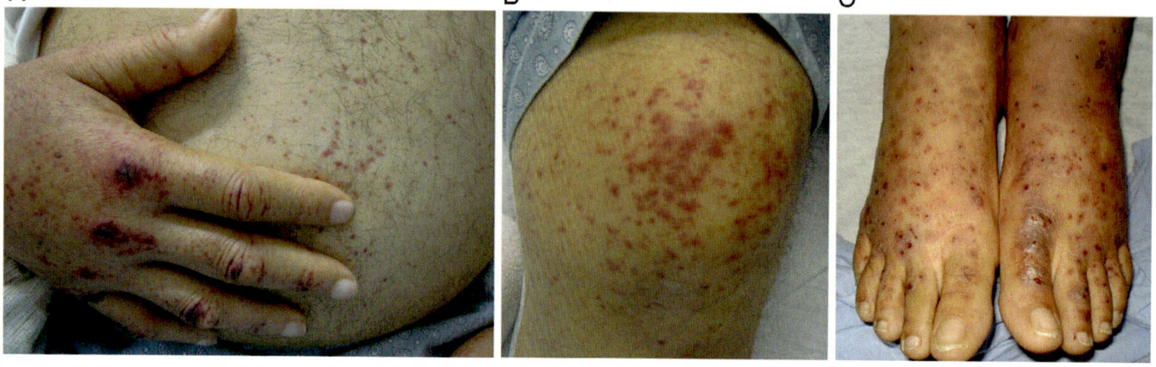

Fig. 8 (a–c) Manifestations of leukocytoclastic vasculitis: palpable purpura in the dependent areas of the body

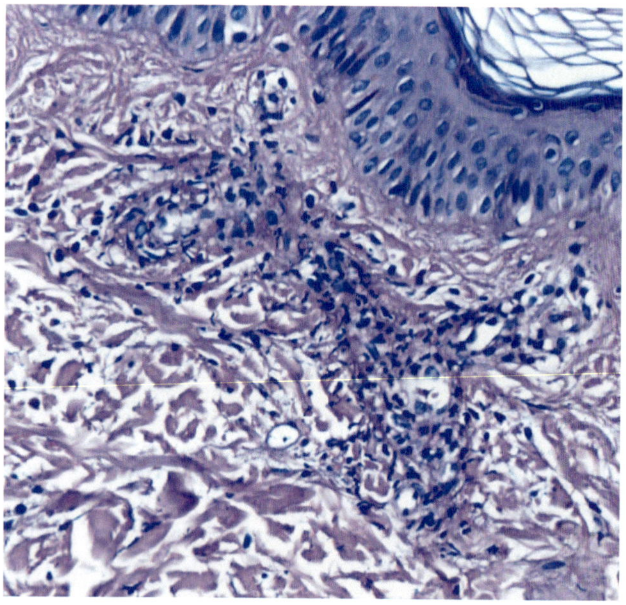

Fig. 9 In the histopathology of LCV, there is a moderate perivascular and interstitial infiltrate with neutrophils, with evidence of "nuclear dust" of neutrophils. There is fibrinization of the walls of venules and a few extravasated erythrocytes

than 70% of cases are due to an underlying pathological process, while 30–50% of cases are idiopathic [51]. However, a diagnosis of idiopathic vasculitis should be made only after all other possible causes have been properly ruled out. Common causes of hypersensitivity vasculitis include, but are not limited to: medication exposure, infection, malignancy, primary systemic vasculitis, or connective tissue disease [54]. Drugs are of the most common causes, acting as haptens that stimulate an immune response. However, drug-induced vasculitis is a weekly defined disorder, since proving causality is difficult. Beta-lactam antibiotics are the most common type of drugs implicated in this disease, but NSAIDs and diuretics are also common. However, almost all drugs are potential causes [54].

A good history and physical examination is important for accurately diagnosing hypersensitivity vasculitis because although most patients experience itching, burning, or pain, some may have asymptomatic lesions [54]. Physicians should assess all possible risk factors such as medication intake, intravenous drug abuse, systemic diseases (particularly connective tissue diseases), and recent infections. The physician must rule out any underlying systemic disease because of its implications on the patient's prognosis. No routine diagnostic test has been established, but should include complete blood cell count, erythrocyte sedimentation rate, urinalysis, and a blood chemistry panel for all adults. Also a stool guaiac test should be obtained in patients with cutaneous vasculitis. Additionally, serologic studies, such as for antinuclear antibodies, ANCA (cytoplasmic ANCA, perinuclear ANCA, or atypical ANCA), and rheumatoid factor, should be obtained in patients without an obvious cause for their condition. A skin biopsy of a reasonably new lesion should be obtained in most, if not all, adult patients [54]. In cases of severe vasculitis, muscle, nerve, or visceral organ biopsies may be required. However, patients with drug-induced vasculitis do not commonly require these tests.

The differential diagnoses of drug-induced vasculitis in the case that there is no previous history of an offending drug includes all the aforementioned risk factors: infection, malignancy, primary systemic vasculitis, or connective tissue disease (Fig. 10). The differential diagnosis of hypersensitivity vasculitis also includes systemic vasculitis conditions such as Wegener's granulomatosis, polyarteritis nodosa, and microscopic polyarteritis. The presence of systemic signs and symptoms, evidence of internal visceral target organ involvement, and ANCA positivity, in combination with the lack of evidence of immune deposits, may be helpful in identifying these syndromes [54].

As with all drug-induced cutaneous reactions, discontinuation of the inciting drug should lead to resolution. The signs and symptoms should disappear in approximately 2 weeks.

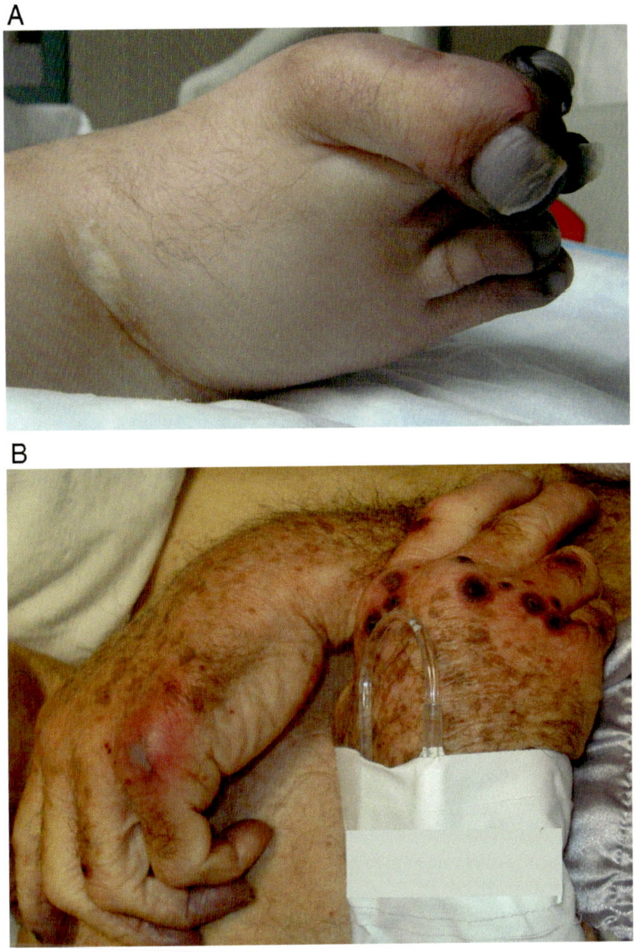

Fig. 10 Septic vasculitis in critically ill patients presenting as (**a**) distal necrosis of the toes and (**b**) purpuric plaques with necrotic centers and digital infarction

After the drug has been retired, the diagnosis can be made within a period of days to a few weeks. Patients with urticarial lesions may be treated with antihistamines. If the patient only has a disease of the skin, with or without joint manifestations, colchicine or dapsone may be administered. For patients with severe visceral involvement, high doses of corticosteroids, with or without an immunosuppressive agent, should be administered. The successful treatment in two patients with rituximab, who had severe, progressive, cutaneous, small-vessel vasculitic conditions, was recently reported [55]. Further studies of rituximab treatment in well-defined patient groups are necessary.

The prognosis of LCV is generally good, but if the kidneys, gastrointestinal tract, lungs, heart, or central nervous system become involved, death is possible.

Conclusion

Skin disorders are a significant component of the diseases occurring in patients in the ICU. Common dermatological conditions seen in the ICU can arise from direct fungal, bacterial, or viral invasion of the skin, or as adverse reactions to drugs administered to patients in the ICU. Additional skin manifestations, beyond the scope of this chapter, can also be observed in the ICU: allergic contact dermatitis reactions, preexisting dermatological conditions not associated to the cause of admission, pressure ulcers, and burns. Skin disorders in the ICU can be due to a wide range of factors and present in multiple modalities. It is essential that careful inspection and effective treatment of skin manifestations in critically ill patients become an integral part of patient management in the ICU.

References

1. Dunnill MG, Handfield-Jones SE, Treacher D. Dermatology in the intensive care unit. Br J Dermatol. 1995;132:226–35.
2. Badia M, Trujillano J, Gasco E. Skin lesions in the ICU. Intensive Care Med. 1999;25:1271–6.
3. Campos-Fernández M, Ponce-De-León-Rosales S, Archer-Dubon C, Orozco-Topete R. Incidence and risk factors for cutaneous adverse drug reactions in an intensive care unit. Rev Invest Clin. 2005;57:770–4.
4. Fischer M, Fischer M, Soukup J, et al. Key dermatological symptoms in the intensive care unit. Int J Dermatol. 2004;43:780–2.
5. Pappas PG. Invasive candidiasis. Infect Dis Clin North Am. 2006;20:485–506.
6. Perlroth J, Perlroth J, Choi B, Spellberg B. Nosocomial fungal infections: epidemiology, diagnosis, and treatment. Med Mycol. 2007;45:321–46.
7. Wisplinghoff H, Bischoff T, Tallent SM, et al. Nosocomial bloodstream infections in US hospitals: analysis of 24,179 cases from a prospective nationwide surveillance study. Clin Infect Dis. 2004;39:309–17.
8. Habif T. Clinical dermatology. 4th ed. Edinburgh: Mosby; 2003.
9. Vazquez JA. Therapeutic options for the management of oropharyngeal and esophageal candidiasis in HIV/AIDS patients. HIV Clin Trials. 2000;1(1):47–59.
10. Lipsett P. Surgical critical care: fungal infections in surgical patients. Crit Care Med. 2006;34:9.
11. Pappas PG, Rex JH, Sobel JD, et al. Guidelines for treatment of candidiasis. Clin Infect Dis. 2004;38:161.
12. Stulberg D, Penrod M, Blatny R. Common bacterial skin infections. Am Fam Physician. 2002;66:119–24.
13. Cole C, Gazewood J. Diagnosis and Treatment of Impetigo. Am Fam Physician. 2007;75(6):859–64.
14. Allen C, Patel B, Endom E. Primary bacterial infections of the skin and soft tissues, changes in epidemiology and management. Clin Ped Emerg Med. 2004;5:246–55.
15. Zetola N, Francis JS, Nuermberger EL, Bishai WR. Community-acquired methicillin-resistant *Staphylococcus aureus*: an emerging threat. Lancet Infect Dis. 2005;5:275–86.
16. Johnston GA. Treatment of bullous impetigo and the staphylococcal scalded skin syndrome in infants. Expert Rev Anti Infect Ther. 2004;2:439–46.
17. Stevens DL, Bisno AL, Chambers HF, et al. Practice guidelines for the diagnosis and management of skin and soft-tissue infections. Clin Infect Dis. 2005;41:1373.
18. Herf C, Nichols J, Fruh S, et al. Meningococcal disease: recognition, treatment, and prevention. Nurse Pract. 1998; 23:30, 33–6, 39–40.
19. Rajapaksa S, Starr M. Meningococcal sepsis. Aust Fam Physician. 2010;39(5):276–8.

20. Rosenstein N, Perkins B, Stephens D, et al. Meningococcal disease. N Engl J Med. 2001;344:1378–88.
21. Hazelzet JA. Diagnosing meningococcemia as a cause of sepsis. Pediatr Crit Care Med. 2005;6(3 Suppl):S50–4.
22. Marzouk O, Thomson AP, Sills JA, et al. Features and outcome in meningococcal disease presenting with maculopapular rash. Arch Dis Child. 1991;66:485.
23. Ramesh V, Mukherjee A, Chandra M, et al. Clinical, histopathologic & immunologic features of cutaneous lesions in acute meningococcaemia. Indian J Med Res. 1990;91:27.
24. Gardner P. Prevention of meningococcal disease. N Engl J Med. 2006;355:1466.
25. Rhody C. Bacterial infections of the skin. Prim Care. 2000;27: 459–73.
26. Singh TN, Devi KM, Devi KS. Ecthyma gangrenosum: a rare cutaneous manifestation caused by pseudomonas aeruginosa without bacteraemia in a leukaemic patient – a case report. Indian J Med Microbiol. 2005;23:262–3.
27. Vinh D, Embil J. Rapidly progressive soft tissue infections. Lancet Infect Dis. 2005;5:501–13.
28. Fast M, Woerner S, Bowman W, et al. Ecthyma gangrenosum. Can Med Assoc J. 1979;120(3):332–4.
29. Vidal F, Mensa J, Almela M, et al. Epidemiology and outcome of Pseudomonas aeruginosa bacteremia, with special emphasis on the influence of antibiotic treatment. Analysis of 189 episodes. Arch Intern Med. 1996;156:2121.
30. Chan Y, Chong C, Puthucheary J, et al. Ecthyma gangrenosum: a manifestation of Pseudomonas sepsis in three paediatric patients. Singapore Med J. 2006;47:1080–3.
31. Bottone E, Maria R, Janda J, et al. Pseudomonas maltophilia exoenzyme activity as correlate in pathogenesis of ecthyma gangrenosum. J Clin Microbiol. 1996;24:995–7.
32. Greene S, Daniel S, Muller S. Ecthyma gangrenosum: report of clinical, histopathologic, and bacteriologic aspects of eight cases. J Am Acad Dermatol. 1984;11:781.
33. Svensson C, Cowen E, Gaspari A. Cutaneous drug reactions. Pharmacol Rev. 2000;53:357–9.
34. Sullivan JR, Shear NH. The drug hypersensitivity syndrome: what is the pathogenesis? Arch Dermatol. 2001;137:357–64.
35. Tas S, Simonart T. Management of drug rash with eosinophilia and systemic symptoms (DRESS Syndrome): an update. Dermatology. 2003;206:353–6.
36. Descamps V, Valance A, Edlinger C, et al. Association of human herpes virus 6 infection with drug reaction with eosinophilia and systemic symptoms. Arch Dermatol. 2001;137:301–4.
37. Tennis P, Stem RS. Risk of serious cutaneous disorders after initiation of use of phenytoin, carbamazepine, or sodium valproate: a record linkage study. Neurology. 1997;49:542–6.
38. Burns JC, Glode MO. Kawasaki syndrome. Lancet. 2004;364: 533–44.
39. Ghislain PD, Roujeau JC. Treatment of severe drug reactions: Stevens-Johnson syndrome, toxic epidermal necrolysis and hypersensitivity syndrome. Dermatol Online J. 2002;8:5.
40. Rzany B, Mockenhaupt M, Baur S, et al. Epidemiology of erythema exsudativum multiforme majus, Stevens-Johnson syndrome, and toxic epidermal necrolysis in Germany (1990–1992): structure and results of a population-based registry. J Clin Epidemiol. 1996;49:769–73.
41. Harr T, French L. Toxic epidermal necrolysis and Steven-Johnson syndrome. J Rare Dis. 2010;5(39):1–11.
42. Bastuji-Garin S, Rzany B, Stern RS, et al. Clinical classification of cases of toxic epidermal necrolysis, Stevens-Johnson syndrome, and erythema multiforme. Arch Dermatol. 1993;129:92–6.
43. Knowles S, Shear N. Recognition and management of severe cutaneous drug reactions. Dermatol Clin. 2007;25:245–53.
44. Choy AC, Yarnold PR, Brown JE, et al. Virus induced erythema multiforme and Stevens-Johnson syndrome. Allergy Proc. 1995;16:157–61.
45. Roujeau JC, Huynh TN, Bracq C, et al. Genetic susceptibility to toxic epidermal necrolysis. Arch Dermatol. 1987;123:1171–3.
46. Lamoreux M, Sternbach M. Erythema multiforme. Am Fam Physician. 2006;74:1883–8.
47. Stanley JR, Amagai M. Pemphigus, bullous impetigo, and the staphylococcal scalded-skin syndrome. N Engl J Med. 2006;355: 1800–10.
48. Todd J, Fishaut M, Kapral F, Welch T. Toxic-shock syndrome associated with phage-group-I Staphylococci. Lancet. 1978;2(8100): 1116–8.
49. Revuz J, Penso D, Roujeau JC, et al. Toxic epidermal necrolysis: clinical findings and prognosis factors in 87 patients. Arch Dermatol. 1987;123:1160–5.
50. Kumar V, Abbas A, Fausto N. Robbins and Cotran pathologic basis of disease. 7th ed. Philadelphia, PA: Saunders; 2005.
51. McKenna J, Leiferman K. Dermatologic drug reactions. Immunol Allergy Clin N Am. 2004;24:399–423.
52. Hynes A, Kafkala C, Daoud Y, Foster C. Controversy in the use of high-dose systemic steroids in the acute care of patients with Stevens-Johnson syndrome. Int Ophthalmol Clin. 2005;45:25–48.
53. Calabrese LH, Michel BA, Bloch DA, et al. The American College of Rheumatology 1990 criteria for the classification of hypersensitivity vasculitis. Arthritis Rheum. 1990;33:1108–13.
54. Harris ED, Budd RC, Genovese MC, Firestein GS, Sargent JS, Sledge CB, eds. *Kelley's Textbook of Rheumatology*. 7th ed. Philadelphia, Pa: Saunders Elsevier; 2005:chap 45.
55. Chung L, Funke AA, Chakravarty EF, et al. Successful use of rituximab for cutaneous vasculitis. Arch Dermatol. 2006;142: 1407–10.

Index

A
Acanthosis nigricans, 55, 64–65
Accelerated rheumatoid nodulosis (ARN), 11–12
Ackerman, A.B., 14
Acquired ichthyosis, 71
Acquired immunodeficiency syndrome (AIDS), 44
Acrochordons, 27
Acrokeratosis paraneoplastica. *See* Bazex's syndrome
Acute cutaneous lupus erythematosus (ACLE), 1
Acute febrile neutrophilic dermatosis. *See* Sweet's syndrome
Acute miliary tuberculosis, 24
Acute myelogenous leukemia (AML), 70
Addison's disease, 57–58
Adenomatous polyposis coli (APC), 47
Adrenal disorders
  Addison's disease, 57–58
  Cushing's syndrome, 56–57
Adrenocorticotropic hormone (ACTH), 57
Altun, E., 34
American College of Rheumatology (ACR) classification of SLE, 3–4
Anhalt, G.J., 71
Atypical mycobacteriosis
  clinical features, 103
  clinical manifestation, 101
  diagnosis, 103
  etiology, 102
  incidence and prevalence, 102
  treatment, 103

B
Bacillary angiomatosis (BA), 121–122
Badia, M., 129
Bailey, W., 61
Bastuji-Garin, S., 137, 139
Bazex's syndrome, 49, 66
Bazin, E., 26
Becker, S.W., 66
Besnier, 18
Besnier–Boeck–Schaumann disease. *See* Lupus pernio
Birt, A., 17, 26
Birt–Hogg–Dubé syndrome (BHDS), 26–27
Blistering distal dactylitis (BDD), 91
Boeck, C., 17, 19
Braverman, 21
Bullous disease of hemodialysis
  PCT, 35
  pseudoporphyria, 35–36
Bullous impetigo, 131
Bullous systemic lupus erythematosus, 3
Bywaters, E.G., 12

C
Calcinosis cutis, 5, 32–33
Calciphylaxis, 33–34
Camisa, C., 71
Candidal paronychia, 125
Castro-Santana, L.E., 1
Cellulitis
  clinical features, 83
  complications, 83
  diagnosis, 83
  differential diagnosis, 83
  etiology, 81–82
  incidence and prevalence, 81
  pathology, 83
  treatment, 83–84
Chávez, J.G., 1
Chiesa-Fuxench, Z.C., 59
Chilblain lupus, 3
Chiqués Colón, L.S., 31
Chronic cutaneous lupus erythematosus (CCLE), 2–3
Chronic kidney disease (CKD), 31
Classic rheumatoid nodules (CRN), 10–11
Common endocrine disease
  adrenal disorders
    Addison's disease, 57–58
    Cushing's syndrome, 56–57
  diabetes mellitus
    acanthosis nigricans, 55
    diabetic dermopathy, 56
    diabetic thick skin, 56
    necrobiosis lipoidica diabeticorum, 55–56
    scleredema, 56
  thyroid disease
    hyperthyroidism, 53–54
    hypothyroidism, 54–55

N.P. Sánchez (ed.), *Atlas of Dermatology in Internal Medicine*,
DOI 10.1007/978-1-4614-0688-4, © Springer Science+Business Media, LLC 2012

Connective tissue diseases
  dermatomyositis
    categories, 4
    characteristic findings, 4–5
    classification and treatment, 6
    Gottron's papules and Gottron's sign, 4, 5
  rheumatoid arthritis (*see* Rheumatoid arthritis)
  scleroderma
    classification and treatment, 9–10
    morphea or localized scleroderma, 8–9
    systemic sclerosis, 6–8
  SLE
    ACLE, 1
    bullous systemic lupus erythematosus, 3
    CCLE, 2–3
    classification and treatment, 3–4
    SCLE, 1–2
Cortisol deficiency. *See* Addison's disease
CREST syndrome, 7–8
Crohn's disease (CD), 41, 42
Curth, H.O., 64
Cushing's syndrome, 56–57
Cystic fibrosis, 27
Cystic fibrosis nutrient deficiency dermatitis (CFNDD), 27

D

Darier, J., 19, 25
Darier–Roussy disease. *See* Subcutaneous nodules
de Jesús-Monge, W.E., 41
Dermatitis herpetiformis (DH), 45–46
Dermatomyositis
  categories, 4
  characteristic findings, 4–5
  classification and treatment, 6
  Gottron's papules and Gottron's sign, 4, 5
Dermatophytoses, 104–106
Diabetes mellitus
  acanthosis nigricans, 55
  diabetic dermopathy, 56
  diabetic thick skin, 56
  necrobiosis lipoidica diabeticorum, 55–56
  scleredema, 56
Diabetic dermopathy, 56
Diabetic thick skin, 56
Discoid lupus erythematosus (DLE), 2–3
Disseminated intravascular coagulation (DIC), 133
Drug reaction, 134–135
Drug reaction with eosinophilia and systemic symptoms (DRESS), 135–136
Dubé, W., 17, 26
Ductal carcinoma in situ (DCIS), 63
Duhring, L., 45
Dykman, C.J., 14

E

Ecthyma, 85–86, 131
Ecthyma gangrenosum (EG), 86–87, 133–134
Erysipelas
  complications, 85
  differential diagnosis, 85
  etiology, 85
  pathology, 85
  treatment, 85
Erythema gyratum repens, 68
Erythema induratum of bazin (EIB), 26
Erythema nodosum (EN), 21, 41–43
Extramammary Paget's disease, 63

F

Familial adenomatous polyposis (FAP), 47
Fibrofolliculoma, 27
Folliculitis
  clinical features, 77–78
  complications, 78
  diagnosis, 78
  differential diagnosis, 78
  etiology, 77
  hair follicles, 77
  incidence and prevalence, 77
  pathology, 78
  treatment, 79–80
Furuncles and carbuncles
  clinical features, 80
  complications, 81
  diagnosis, 80
  differential diagnosis, 81
  etiology, 80
  pathology, 81
  treatment, 81

G

Gardner's syndrome, 47–48
Gastrointestinal diseases
  dermatitis herpetiformis, 45–46
  gastrointestinal hemorrhage, 47
  gastrointestinal neoplasias
    Bazex's syndrome, 49
    Gardner's syndrome, 47–48
    MTS, 48–49
    necrolytic migratory erythema, 49–50
    Peutz–Jeghers syndrome, 49
  inflammatory bowel disease
    EN, 41–43
    PG, 43–44
    Sweet's syndrome, 44–45
  Kaposi's sarcoma, 47, 48
  lichen planus, 46–48
  nutritional and metabolic disorders, 45
Gastrointestinal neoplasia
  Bazex's syndrome, 49
  Gardner's syndrome, 47–48
  MTS, 48–49
  necrolytic migratory erythema, 49–50
  Peutz–Jeghers syndrome, 49
Ginsberg, M.H., 12
Glucagonoma syndrome, 66–67
Gomm–Button's disease, 68
González Rivera, R., 31, 121
González Santiago, T.M., 129
Gottron's papules and Gottron's sign, 4, 5
Gougerot, 66
Granulocytic sarcoma, 69
Graves disease, 53
Guiot, H.M., 121

H

Hansen's disease
  characteristics, 99

clinical features, 98
complications, 100, 103
diagnosis, 98, 100
differential diagnosis, 100
etiology, 98
incidence and prevalence, 98
treatment, 101
Hara, K., 26
Hebra, F., 26
Hemodialysis (HD), 31
Hernández, I.M., 53
Hirsutism, 57
Histiocytoid Sweet syndrome, 69
Hodgkin's lymphoma, 62
Hogg, G., 17, 26
Human immunodeficiency virus (HIV)
bacillary angiomatosis, 121–122
exanthem, 121
Kaposi's sarcoma, 125–126
molluscum contagiosum, 126–127
onychomycosis, 125
oral hairy leukoplakia, 124
oral thrush, 124–125
seborrheic dermatitis, 123–124
varicella-zoster virus, 122–123
Hutchinson, J., 17
Hypersensitivity syndrome, 135–136
Hypersensitivity vasculitis, 139–141
Hyperthyroidism
Graves disease, 53
infiltrative thyroid dermopathy, 53–54
onycholysis, 53
pretibial myxedema, 53–54
sign and symptoms, 53
thyroid achropachy, 54
Hypothyroidism, 54–55

I
Impetigo, 131–132
Infiltrative thyroid dermopathy, 53–54
Intensive care unit (ICU)
dermatomycoses, 130–131
drug reaction, 134–135
ecthyma gangrenosum, 133–134
hypersensitivity syndrome, 135–136
hypersensitivity vasculitis, 139–141
meningococcal septicemia, 132–133
pathogen-related skin disorders, 130
peripheral vascular disease, 132
pyoderma, 131–132
Steven-Johnson syndrome, 137–139
toxic epidermal necrolysis, 137–139
Internal malignancy
breast metastases, 59–61
disease entities, 62
inflammatory carcinoma, 60, 61
ocular melanoma, 61
Paget's disease
breast, 62–63
extramammary Paget's disease, 63
treatment, 63–64
prevalence, 59
sign and symptoms, 62
Sister Mary Joseph's nodule, 61–62
Interstitial granulomatous dermatitis with arthritis (IGDA), 14

J
Jeghers, H.J., 49

K
Kaposi's sarcoma (KS), 47, 48, 125–126
Karyorrhexis, 69
Koch, R., 22
Kramer, 11

L
Laennec, T., 22
Lee, 11
Lepromatous leprosy, 101, 102
Leprosy. *See* Hansen's disease
Leptospirosis, 94–96
Leukocytoclasia, 69
Leukocytoclastic vasculitis (LCV), 139–141
Lichen planus, 46–48
Lichen scrofulosorum (LS), 26
Lofgren, 21
Lundback, 21
Lupus erythematosus tumidus, 3
Lupus panniculitis, 3
Lupus pernio, 18
Lupus vulgaris (LV), 23–24
Lyme disease, 96–97

M
Malar erythema, 1
Marrero, Y., 53
Mayo, W., 61
Melanin, 58
Meningococcal septicemia, 132–133
Methicillin-resistant *S. aureus* (MRSA), 84
clinical features, 84
diagnosis, 84
etiology, 84
treatment, 84–85
Miró, E.M., 77
Molluscum contagiosum (MC), 126–127
Morphea, 8–9
Mucocutaneous candidiasis, 130–131
Mucocutaneous infections
atypical mycobacteriosis, 101–103
blistering distal dactylitis, 91
cellulitis
clinical features, 83
complications, 83
diagnosis, 83
differential diagnosis, 83
etiology, 81–82
incidence and prevalence, 81
pathology, 83
treatment, 83–84
dermatophytoses, 104–106
ecthyma, 85–86
ecthyma gangrenosum, 86–87
erysipelas
complications, 85
differential diagnosis, 85
etiology, 85
pathology, 85
treatment, 85

Mucocutaneous infections (*cont.*)
  folliculitis
    clinical features, 77–78
    complications, 78
    diagnosis, 78
    differential diagnosis, 78
    etiology, 77
    hair follicles, 77
    incidence and prevalence, 77
    pathology, 78
    treatment, 79–80
  furuncles and carbuncles
    clinical features, 80
    complications, 81
    diagnosis, 80
    differential diagnosis, 81
    etiology, 80
    pathology, 81
    treatment, 81
  Hansen's disease, 98–101
  leptospirosis, 94–96
  Lyme disease, 96–97
  methicillin-resistant *S. aureus*
    clinical features, 84
    diagnosis, 84
    etiology, 84
    incidence and prevalence, 84
    treatment, 84–85
  mucocutaneous candidiasis, 106–108
  necrotizing soft tissue infections, 91–94
  pityriasis versicolor, 108–110
  rhinoscleroma, 94
  sporotrichosis, 110–112
  staphylococcal scalded skin syndrome, 87–89
  superficial mycoses, 103–104
  systemic mycoses, 112–115
  toxic shock syndrome, 89–91
  varicella-zoster virus, 112–116
Müir–Torre syndrome (MTS), 48–49

N
Necrobiosis lipoidica diabeticorum (NLD), 55–56
Necrolytic migratory erythema (NME), 49–50
  glucagonoma syndrome, 66–67
  histological findings, 67
  pathophysiology, 67–68
  skin lesions, 67
  treatment, 68
Necrotizing soft tissue infections (NSTI), 91–94
Neisseria meningitidis, 132–133
Nephrogenic systemic fibrosis (NSF), 34–35
Nodular tuberculid, 26
Nodular vasculitis. *See* Erythema induratum of bazin (EIB)
Nonbullous impetigo, 131
Nutritional and metabolic disorders, 45

O
Onycholysis, 53
Onychomycosis, 125
Ophthalmic herpes-zoster, 124
Oral candidiasis, 130
Oral hairy leukoplakia (OHL), 124
Oral lichen planus, 47
Oral thrush, 124–125
Orenstein Cardona, J.M., 129
Orificial tuberculosis, 24, 25

P
Pachydermatoglyphy. *See* Tripe palms
Paget, J., 62
Paget's disease
  breast, 62–63
  extramammary Paget's disease, 63
  treatment, 63–64
Palisaded neutrophilic granulomatous dermatitis, 14–15
Papulonecrotic tuberculid, 26
Paraneoplastic acrokeratosis of Bazex. *See* Bazex's syndrome
Paraneoplastic pemphigus, 71–72
Paraneoplastic syndrome
  acanthosis nigricans, 64–65
  acquired ichthyosis, 71
  acrokeratosis paraneoplastica, 66
  acute febrile neutrophilic dermatosis
    classical Sweet's syndrome, 69–70
    histopathological findings, 69
    malignancy-associated Sweet's syndrome, 70
    skin manifestations, 68–69
    treatment, 70–71
  clinical manifestation, 64
  erythema gyratum repens, 68
  NME
    glucagonoma syndrome, 66–67
    histological findings, 67
    pathophysiology, 67–68
    skin lesions, 67
    treatment, 68
  paraneoplastic pemphigus, 71–72
  sign of Leser–Trélat, 65
  tripe palms, 65–66
Peripheral vascular disease, 132
Peutz–Jeghers syndrome, 49
Peutz, J.L., 49
Pityriasis versicolor, 108–110
Poikiloderma atrophicans vasculare, 5
Polycystic ovary syndrome (PCOS), 57
Porphyria cutanea tarda (PCT), 35
Pretibial myxedema, 53–54
Proximal subungual onychomycosis, 125
Pseudomonas aeruginosa, 133–134
Pseudoporphyria, 35–36
Pulmonary disease
  Birt–Hogg–Dubé syndrome, 26–27
  cystic fibrosis, 27
  sarcoidosis
    alopecia, 21
    childhood sarcoidosis, 21–22
    classification, 17–18
    clinical manifestation, 17
    erythema nodosum, 21
    hypopigmentation, 21
    ichthyosiform sarcoidosis, 21
    lupus pernio, 18
    macules, 18–19
    mucosal sarcoidosis, 21–22
    nail sarcoidosis, 21–22
    nodules and plaques, 18–19
    papules, 18–20

scar sarcoidosis, 19–20
subcutaneous nodules, 19, 20
treatment, 22
tuberculids, 25–26
tuberculosis
clinical manifestation, 22–23
endogenously acquired disease, 23–25
exogenously acquired disease, 25
medical history, 22
primary infection, 22–23
systemic infection, 23
Purple striae, 57
Pyoderma, 131–132
Pyoderma gangrenosum (PG), 13, 43–44

R
Ramírez, L., 59
Renal disease
bullous disease of hemodialysis
PCT, 35
pseudoporphyria, 35–36
calcinosis cutis, 32–33
calciphylaxis, 33–34
nail changes, 31
NSF, 34–35
pigmentation changes, 31
uremic pruritus, 31–32
xerosis changes, 31
Renal insufficiency, 31
Rheumatoid arthritis (RA)
ARN, 11–12
clinical manifestations, 10
CRN, 10–11
IGDA, 14
palisaded neutrophilic granulomatous dermatitis, 14–15
PG, 13
RN, 12
RV, 12–13
Rheumatoid nodulosis (RN), 12
Rheumatoid vasculitis (RV), 12–13
Rhinoscleroma, 94
Ridley–Jopling classification of Leprosy, 98, 99
Roussy, 19
Rullán, J., 1, 17
Rupp, 66

S
Sánchez, N.P., 17, 59, 77
Sánchez Rivera, C.J., 121
Sánchez Sergenton, C.G., 121
Sangueza, O.P., 14
Sarcoidosis
alopecia, 21
childhood sarcoidosis, 21–22
classification, 17–18
clinical manifestation, 17
erythema nodosum, 21
hypopigmentation, 21
ichthyosiform sarcoidosis, 21
lupus pernio, 18
macules, 18–19
mucosal sarcoidosis, 21–22
nail sarcoidosis, 21–22
nodules and plaques, 18–19
papules, 18–19
scar sarcoidosis, 19–20
subcutaneous nodules, 19, 20
treatment, 22
Scar sarcoidosis, 19–20
Schmidt, E., 72
Scleredema, 56
Sclerodactyly, 8
Scleroderma
classification and treatment, 9–10
morphea or localized scleroderma, 8–9
systemic sclerosis, 6–8
Scrofuloderma, 24
Seborrheic dermatitis, 123–124
Seijo-Montes, R.E., 1, 17
Sevensson, C., 134
Sign of Leser–Trélat, 65
Sister Mary Joseph's nodule, 61–62
Sporotrichosis, 110–112
Staphylococcal scalded skin syndrome (SSSS), 87–89
Staphylococcus aureus, 131–132
Steven–Johnson syndrome (SJS), 137–138
Subacute cutaneous lupus erythematosus (SCLE), 1–2
Subcutaneous nodules, 19, 20
Sullivan, J.R., 136
Superficial mycoses, 103–104
Sweet, R.D., 44, 68
Sweet's syndrome, 44–45
classical Sweet's syndrome, 69–70
histopathological findings, 69
malignancy-associated Sweet's syndrome, 70
skin manifestations, 68–69
treatment, 70–71
Systemic lupus erythematosus (SLE)
ACLE, 1
bullous systemic lupus erythematosus, 3
CCLE, 2–3
classification and treatment, 3–4
SCLE, 1–2
Systemic mycoses, 112–115
Systemic sclerosis (SSc)
atrophic phase, 7
classification and treatment, 9–10
clinical manifestation, 6
edematous phase, 7
indurative phase, 7
limited and diffuse disease, 7–8
Raynaud's phenomenon, 7–8

T
Thomas, R.H., 21
Thyroid achropachy, 54
Thyroid disease
hyperthyroidism (*see* Hyperthyroidism)
hypothyroidism, 54–55
Thyrotoxicosis. *See* Hyperthyroidism
Tinea unguium. *See* Onychomycosis
Toxic epidermal necrolysis (TEN), 137–138
Toxic shock syndrome, 89–91
Trichodiscomas, 27
Tripe palms, 65–66
True cutaneous tuberculosis, 23–25

Tuberculids
clinical manifestation, 25
erythema induratum of bazin, 26
lichen scrofulosorum, 26
nodular tuberculid, 26
papulonecrotic tuberculid, 26
treatment, 26
Tuberculoid leprosy, 100
Tuberculosis
clinical manifestation, 22–23
endogenously acquired disease
acute miliary tuberculosis, 24
lupus vulgaris, 23–24
orificial tuberculosis, 25
scrofuloderma, 24
exogenously acquired disease
tuberculosis verrucosa cutis, 25
tuberculous chancre, 25
medical history, 22
primary infection, 22–23
systemic infection, 23
Tuberculosis verrucosa cutis (TVC), 23, 25
Tuberculous chancre, 25
Twycross, R., 62
Tzanck smear, 123

U
Ulcerative colitis (UC), 41
Uremic frost, 31
Uremic pruritus, 31–32

V
Vaillant, A., 17
Valdivielso, M., 66
Varicella–zoster virus (VZV)
clinical features
herpes zoster, 114–115
varicella, 114, 115
complications, 115–116
diagnosis, 115
differential diagnosis, 115
etiology, 112
human immunodeficiency virus, 122–123
incidence and prevalence, 112
treatment, 116
Vázquez-Roque, M.I., 41

W
Whittle, C.H., 44

GPSR Compliance

The European Union's (EU) General Product Safety Regulation (GPSR) is a set of rules that requires consumer products to be safe and our obligations to ensure this.

If you have any concerns about our products, you can contact us on ProductSafety@springernature.com

In case Publisher is established outside the EU, the EU authorized representative is:

Springer Nature Customer Service Center GmbH
Europaplatz 3
69115 Heidelberg, Germany

Batch number: 10683953

Printed by Printforce, the Netherlands